Nutrition

Nutrition

Science, Issues, and Applications

Volume 1: A–H

Barbara A. Brehm, Editor

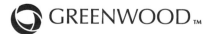

GREENWOOD™

An Imprint of ABC-CLIO, LLC

Santa Barbara, California • Denver, Colorado

Library of Congress Cataloging-in-Publication Data

Nutrition : science, issues, and applications / Barbara A. Brehm, editor.
  volumes cm
  Includes index.
  ISBN 978-1-4408-2849-2 (alk. paper : v. 1) – ISBN 978-1-4408-2850-8 (ebook)
1. Diet.   2. Nutrition.   3. Dietary supplements.   I. Brehm-Curtis, Barbara, editor.
  RA784.N94 2015
  613.2–dc23   2014038576

ISBN: 978-1-4408-2849-2
EISBN: 978-1-4408-2850-8

19   18   17   16   15   1   2   3   4   5

This book is also available on the World Wide Web as an eBook.
Visit www.abc-clio.com for details.

Greenwood
An Imprint of ABC-CLIO, LLC

ABC-CLIO, LLC
130 Cremona Drive, P.O. Box 1911
Santa Barbara, California 93116-1911

This book is printed on acid-free paper ∞
Manufactured in the United States of America

This book discusses treatments (including dietary therapies, dietary supplements, medications, and mental health therapies) for a variety of symptoms and disorders, and a variety
of organizations. The authors have made every effort to present accurate and up-to-date
information. However, the information in this book is not intended to recommend or
endorse particular treatments or organizations, or substitute for the care or medical advice
of a qualified health professional, or used to alter any medical therapy without a medical
doctor's advice. Specific situations may require specific therapeutic approaches not
included in this book. For those reasons, we recommend that readers follow the advice of
qualified health care professionals directly involved in their care. Readers who suspect they
may have specific medical problems should consult a physician about any suggestions
made in this book.

Contents

List of Entries

Guide to Related Topics

Intestinal Gas
Irritable Bowel Syndrome
Lactose Intolerance
Large Intestine
Lipoproteins
The Liver
Metabolism
Microbiota and Microbiome
The Mouth
Pancreas
Parenteral Nutrition
Peptic Ulcers
Prebiotics
Probiotics
Salivary Glands and Saliva
Small Intestine
Stomach
Water Needs; Water Balance

Environmental Issues

Arsenic
Bottled Water
Climate Change and Global Food
    Supply
Food Gardens
Food Security and Food Insecurity
Foodborne Illness and Food Safety
Genetically Modified Organisms
Global Hunger and Malnutrition
Insects as Food
Irradiation
Lead
The Locavore Movement
Mercury
Obesity, Causes
Organic Food and Farming
Sustainable Agriculture

Foods and Food Ingredients

Agave Syrup
Alcohol
Alternative Sweeteners (Sugar
    Substitutes)
Artificial Sweeteners

Caffeine
Carrageenan
Chamomile
Chlorella
Chocolate
Cholesterol
Coffee
Colostrum
Cordyceps Sinensis
Curcumin
Dairy Foods
Dietary Supplements
Echinacea
Energy Drinks
Fermentation and Fermented Foods
Fiber
Food Additives
Fructose
Functional Foods
Garlic
Ginger
Ginkgo Biloba
Ginseng
Grains
Herbs and Herbal Medicine
High-Fructose Corn Syrup
Honey
Hydrogenation
Insects as Food
Legumes
Margarine and Vegetable Oil Spreads
Marine Omega-3 Fatty Acids
Phospholipids
Prebiotics
Probiotics
Quorn
Raw Milk
Seafood
Sodium and Salt
Soybeans and Soy Foods
Spirulina
Stevia
Sugar Alcohols
Sugar-Sweetened Beverages
Taurine

Tea
Trans Fatty Acids
Triglycerides
Valerian
Wheatgrass
Whey Protein
Yerba Mate

Health Issues and Nutrition

Acne
Alcohol
Alzheimer's Disease and Nutrition
Arthritis and Nutrition
Attention-Deficit Hyperactivity
    Disorder and Nutrition
Autism and Nutrition
Blood Sugar Regulation
Caffeine
Cancer and Nutrition
Cardiometabolic Syndrome
Cardiovascular Disease and Nutrition
Celiac Disease
Cholesterol
Diabetes, Type 1
Diabetes, Type 2
Energy Drinks
Enteral Nutrition
Eye Health
Fetal Alcohol Syndrome and
    Disorders
Food Allergies and Intolerances
The French Paradox
Functional Foods
Gallbladder and Gallbladder Disease
Gastro-esophageal Reflux Disease
Glycemic Index and Glycemic Load
Hyperglycemia
Hypertension and Nutrition
Hypoglycemia
Inflammation
Inflammatory Bowel Disease
Insulin
Iron-Deficiency Anemia
Irritable Bowel Syndrome

Ketosis and Ketogenic Diets
The Kidneys
Lactose Intolerance
Lipoproteins
Megaloblastic Anemia
Nutritional Genomics
Obesity, Causes
Obesity, Definition and Health
    Effects
Obesity, Treatment
Osteoporosis
Peptic Ulcers
Phenylketonuria
Premenstrual Syndrome
Underweight
Upper Respiratory Tract Infections

Life Cycle

Adolescence and Nutrition
Breast-Feeding
Childhood Nutrition
Colostrum
Creatine
Electrolytes
Energy Drinks
Enrichment and Fortification
Female Athlete Triad
Fetal Alcohol Syndrome and
    Disorders
Infant Formula
Iron-Deficiency Anemia
Lactation
Older Adults, Nutrition
    Needs
Pregnancy and Nutrition
Premenstrual Syndrome

Nutrients

Alpha-Linolenic Acid
Amino Acids
Biotin
Boron
Calcium
Carbohydrates

Obesity

Organizations and Programs

Phytochemicals and Other Compounds in Foods and Dietary Supplements

Allyl Sulfides (Organosulfurs)
Alpha-Lipoic Acid
Anthocyanins
Antioxidants
Arginine
Astaxanthin
Berberine
Beta-Carotene
Black Cohosh
Caffeine
Capsaicin
Carnitine
Carotenoids
Catechins
Choline
Coenzyme Q10
Creatine
Curcumin
Dietary Supplements
Ellagic Acid
Fiber
Functional Foods
Gamma Linolenic Acid
Glucosamine
Glutamine
Glutathione
Indoles
Inositol
Isothiocyanates
Lecithin
Lutein
Lycopene
Lysine
Marine Omega-3 Fatty
    Acids
Melatonin
Milk Thistle
Monoterpenes
N-Acetylcysteine
Nitrates and Nitrites, Dietary
Phytochemicals
Phytoestrogens
Polyphenols
Pyruvate and Pyruvic Acid
Quercetin
Resveratrol
S-Adenosylmethionine
Saponins
St. John's Wort
Zeaxanthin

Psychological Issues

Appetite
Attention-Deficit Hyperactivity
    Disorder and Nutrition
Autism and Nutrition
"Brain Foods"
Cognitive Restructuring
Depression and Nutrition
Detoxification
Eating Disorders
Feeding Disorders
Female Athlete Triad
Food Addiction
Food Cravings
Hunger, Biology of
Mood and Food
Obesity, Causes
Obesity, Definition and Health
    Effects
Obesity, Treatment
Orthorexia
Premenstrual Syndrome

Sports Nutrition

Creatine
Electrolytes
Female Athlete Triad
Glycemic Index and Glycemic
    Load
Iron-Deficiency Anemia
Sports Beverages
Sports Nutrition
Sports Supplements

Toxins

Alcohol
Arsenic
Copper
Detoxification
Fluoride
Foodborne Illness and Food Safety
Heterocyclic Amines and Polycyclic
    Aromatic Hydrocarbons
Hydrogenation
Lead
Mercury
Nickel
Raw Milk
Trans Fatty Acids

Preface

Nutrition news is everywhere. Opinions on the best way to eat often clash with one another, however, which bewilders and frustrates consumers. Nutrition-related health problems can prompt patients and family members to seek more information on healthful eating—but the search often leads to more questions than answers. The purpose of this encyclopedia is to provide the information needed for a deeper understanding of today's most thought-provoking topics in nutrition, and to help readers make more informed decisions about food choices and dietary patterns.

Human nutrition is a broad and multidisciplinary subject that combines physiology, biochemistry, psychology, and sociology. The entries in this encyclopedia give a basic overview of the most important and relevant nutrition topics for which readers are likely to seek information. This encyclopedia also provides a foundation for students taking introductory nutrition courses. It discusses the most common and interesting topics regarding human nutrition, provides solid background on the topics, and is a starting point for further research. The entries include relevant definitions, background, and a balanced perspective of current knowledge. The essays are written at a level accessible to upper-grade high school students, college students, as well as other readers. Each entry offers suggestions for further reading and research.

The material provided by this encyclopedia is helpful for students studying nutrition and other fields in which nutrition is important, such as medicine and health. Consumers will find the information helpful for making decisions about diet, and for understanding current controversies in nutrition and health.

Scope: Science, Issues, and Applications

People often seek information about nutrition because they wish to understand nutrition issues currently in the news, and want information to make decisions about what to eat to be healthy and to prevent or treat health problems. Nutrition issues are best understood in the context of relevant scientific information. Each entry presents a scientific background to illuminate some of the current issues related to the topic. Health applications are outlined conservatively so as to discourage readers from trying potentially useless, expensive, or harmful nutrition remedies that lack sufficient research support.

This encyclopedia contains 281 entries that encompass the most interesting and current topics in nutrition. Topic areas include the following:

- Nutrition-related health issues, including acne; Alzheimer's disease; arthritis; cancer; cardiovascular disease; food allergies and intolerances; inflammation; and osteoporosis.
- Obesity-related issues including approaches to weight control; body composition; body mass index (BMI); energy balance; and obesity-related health problems (e.g., type 2 diabetes).
- Psychological issues and the role played by nutrition in each area, including autism; attention deficit hyperactivity disorder; brain foods; depression; eating disorders; and food addiction.
- Basic human nutrition, including the digestive system and the major organs of digestion; and each nutrient and class of nutrients, including proteins, carbohydrates, fats, vitamins, minerals, and water.
- Phytochemicals in foods and dietary supplements, from alpha lipoic acid to zeaxanthin.
- Toxins that can contaminate food, including arsenic, lead, and mercury; and those caused by foodborne illnesses.
- Environmental issues and their interaction with nutrition and the food supply, including climate change; genetically modified foods; organic foods and farming; and sustainable agriculture.
- Ideas about eating, such as detoxification; the Locavore Movement; the Paleolithic diet; the Slow Food Movement; and public policy and nutrition.

Special Features

In addition to entries covering a wide range of nutrition topics, this encyclopedia includes special features to assist readers in the search for information and understanding. Students completing class assignments such as research papers also will find these features helpful.

- **Introduction to information literacy**. Nutrition topics often are fraught with controversy and one-sided, sensational media coverage that blows the results of a single study out of proportion. The introduction to this encyclopedia—"Fact or Fiction? Evaluating Nutrition Information"—provides a brief overview of the scientific methods used by researchers studying topics in nutrition. The overview can help readers evaluate research findings described in the popular media.
- **Further reading**. Each entry lists at least two easily accessible articles or authoritative websites for readers seeking more information.
- **Research issues**. Many entries include guidance on research areas for students seeking project topic ideas. These issues might stimulate further reading and research for school presentations or papers, or simply spur on the curious reader to find more information about a nutrition topic.

- **Sidebars**. Sidebars (boxed text) accompany some entries to provide noteworthy and relevant applications for entry information. A sidebar accompanying the topic "Eating Disorders," for example, provides suggestions for helping someone who might have an eating disorder.
- **Recommended resources**. At the end of volume 2 of the encyclopedia, a list of general resources provides a list of well-respected accessible sources of nutrition information for readers seeking more information. It also includes pertinent websites and a note about some websites to avoid.

Additionally, these features can help readers find information in *Nutrition: Science, Issues, and Applications*.

- Cross-references to other essays in the encyclopedia that can provide relevant information are included in each entry.
- A comprehensive index to the entire work is located at the end of volume 2.
- A "Guide to Related Topics" at the front of each volume lists all of the entries in the book categorized under broad topics.

Acknowledgments

I am deeply grateful to Smith College for funding several valuable research assistants, especially two of my graduate students, Patricia Cipicchio and Lisa P. Ritchie, who helped extensively with research, writing, and editing this encyclopedia. The students I have worked with over my 30-plus years of teaching nutrition have helped me understand the interests of young people and how to best guide them in productive research. Their interests helped inform the topic selection for the encyclopedia, and many of my advanced students also helped with research and writing. Smith College truly strives to remain true to its mission of educating women of promise for lives of distinction.

Special thanks to the many writers—including many former students—who contributed to this encyclopedia. Your extensive research, interdisciplinary perspectives, and willingness to write second and third drafts helped to shape the quality of this encyclopedia. Thank you.

I would also like to thank my developmental editor, Anne Thompson, for her advice and guidance throughout the planning and writing of this work. Her experience, knowledge, insight, and good humor have been invaluable.

Introduction: Fact or Fiction? Evaluating Nutrition Information

Is milk bad for you? Are low-carb diets or low-fat diets better for losing weight? Should you eat more turmeric to prevent cancer? Does red wine reduce risk for heart disease? These deceptively simple questions are difficult to answer. Often, the answer begins with the phrase, "It depends . . . " followed by a mile-long list of issues to consider. Most people lose interest before hearing the full response.

Why can't scientists figure out the answers to these and other nutrition questions? Why do the experts seem to disagree on everything—from how much vitamin D people need each day to whether genetically modified foods are risky? Answers to these questions are elusive for several reasons. A brief overview of the research process helps to explain why.

The Goal of Science: Determining Relationships among Variables

Scientists use logic, observation, and reasoning to determine relationships among variables. A variable is something that can take on two or more values. Body weight, daily calorie intake, and blood cholesterol levels are examples of variables. Scientists conduct investigations to try to understand how the change in one variable—typically called an "independent variable" or "treatment variable"—is related to or causes change in another variable, the dependent variable. To untangle these relationships, scientists use established research practices to identify the underlying truth as effectively as possible. In the study of nutrition, the most common of these practices include experimental studies and correlational studies.

Experimental Studies

Experimental studies have the most control over the subjects and variables involved. Typically, an experimental situation is designed and administered, and the results are observed. Some of the ways that scientists conducting experimental studies strive to achieve accuracy in the results include the following.

Isolate the Effect of Independent Variables

To observe and understand the relationships between variables, researchers try to hold all nonexperimental variables as constant as possible. Thus, the independent and dependent variables are the variables that change during the experiment. An example is researchers that are interested in the effect of omega-3 fatty acid intake on certain chemicals in the brain. They design an experiment that uses two groups of rats; one group is given a diet enriched with omega-3 fatty acids, and the other group receives a control diet. To make the differences in diet the only independent variable, researchers attempt to keep all other conditions the same. They use exactly the same strain, age, and sex of rat for both groups, and house, feed, handle, and care for all rats identically. At the end of the experiment, when the brain chemical levels are compared, the scientists are more certain that any changes in these chemicals were caused by differences in activity level.

Experiments with humans tend to present a different set of challenges. Sometimes researchers have little or no control over the variables in their studies. Therefore, instead of controlling outside variables, they simply try to keep the variance of values for the outside variables as similar as possible for all groups. For example, if researchers want to find out whether students who consume more servings of fruits and vegetables report less stress and greater levels of well-being than other students, they might solicit a large group of volunteers. Obviously, the students will not be littermates with identical genetic material. Participants will have many other differences as well. To try to make the groups as similar as possible, investigators use a process called random assignment. Random assignment to groups or treatments means that each subject has the same chance of getting into a given group. By assigning students randomly to groups (one group consumes more fruits and vegetables, another gets an alternative treatment as similar as possible to the other group, perhaps a diet focused on whole grains), researchers hope the groups vary in similar ways on factors such as health, sleep habits, exercise, or anything else that might affect feelings of stress and well-being. Some students in each group will not be getting enough sleep, some will be breaking up with their romantic partners, and some will have parents going through a divorce. The researchers, however, hope that the level of background emotional distress will be similar for each group.

Control for the Expectations of Subjects and Researchers

Expectations strongly influence the way humans experience life, therefore science tries to control these as much as possible. Subjects in the experiment should not know whether they are receiving a treatment that might cause a certain effect. The group receiving the actual experimental variable of interest is called the "treatment group." A "control group" does not receive or undergo the treatment or variable being tested. Ideally, the subjects in the control group receive a "placebo." A placebo closely matches the treatment condition but lacks the ingredient believed to be exerting an effect. This group "controls for" the placebo effect. The "placebo effect" refers to the fact that subjects in a study might demonstrate changes in the dependent variable simply because they are getting attention or expecting an effect, rather than because the independent variable itself is causing the change. In some nutrition studies, inert pills that look the same as the nutrient or supplement being tested are given. Both groups think they are getting "the real thing." Even in animal studies the control group receives a placebo. If the treatment group receives injections of a nutrient, then the control group receives injections of an inert substance to control for the effect of the injection procedure.

The expectations of the researchers performing the experiment also can get in the way of accurate results. Even the most careful and well-meaning people tend to see what they expect or want to see. (This expectation can be strengthened when the researcher's income or grant money is dependent upon experimental results.) Experimenters might throw out data that do not conform, thinking that an error has occurred. They could miss certain observations that they were not expecting to see. In the best type of testing—a double-blind study—neither the researchers running the tests nor the subjects know who is in the experimental group or who is in the placebo treatment group. Of course, someone knows, but that person assigns numbers to subjects and is not directly involved in administering the study. In the health sciences, a double-blind experimental study usually is used to test medical treatments or drugs. Many of these are called double-blind randomized control trials, meaning that they use double-blind methods with subjects that are randomly assigned to groups. Such studies are considered the "gold standard" of experimental methods, as they have the most experimental control.

Use Statistical Methods to Evaluate the Probability That Results Were Due to Chance

Statistical methods are based on mathematical models of probability. Statisticians use these methods to examine experimental data. They compare groups and examine how the values of one variable change in relationship to other variables or treatments. Because most variables vary somewhat, there always is the possibility that the variance observed between groups is due to random chance, rather than being an effect of the independent variable. Scientists using statistical methods can calculate the likelihood that differences observed in experimental data are significant—which means that the results have a low likelihood of occurring purely by chance. Statistical methods also are used in correlational research.

Correlational Research

Experimental study designs often are not feasible. For example, it might be unethical to administer the treatment variable of interest to subjects—such as asking people to consume trans-fatty acids or increased levels of salt—because health risks are associated with these behaviors. Instead, scientists must just observe what naturally occurs in people who choose these behaviors. Sometimes it is not possible for subjects or experimenters to be blind to the treatment: Participants can determine whether they are consuming a low-calorie diet. The time course of the development of chronic disease often is an issue, as is the cost of following participants for several years.

Correlational research methods commonly are employed by scientists when a true experiment is not feasible or might not yield the best information. In correlational research, values on variables of interest are observed and recorded, and statistical methods are used to evaluate the relationship—or correlations—among variables. Such research methods enable investigators to draw conclusions about how the behavior of one variable is related to another. When two variables are associated with each other (correlated), they vary together. When one variable increases, the other variable either increases or decreases. For example, because intake of red meat is correlated with heart disease, epidemiological data should show that as the amount of red meat consumed per day increases so does likelihood of heart disease occurring.

Epidemiological studies collect data on free-living populations and use statistical methods to observe associations and draw conclusions. Such studies can take several forms. Case-control studies are a type of correlational research commonly used by epidemiologists and medical researchers, in that naturally occurring disease patterns are observed. In case-control studies, researchers examine people who have the variable of interest; for example, colon cancer. Researchers then select a comparable group of people who do not have colon cancer as the "control" group. The researchers try to match the control group to the other group on as many variables as possible, including age, gender, and socioeconomic status. The groups then are compared on variables of interest to the researchers; for example, the intake of fruits, vegetables, and dietary fiber.

Most case-control studies are retrospective—they look back in time. Evidence and conclusions drawn from such studies are not considered to be as strong as that of prospective research, in which investigators gather data about the present, recording answers over time. This is because time—along with a disease diagnosis—can blur the memory. People trying to answer questions about what they ate many years ago can err. Prospective research measures variables as they occur. People usually are more accurate when reporting how much fish they ate this week, or how much alcohol they drank yesterday, than when recalling consumption patterns from many years ago.

Sometimes epidemiological studies simply collect a large amount of information on a great number of people and analyze the data without forming case-control comparisons. In 1948, for example, researchers performing a new study called the "Framingham Heart Study" began collecting data on a group of 5,209 men and women who were between the ages of 30 and 62 and from the town of Framingham, Massachusetts. The study's goal was to determine major risk factors for heart disease. This study was one of the first to find an association between lifestyle factors—including diet, smoking, physical activity—and heart disease. The original volunteers still are being followed, and new groups have been added to this exciting study. More information about the Framingham Heart Study can be found on its website (https://www.framinghamheartstudy.org/about-fhs/history.php).

When evaluating the results of epidemiological studies, or other studies that generate correlations, it is important to remember that correlations might not necessarily have a cause-and-effect relationship. Correlations only show that two (or more) variables vary together; they cannot demonstrate that one is causing the other to change. Sometimes there is a cause-and-effect relationship, but other times another factor could be causing both of the other variables to change together. For example, it has been observed that countries with populations that have a greater daily average intake of fat tend to have increased rates of breast cancer. As further studies have been conducted, however, the total daily fat intake does not appear to cause most breast cancer. It is possible that a third factor, for example, increased intake of meat, reduced intake of fruits and vegetables, or living in a polluted, industrialized country, is linked to both fat intake and breast cancer rate.

Epidemiological studies, however, can suggest causative relationships which then are explored with other studies. Experimental studies in laboratory animals could demonstrate a biologically plausible mechanism for causation. When a large number of epidemiological studies all find a similar association between two variables, scientists take note, especially when studies find the same result for different groups of people. Case-control studies also can strengthen an observation. Often statistical techniques combine the data from several studies into one large analysis, called a meta-analysis, to get a clearer picture of a correlation. In the end, however, take care to never assume causation in correlational data.

Research Ethics

The ethical conduct of scientists and their institutions sometimes comes under intense scrutiny when reports of fraudulent data or inaccurate statistical calculations come to light. It usually is other scientists who uncover the unethical behavior of their peers. Such behavior fortunately is fairly rare. Although scientists are human and do make mistakes—and even lie from time to time—on the whole, the process of science is eventually self-correcting and leads to improvements in long-term understanding.

All research institutions have strict guidelines concerning research ethics, and researchers are punished when the rules are broken—often losing their research funding and even their jobs. Guidelines spell out every detail of the research process. Especially important are the rules concerning the use of human subjects. Every institution has an independent board that reviews research proposals to make sure that people are treated ethically, that experimental protocols are not harmful, and that subjects are given as much information as possible about the potential benefits and costs of their participation. Additionally, use of laboratory animals is strictly regulated. Ethical guidelines provide protocols and training for researchers to ensure that they treat their subjects appropriately.

Most journals and professional meetings ask researchers to give full disclosure of all special interests that might influence their work. For example, sources of funding from grants and the researcher's participation in other relevant organizations must be listed in the article.

Continued Questioning, Analysis, and Research

For scientists, the research process is never over because the results from one study always suggest more questions that lead to more thinking, hypotheses, testing, and analysis. Scientists avoid the use of the words "prove" or "proof," which imply that conclusions are unquestionable and beyond the shadow of a doubt. Science is built upon doubt and critical analysis. When scientists evaluate the conclusions of their studies, they use a softer language. They say, "Our studies support the idea that . . ." or "Our data suggest that . . ." even when the results are very strong and meaningful.

Peer Review, Publication Bias, and Science Reporting

Results of a study are not accepted by the scientific community until the research reporting the findings has gone through the peer-review process (in which other scientists evaluate the study) and have been accepted for publication. Even after publication, other scientists question the experimental methods, the statistics, and the results.

Although the peer-review process is designed to ensure that scientific research is as accurate as possible, it has been shown that journals are more likely to publish "interesting" studies—in which an independent variable is shown to influence a dependent variable—rather than studies in which no effect is found. This means that important studies showing no relationship are less likely to be published, thus confounding understanding. A study finding that a higher vitamin D intake in laboratory rodents leads to lower cancer rates, for example, probably would be more likely to be published than a study that does not find an effect. Over time an accurate picture of relationships generally emerges as more studies are conducted, but this can take several years. Publication bias reminds readers that exciting results of a single study should be taken with a grain of salt (or something more healthful), until additional studies support that relationship.

People should be cautious when reading scientific reports about research in the popular media. Even though the research could be very interesting, science reporters might overstate a study's conclusions to attract readers. Years ago when researchers found a link between consumption of tomato products and reduced risk of prostate cancer, for example, headlines blared, "Pizza reduces cancer risk." Such news stories and headlines are misleading.

Food Consumption and Dietary Patterns

The human diet is a complicated variable. Identifying helpful and harmful foods, food components, and dietary patterns is difficult for a variety of reasons, including those listed below.

- People consume a wide variety of foods each day, and diets also can vary considerably from day to day; simply obtaining accurate food records from people is challenging.
- Individuals generally consume more than 25,000 bioactive food constituents—including nutrients and phytochemicals—in any given diet, therefore it is not easy to determine the influence of any given compound (WCRF/AICR, 2007).

- Results obtained in the laboratory with in vitro cell cultures could have little relevance to human beings. For example, although beta-carotene slows cancer cell growth in vitro, use of beta-carotene supplements by former smokers is associated with an increased risk of lung cancer.
- Dietary compounds interact with the digestive system and other constituents from food as food is broken down and absorbed. Therefore even though a dietary constituent attacks cancer cells in vitro, this effect might not occur in the body. Digestive enzymes can alter and inactivate the constituent's chemical structure. Active constituents could bind to dietary fiber and not be absorbed, or might not be absorbed from the diet in amounts sufficient to produce a significant effect. If they are absorbed, nutrients and phytochemicals then must travel in the bloodstream, where they can be influenced by various biochemical pathways in the liver, kidney, and other organs. The constituents might never even come into contact with cancerous cells; and if they do, they could behave differently in the body than in the lab.
- Animal studies can be helpful but they do not always apply to humans.
- Dietary components can influence different people in different ways depending upon their genetics, as demonstrated by the fields of nutrigenomics and nutrigenetics.
- Influence of a nutrient or other phytochemical often depends upon the dosage of the substance. Many compounds are ineffective at low doses, helpful at moderate doses, and harmful at high doses.
- Timing in a person's life cycle can shape the influence of particular dietary factors on cancer risk. For example, women who experience famine before age 10 have a reduced risk of developing precancerous breast tissue later in life, and women who experience famine after age 18 have an increased risk (WCRF/ AICR, 2007).

Evaluating Nutrition Information

People should use a cautious, critical approach when evaluating nutrition information. The following strategies can help readers separate fact from fiction.

- Before adopting information gleaned from a book or article about nutrition, always consider the source. Television shows, websites, blogs, books targeting the general public, and articles published in the popular media often blow research results out of proportion. If the sources cite studies, then try to find and read the peer-reviewed studies to determine whether the media reports actually match the study findings.
- Is the information source selling products that are supported by the reported research results? For example, a website that sells dietary supplements might overstate the results of studies on a given supplement.
- Search well-respected journals, professional organizations, and websites (see the "Recommended Resources" included in this book). What do these sources say about the subject?

- Look for studies produced by experts in the area of interest. Especially helpful are review articles and meta-analyses that examine the big picture, and that discuss the evidence on both sides of the issues.
- Seek the advice of a nutrition professional or health care provider before taking dietary supplements, especially when being treated for a health problem.
- Healthy young people should strive for good intake of nutrients and phytochemicals through good food choices rather than from dietary supplements, unless otherwise directed by a health care provider. (For example, people with iron-deficiency anemia might be directed by a health professional to take iron supplements.)

Reference

World Cancer Research Fund/American Institute for Cancer Research (WCRF/AICR). 2007. *Food, Nutrition, Physical Activity, and the Prevention of Cancer: A Global Perspective*. Washington, DC: AICR. Accessed November 12, 2014, http://www.dietand cancerreport.org/cancer_resource_center/downloads/Second_Expert_Report_full.pdf.

Academy of Nutrition and Dietetics

The Academy of Nutrition and Dietetics (AND) is the world's largest organization of certified nutrition specialists, and includes registered dietitians (RD) and registered dietetic technicians (DTR). This organization began life as the American Dietetics Association (ADA) but was renamed in 2012. Lenna F. Cooper founded the ADA in Ohio during World War I in 1917. The ADA's focus originally was on assisting the government's emergency food conservation initiative (Barber, 1959). Today, however, the Academy's objective is to improve national health through empowering dietetic professionals, providing education, and performing research and advocacy work. The AND manages *The Journal of the Academy of Nutrition and Dietetics*, a monthly peer-reviewed publication for members, educators, and scholars. The AND website (EatRight.org) is maintained by the AND to provide evidence-based scientific information on disease, exercise, and general health concerns; it also includes healthy recipes and daily tips for maintaining a healthy lifestyle.

The Academy maintains several offshoot organizations, including the AND Foundation, the Accreditation Council for Education in Nutrition and Dietetics (ACEND), and the Commission on Dietetic Registration (CDR). The AND Foundation is a charity organization that incorporates scholarships, awards, and the "Kids Eat Right" initiative. The Accreditation Council for Education in Nutrition and Dietetics oversees accreditation for educational programs completed prior to RD and DTR certification. The Commission on Dietetic Registration provides independent board certification for nutrition, dietetics, and specialties administering the RD and DTR legally protected titles. This protection is suggested to prevent the dissemination of inaccurate nutritional information by less qualified or less educated individuals in the field. Approximately 72% of the Academy's 75,000+ members are registered dieticians. The Academy of Nutrition and Dietetics has legal control over titles describing expert or professional nutritional practice, thus acquiring the title is an elaborate and highly regulated process. The general process is described below.

Registered Dietitian Certification Process

- Bachelor's degree in nutrition from ACEND-accredited university
  - Coordinated Program (CPD)
  - Dietetic Program (DPD)

- 1,200 hours of a ACEND-accredited internship
  - Offered through CPD program, and independently through health care facilities and the foodservice industry
  - Approximately 6 to 12 months needed to complete the program
- Pass national RD examination through CDR (additional specialization certifications in sports, pediatrics, and others is offered by CDR)
- Maintain professional certification through continuing education program

The Academy of Nutrition and Dietetics is not associated with the government; however, the AND maintains strong communication with the government through its Washington, DC, headquarters. The ADA's 2010 Kids Eat Right initiative works in conjunction with White House efforts to end childhood obesity by mobilizing members in community nutrition education and through policy-based advocacy (Academy of Nutrition and Dietetics, 2013; Academy of Nutrition and Dietetics, 2010).

The AND is not without criticism from members and the public. Many members are frustrated by the Academy's conflicting nutrition messages, and are concerned about possible influence of the AND's corporate sponsors, such as Coca-Cola and McDonald's. Critics have charged that the AND's core stance, "there is no 'good' or 'bad' food," could be tainted by monetary gain—thus risking the Academy's reputation as a science-based organization (Burros, 1995). The Academy also maintains strong, highly criticized financial affiliations with the pharmaceutical industry (Babjak, 2009). Despite criticism, however, the AND's membership continues to grow steadily and its publication remains the most often-read journal among Academy members (Lipscomb, 2011).

Allison R. Ferreira

See Also: Nutritionists and dietitians.

Further Reading

Academy of Nutrition and Dietetics. (n.d.). Eat Right Initiative. Retrieved from http://www.eatright.org/

Academy of Nutrition and Dietetics. (2010, February 9). *Finding causes and solutions: American Dietetic Association supports First Lady's childhood obesity initiative* [Press release]. Retrieved November 18, 2014, from http://www.eatright.org/Media/content.aspx?id=4294968094&terms=michelle%20obama#

Academy of Nutrition and Dietetics. (2013, October 2). Kids Eat Right Initiative. Addressing the "hungry and overweight paradox" across the nation. Retrieved from http://www.newswise.com/articles/kids-eat-right-addressing-the-hungry-and-overweight-paradox-across-the-nation

Babjak, P. (2009). Correspondence with the American Dietetic Association. *ProPublica*. Retrieved November 18, 2014, from http://www.propublica.org/documents/item/87299-american-dietetic-association

Barber, M.I. (1959). *History of the American Dietetic Association, 1917–1959*. Philadelphia: Lippincott.

Burros, M. (1995, December 6). Group's pursuit of cash draws fire. *Milwaukee Journal Sentinel*, p. 27.

Lipscomb, R. (2011). 2010 Journal reader survey results. *Journal of the American Dietetic Association, 111* (2): 206, 209–11. doi:10.1016/j.jada.2010.12.012.

Acne

Acne (*Acne vulgaris*) is the most prevalent chronic skin disorder. It occurs when hair follicles become blocked by dead skin cells and oils—leading to the development of blackheads, pimples, infection, and inflammation. The most severe form of acne—cystic acne—includes infection of the hair follicles and associated structures in the deeper skin layers, forming cysts and deep scarring. Acne occurs most commonly on the face, neck, shoulders, chest, and back, and is most likely to appear during periods of hormonal change, such as adolescence.

Throughout the years, the dermatological community has strongly disputed the relationship between acne and nutrition. Recent studies, however, indicate that certain dietary components—especially food with a high glycemic load, and possibly dairy products—can increase acne severity. Anti-inflammatory foods and supplements might reduce the inflammation associated with acne. Although not everyone with acne responds to dietary changes, some people with acne who adhere to the dietary changes do experience some improvement in the condition.

Skin is lubricated by oil called "sebum," which is produced by microscopic sebaceous glands. These glands open into the hair follicle. The concentration of sebaceous glands is greater on the face and scalp. Acne is associated with overproduction of sebum, which appears to interfere with the normal shedding of dead skin cells. An accelerated turnover of skin cells (more shedding of dead skin cells) also can exacerbate acne. Bacteria from the skin can thrive in the hair follicle, stimulating the body's inflammatory response as immune cells attempt to rid the body of infection.

Treatment for acne includes medications—some applied topically and others taken internally—which reduce bacteria concentrations, slow the production of sebum, and open pores. Some medications influence the levels of the sex hormones, which seem to exacerbate acne development. Nutrition is not considered a primary factor in acne causation or treatment, although dietary changes can be moderately helpful for some people.

Medical reports associating acne and nutrition persisted from the late 19th century until the late 1960s, and dietary restriction was part of standard acne therapy throughout those years. Foods high in sugars and fats, including chocolate, generally were believed to exacerbate acne symptoms. Studies conducted from the 1960s onward, however, failed to find associations between these foods and acne; and suggesting dietary alterations to improve acne in patients became controversial. Recently, interesting evidence linking acne symptoms to a variety of dietary components has revived the acne-nutrition discussion. Another interesting nutrition-related component of acne treatment is the development of medications derived from vitamin A.

Diet and Acne

As a general rule regarding acne and nutrition, what is good for one's health is good for one's skin. Consuming a healthful diet provides skin with the nutrients needed for its good health. Adequate hydration also is important for healthy skin. Acne involves high levels of inflammation, therefore consuming foods high in antioxidants might be helpful in some cases. Important antioxidant nutrients include the vitamins C and E, the mineral selenium, and phytochemicals such as the carotenoids. Some researchers have explored potential diet-related mechanisms that might influence the acne-development process. Early evidence, for example, suggests that microorganisms inhabiting the gastrointestinal tract could influence levels of inflammatory activity throughout the body (Bowe & Logan, 2011).

Some researchers have argued that epidemiological evidence suggests that acne is a phenomenon of Western civilizations having populations that consume a high concentration of foods that have a high glycemic index (Melnik, 2012). Dairy and high-glycemic carbohydrates have been theorized to contribute to insulin resistance and to an increase in blood insulin levels (Liakou, Liakou, & Zouboulis, 2012). Chronically elevated blood insulin levels appear to influence cellular activity in a number of ways that could contribute to acne occurring in vulnerable individuals (Melnik, 2012). Prescribing a low-glycemic index diet to treat acne patients, however, has not yet been explored in a systematic fashion.

What is a person with acne to do? Dermatologists suggest that people with acne keep a food diary to use in developing a healthful, well-balanced diet that reduces or eliminates potential problematic foods—such as dairy and wheat—and increases servings of vegetables high in antioxidants and servings of fish containing healthy oils that can help combat inflammation. Meeting with a dietitian for meal-planning advice also is recommended, especially for growing adolescents. Eliminating foods must not lead to poor diets. It can take several weeks for dietary change to have an effect. Although dietary change alone does not appear to be a fully effective treatment for acne, it might be helpful when used in combination with prescribed skin care and medications.

Vitamin A Medications for Acne

Vitamin A, also called "retinol," is found naturally in fish oils such as cod liver oil. Precursors to vitamin A, carotenoids, are found in many fruits and vegetables. Prescription medications derived from vitamin A compounds reduce inflammation in mild to moderate acne. Tretinoin ("Retin-A"), adapalene ("Differin"), and other topical retinoid products work to prevent oil and skin-cell trapped pores. Severe acne—especially the type of acne that involves deep inflammation in the sebaceous glands that is not responsive to any other treatment—sometimes is treated with a vitamin A derivative, isotretinoin ("Accutane"), that is taken internally. Isotretinoin can have serious side effects, therefore patients using the drug must be monitored closely. Serious birth defects can result when pregnant women take isotretinoin, however; therefore women of childbearing age must be especially careful to avoid conceiving while taking this drug.

Allison R. Ferreira and Barbara A. Brehm

See Also: Antioxidants; Glycemic index and glycemic load.

Further Reading

American Academy of Dermatology (2014). *Acne*. Retrieved November 18, 2014, from http://www.aad.org/dermatology-a-to-z/diseases-and-treatments/a---d/acne

Andrews, R. (2014). Fighting acne with food: Can what you eat worsen or help your acne? *Precision Nutrition*. Retrieved November 18, 2014, from http://www.precisionnutrition .com/all-about-acne-nutrition

Bowe, W. P., & Logan, A. C. (2011). Acne vulgaris, probiotics and the gut-brain-skin axis—back to the future? *Gut Pathogens 3* (1). Retrieved from http://www.gutpathogens .com/content/3/1/1. doi:10.1186/1757-4749-3-1.

Bowers, J. (2012, May 1). *Diet and acne; role of food remains controversial*. American Academy of Dermatology. Retrieved from http://www.aad.org/dw/monthly/2011/september /diet-and-acne#page5

Burris, J., Rietkerk, W., & Woolf, K. (2013). Acne: The role of medical nutrition therapy. *Journal of the Academy of Nutrition and Dietetics, 113* (3), 416–430. doi: 10.1016/j. jand.2012.11.016.

Liakou, A. I., Liakou, C. I., & Zouboulis, C. C. (2012). Acne and nutrition. In V. R. Preedy (Ed.), *Handbook of diet, nutrition and the skin*. Wageningen Academic Publishers, 414–422.

Melnik, B. C. (2012). Diet in acne: Further evidence for the role of nutrient signaling in acne pathogenesis. *Acta Dermato-Venereologica*, 92 (3), 228–231. doi:10.2340/000 15555-1358.

Adipose Tissue

Adipose tissue refers to body tissues composed primarily of fat storage cells, called "adipocytes." Adipocytes are specialized for storing energy in the form of triglyceride molecules. Triglyceride is manufactured by the liver from excess fuel substrates, which are the nutrients that provide the body with energy: carbohydrates, proteins, and fats. (Alcohol also supplies calories, but it is not considered to be a nutrient.) After the liver manufactures triglycerides from excess energy the triglycerides are sent into the bloodstream, primarily in the form of chylomicrons and other lipoprotein compounds. From the bloodstream the triglyceride is picked up by adipocytes and shuttled into storage.

In addition to their energy storage functions, adipose tissue, adipocytes, and triglyceride molecules perform several other vital physiological and anatomical

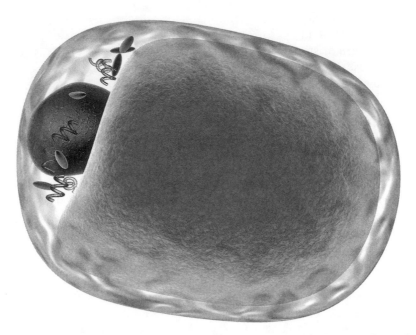

Fat cells, or adipocytes, are specialized cells capable of synthesizing and storing fat, in the form of triglycerides. Up to 90% of an adipocyte's volume may be composed of triglycerides. (Spectral-design/Dreamstime.com)

functions in the body. Pads of adipose tissue help to cushion vital organs, such as those in the abdomen. Adipose tissue pads also serve as shock absorbers throughout the body, including in the synovial joints. Many important body structures are composed of fats, including the cell membranes, the sheath surrounding many nerve cells, and some components of bone marrow. Fat located in these places is referred to as "essential fat" because it is essential for health. Essential fat contributes about 3% to 5% of total body weight.

Sex-Specific Adipose Stores

Women have an additional category of essential fat called "sex-specific fat." It is found in the breasts, hips, and thighs. Sex-specific fat explains why the leanest of females has more body fat than the leanest of males. A great deal of energy is required to run the menstrual cycle and to grow and nurse a baby, hence the extra energy stores. Sex-specific fat stores contribute about 5% to 9% of body mass in women.

Intramuscular Triglycerides

Some fat is found in muscle tissue, in the form of intramuscular triglycerides (IMTG). This fat stores energy and can be used to support muscular contraction during physical activity. In general, IMTG are most commonly used during submaximal exercise of medium intensity. IMTG also are used along with muscle glycogen (a form of starch storage) during resistance exercise. Research indicates that women use about twice as much IMTG as men do during exercise, and that exercise training improves skeletal muscle's ability to metabolize IMTG for fuel. The ability to use IMTG for fuel can vary with glucose tolerance—an indication of how well blood sugar is regulated by the body.

One study, for example, examined the use of IMTG in obese subjects having normal or impaired glucose tolerance, thus qualifying subjects for a diagnosis of prediabetes (Perreault, Bergman, Hunerdosse, Playdon, & Eckel, 2010). The average BMI of the men and women participating in the study was about 31.5, and the average body composition was about 36% fat. The subjects were 45 to 70 years old and fairly sedentary. The researchers found subjects with prediabetes had greater levels of IMTG and showed a lower rate of IMTG use at rest as compared with subjects who had normal glucose tolerance. This research supports the observation that prediabetes has a wide range of effects upon energy-production systems and not simply blood-sugar regulation.

So are IMTG a good thing? Young, lean endurance athletes seek to maximize their utilization of IMTG stores to supply fuel for activities such as endurance running, cycling, and swimming. Trained muscles effectively draw on these stores, and IMTG stores contribute to performance. These stores, however, are higher in older adults and not linked to improved performance. In fact, in older adults, the IMTG stores increase and the number of mitochondria decline. The triglycerides must get into mitochondria to be metabolized into energy. One study found that older men and women had more IMTG not in contact with mitochondria (Crane, Devries, Safdar, Hamadeh, & Tarnopolsky, 2010). Both old and young subjects had similar levels of daily physical activity, therefore the researchers concluded that, with age, muscle cells become less efficient at producing energy from IMTG. And, as noted, obese individuals also have higher IMTG stores. Therefore whether IMTG is good or bad depends upon the amount, a person's age, a person's training status, the BMI, and glucose tolerance.

Subcutaneous Fat

Approximately a third of a person's body fat is stored under the skin. These fat stores are called "subcutaneous fat." Some subcutaneous fat is helpful as insulation, keeping warmth within the body in cold weather. People who have observed (or remember being part of) a pool or lake full of children probably recall the thinner children having less tolerance for staying in cool water, and the heavier children were comfortable for longer periods. Conversely, people with extra subcutaneous fat lose heat less quickly in hot environments and have increased risk of heat illness, especially during high-intensity and prolonged physical activity. Subcutaneous fat improves the appearance of the face, helping to support the skin. The faces of very thin people usually look older in later life than those of their heavier peers.

Brown Adipose Tissue

Brown adipose tissue (BAT) is a special type of fat that contains a greater density of capillaries and mitochondria than that of white fat. Brown fat cells generate heat and in cool environments help mammals maintain body temperature without shivering. Researchers have speculated that the greater levels of BAT in lean people as compared with obese individuals might partly explain differences in body composition. Higher levels of BAT contribute to a higher resting metabolism and the ability to consume more calories without gaining weight. Once thought to be present in significant amounts only in infants, now—through nuclear imaging techniques—BAT has been shown to be present in adults.

Visceral Adipose Tissue

Visceral adipose tissue (VAT) consists of fat stored around the abdominal organs, including the liver, stomach, intestines, and kidneys. Excess VAT appears to be the link between obesity and negative health effects such as artery disease, type 2 diabetes, hypertension, and inflammatory disorders (Cornier et al., 2011). Although waist circumference gives some information about central obesity (excess fat storage in the torso), it does not reveal whether the excess fat is subcutaneous or VAT. Computerized tomography (CT) scans provide information on the volume of fat inside the abdomen, but such tools are not yet commonly used for diagnosis. Symptoms such as the metabolic syndrome, with disorders of blood sugar and blood pressure regulation, indicate the need for lifestyle change to reduce VAT and restore normal metabolic functions.

Adipose Tissue: More Than a Storage Depot

Adipose tissue participates actively in metabolic regulatory processes, communicating extensively with other cells, tissues, and organs in the body. For example, an interesting messenger affected by adipose stores is called "adiponectin"—a hormone-like molecule produced by adipose tissue as well by as other tissues. Higher levels of body fat have been associated with lower levels of adiponectin (Liu et al., 2012). Adiponectin helps insulin get sugar from the bloodstream into cells, where it can be stored or burned for energy. This observation might help explain the insulin resistance that often develops with obesity (Liu et al., 2012).

Barbara A. Brehm

Research Issues

Scientists have begun to explore what factors influence the location of adipose tissue stores. They are particularly interested in factors that lead to excess storage of visceral fat.

Researchers continue to uncover a variety of health risks associated with visceral adipose tissue (VAT). They are exploring what these health risks are, and the biochemical and physiological mechanisms responsible for these risks. Researchers also are trying to determine why some people with excess VAT develop health problems and others do not.

See Also: Body composition; Brown adipose tissue; Energy balance; Obesity, definition and health effects

Further Reading

Brehm, B. A. (2014). *Psychology of health and fitness*. Philadelphia: F. A. Davis.

Cornier, M.-A., Despres, J.-P., Davis, N., et al. (2011). Assessing adiposity: A scientific statement from the American Heart Association. *Circulation, 124* (18), 1996–2019.

Crane, J. D., Devries, M. C., Safdar, A., Hamadeh, M. J., & Tarnopolsky, M. A. (2010). The effect of aging on human skeletal muscle mitochondrial and intramyocellular lipid ultrastructure. *Journal of Gerontology, Series A: Biological Sciences, 65*(2), 119–128. doi: 10.1093/gerona/glp179

Liu, Y., Turdi, S., Park, T., et al. (2012). Adiponectin corrects high-fat diet-induced disturbances in muscle metabolomic profile and whole-body glucose homeostasis. *Diabetes*, December 13, 2012, [Epub ahead of print].

Nishimura, S., Manabe, I., & Nagal, R. (2009). Adipose tissue inflammation in obesity and metabolic syndrome. *Discovery Medicine, 8* (41), 55—60.

Perreault, L., Bergman, B. C., Hunerdosse, D. M., Playdon, M. C., & Eckell, R. H. (2010). Inflexibility in intramuscular triglyceride fractional synthesis distinguishes prediabetes from obesity in humans. *Integrative Physiology, 18* (8), 1524–1531. doi: 10.1038 /oby.2009.454

Science news articles about "visceral adipose tissue." (n.d.) e!Science News. Retrieved November 18, 2014, from http://esciencenews.com/dictionary/visceral.adipose.tissue

Adolescence and Nutrition

Adolescence refers to the transition from childhood to adulthood, which begins with puberty. On average, girls begin puberty when they are between 10 and 13 years old, and boys begin when they are between 12 and 15 years old. Adolescence frequently is divided into three stages: early adolescence (11 to 14 years of age), which is characterized by increased cognitive development and the physical changes that accompany puberty; middle adolescence (15 to 17 years of age), which is characterized by increased independence; and late adolescence (18 to 21 years of age), when teenagers transition into adulthood.

Puberty is a dynamic period of rapid growth and physical, cognitive, and social/emotional maturation; it is second only to infancy in the rate of change taking place in the body. All this development requires additional calories and nutrients, particularly protein, calcium, and iron. Proper nutrition during this critical time leads to improved mood, enhanced school performance, increased energy, and better health in adulthood. Consequences of inadequate nutrition during adolescence can influence the rest of a person's life and include osteoporosis, anemia, increased risk of heart disease, and type 2 diabetes.

Adolescence also is a period of change in lifestyle, as children transition into more independent teenagers and begin to make decisions—including food decisions—for themselves. Because teenagers often are influenced by a need to fit in, the decisions they make are easily swayed by their peers and the media. Teens frequently succumb to advertisements for fad diets, acne solutions, and other claims to help them look and feel good. They live in a world of conflict, where they are expected to look slim or strong, but they are being encouraged to eat foods full of sugar, fat, and sodium that can contribute to overweight and obesity. This impossible mix encourages eating disorders and poor body image. Schools and caregivers play a critical role in educating and encouraging adolescents to make healthful food decisions, as well as providing healthy, realistic role models for adolescents.

Nutritional Needs

Adolescents' nutritional needs depend on age, sex, height, weight, and activity level. Females generally require between 1,600 and 2,400 calories a day, and males generally require 1,800 to 3,200 calories per day. These calories should come from nutrient-rich foods such as a variety of protein foods, whole grains, vegetables, fruits, and low-fat dairy products. The best meals include an assortment of foods from different food groups. Unfortunately, most adolescents do not eat the 2½ to 6½ cups of fruits and vegetables or the 2 to 3 ounces of whole grains recommended per day, and they eat twice the maximum recommended daily intake of sodium (2,300 mg each day) (CDC, 2013).

Calcium and iron are two nutrients critical for growth and development that adolescents frequently lack. Over the last 20 years, soft drinks have been replacing milk as the preferred beverage of adolescents. The Dietary Reference Intake for calcium is 1,300 mg per day, which corresponds to three servings of milk, yogurt, or cheese. Calcium also can be found in fortified beverages (such as orange juice), leafy greens like kale and broccoli, and almonds. Calcium is necessary for strong bone development, and inadequate intake during adolescence can lead to decreased bone mass, increased bone fractures, and osteoporosis later in life. Iron is another common deficiency, especially among girls. Iron deficiency can lead to fatigue and decreased concentration, both of which can impact school performance. All adolescents are at risk of developing iron deficiency anemia during growth spurts when their bodies need more of all nutrients; however, girls are particularly at risk because they lose iron during menstruation (in menstrual blood). Meat is a rich source of iron, therefore vegetarians can be at risk for iron deficiency if they do not eat enough iron-containing foods (such as leafy greens, fortified cereal, and beans) or take a vitamin supplement. Other nutrients commonly found in meat that vegetarians must be sure to consume include protein, zinc, and vitamin B12.

Healthy and Unhealthy Eating Habits

Adolescent lifestyles can cause irregular eating habits. Teens tend to stay up late, snack often, eat on the go, skip meals, and consume fast food or other highly processed foods. Although these habits are not necessarily unhealthy by themselves, food choices made because of such habits can be very unhealthy. According to the

American Academy of Pediatrics, for example, 20% to 30% of teenagers do not eat breakfast (American Academy of Pediatrics, 2013). Adolescents who eat breakfast regularly have a lower body mass index than teens who do not eat breakfast. Breakfast gives kids more energy and the ability to focus on school. Easy breakfast foods also can be nutritious—a bowl of fortified cereal with milk and a glass of juice provides fiber, calcium, vitamins, and iron. Skipping meals often leads to excess eating later in the day, and adolescents frequently consume foods such as chips and cookies, which are high in calories and low in nutrients.

Adolescents who perceive themselves as being overweight—regardless of whether they actually are overweight—are more likely to have irregular meals and to skip meals. Skipping meals can lead to inadequate nutrition intake, increased snacking on unhealthy foods, and overeating at the next meal. Poor body image also leads to a variety of other unhealthy eating habits and eating disorders. Many adolescents attempt fad diets that require cutting out entire nutrient groups such as fats or carbohydrates, both of which are essential (in healthy amounts) for the body to grow and develop properly. Eating disorders—including anorexia nervosa, bulimia nervosa, and binge eating disorder—are characterized by extreme attitudes and behaviors toward food. The attitudes toward food often coincide with other issues, such as stress, anxiety, depression, and substance use. Eating disorders are serious medical conditions that can lead to the development of life-threatening problems, such as heart conditions and kidney failure, as well as other complications of malnutrition.

One of the best ways to improve adolescent eating patterns is to eat regular meals as a family. Teens who eat with their families are more likely to consume healthier foods and get better grades, and they are less likely to engage in risky behaviors, such as smoking, drinking, and drug use (CDC, 2012).

Acne

Acne affects the majority of teenagers. Myths connecting diet to acne abound, but numerous scientific studies have failed to show a strong connection between the two. The best method for treating acne continues to be eating a balanced diet, exercising regularly, and practicing good hygiene. Although vitamin A and its analogs are ingredients in several acne medications, consuming extra vitamin A will not prevent acne and also can be toxic.

Sugar-Sweetened Beverages and Caffeine

Sugar-sweetened beverages (SSBs) are beverages that contain added caloric sweeteners such as high-fructose corn syrup or sucrose. The SSB category includes soft drinks, fruit drinks, sports drinks, energy drinks, and sweetened coffee and tea drinks. Importantly, SSBs tend to have few nutrients and are thought to be the greatest source of added sugar in North American diets. Adolescents who drink soft drinks regularly drink less juice and milk and consume approximately 200 calories more per day than those children who do not (Temple, 2009).

Caffeine is a stimulant that arouses the central nervous system. Although moderate caffeine consumption among adults (equivalent to 400 mg per day, or 2 to 4 cups of coffee) generally is considered safe, little research has been done on the effects of caffeine on children and adolescents. The American Academy of Pediatrics encourages little to no consumption of caffeine by children or adolescents (AAP, 2011), and Health Canada considers the maximum safe limit to be 2.5 mg per kilogram of body weight (Government of Canada, 2012). Following these guidelines, a 100-pound child (45 kg) should consume no more than 100 mg of caffeine per day, which is less than one cup of coffee.

Caffeine consumption by adolescents is on the rise and has increased by 70% since 1977 (Temple, 2009). In addition to soft drinks and coffee, adolescents are getting their caffeine from less traditional sources, such as energy drinks, gum, mints, and other products to which caffeine has been added. Energy drink advertisements often specifically target adolescents. Energy drinks are not the same as sports drinks. Sports drinks contain carbohydrates, minerals, electrolytes, and flavoring, and are intended to replace water and electrolytes lost through sweat during physical activity. By contrast, energy drinks contain stimulants, such as caffeine, guarana, and taurine, as well as sugar. Some energy drinks contain 500 mg of caffeine—as much as 14 cans of caffeinated soft drinks (AAP, 2011).

Much remains unknown about caffeine's effects on adolescents; however, several trends are apparent. Many adolescents are not getting enough sleep, and sleep disruption is a clear side effect of caffeine. Sleep deprivation can lead to lack of energy and focus, increased moodiness, depression, slower reaction time, and impaired judgment. Additionally, SSBs and energy drinks are high in sugar— contributing to obesity, tooth decay, and other physical problems.

The American Academy of Pediatrics states that energy drinks are never appropriate for children or adolescents. It encourages limited to no consumption of sports drinks, as well. Instead, the Academy recommends that adolescents consume water during exercise and juice and low-fat milk with meals.

Lisa P. Ritchie

See Also: Acne; Caffeine; Eating disorders; Energy drinks; Iron-deficiency anemia; Obesity, causes; Sugar-sweetened beverages.

Further Reading

American Academy of Pediatrics. (2011). *Kids should not consume energy drinks, and rarely need sports drinks, says AAP*. Retrieved from: https://www.aap.org/en-us/about-the-aap/aap-press-room/pages/Kids-Should-Not-Consume-Energy-Drinks,-and-Rarely-Need-Sports-Drinks,-Says-AAP.aspx

American Academy of Pediatrics. (2013). *Healthy living: The case for eating breakfast.* healthychildren.org. Retrieved from http://www.healthychildren.org/English/healthy-living/nutrition/pages/The-Case-for-Eating-Breakfast.aspx?nfstatus=401&nftoken

=00000000-0000-0000-0000-000000000000&nfstatusdescription=ERROR%3a+No+l ocal+token

Centers for Disease Control and Prevention (CDC). (2012). *Child development: Teenagers (15–17 years of age)*. Retrieved from http://www.cdc.gov/ncbddd/childdevelopment /positiveparenting/adolescence2.html

Centers for Disease Control and Prevention (CDC). (2013). *Adolescent and school health nutrition and the health of young people*. Retrieved from http://www.cdc.gov/healthy youth/nutrition/facts.htm

Government of Canada. (2012). *Caffeine in food*. Health Canada. Retrieved from http: //www.hc-sc.gc.ca/fn-an/securit/addit/caf/food-caf-aliments-eng.php#a1

Temple, J. (2009). Caffeine use in children: What we know, what we have left to learn, and why we should worry. *Neuroscience Behavioral Review, 33* (6), 793–806. Retrieved from http://www.ncbi.nlm.nih.gov/pmc/articles/PMC2699625/

Agave Syrup

Agave is a genus of plant found primarily in Mexico, where this edible plant has been used for centuries. In Mexico, Aztecs made pins, thread, rope, and even

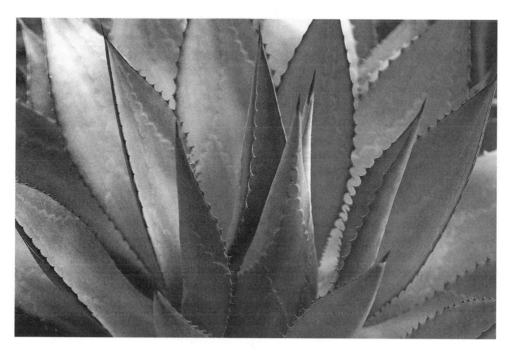

Blue agave plant. Agave plants are characterized by succulent leaves and can tolerate hot, dry climates such as those found in the southern United States and in South America. Agave syrup is produced from the juice taken from the core of the plant once the leaves are removed. (Jorge M. Vargas Jr./Dreamstime.com)

medicine from agave stalks and leaves. The most well-known species is the blue agave, which contains aguamiel—"honey water"—sap that is fermented into tequila. Since the mid-1990s, aguamiel made from the leaves and stalks of blue agave and several other agave species has been processed into syrup and sold commercially as an all-natural sweetener and sugar alternative. Agave syrup is a common choice for vegans looking for a sugar substitute other than honey. Agave syrup labeling has been the subject of debate, as the agave must undergo heating, filtering, and often chemical treatment that can change its molecular structure and yield various amounts of refined fructose.

One tablespoon of agave contains about 60 calories, as compared to 40 calories in a tablespoon of white (table) sugar. Table sugar is composed of an equal ratio of fructose and glucose molecules, and agave syrup is 55% to 90% fructose, giving agave its much sweeter quality. Although glucose and fructose are both absorbed by the small intestine, fructose must be metabolized directly by the liver, but glucose can be carried in the blood stream and metabolized throughout the body. When too much fructose is ingested it cannot be converted for immediate use by the body, and instead is converted by the liver into triglycerides then enters the blood stream or is stored as body fat.

Agave syrup's health benefits are attributed to its low glycemic index (20–30), which means that it provides minimal elevation to blood sugar levels, although this property has not been conclusively determined through scientific research. The American Diabetes Association considers it to be in the same class as other sweeteners such as table sugar, molasses, and high-fructose corn syrup—which should be ingested in limited quantities. Similarly, the American Botanical Council considers agave to be safe in the amounts normally found in food and drink, but does not recommend it for use by pregnant women (Horton, n.d.).

Patricia M. Cipicchio

See Also: Fructose; Glycemic index and glycemic load.

Further Reading

Horton, J. (n.d.). *The truth about agave: Is this "natural" sweetener better than table sugar?* WebMD Expert Column. Retrieved from http://www.webmd.com/diet/features/the-truth-about-agave

Oliff, Heather. (2007). HerbClip, systematic review of agave. American Botanical Council. Retrieved from http://cms.herbalgram.org/herbclip/pdfs/010572-335.pdf

Alcohol

Alcoholic drinks contain ethanol, an organic molecule with the chemical formula C_2H_5OH that can cause alcohol intoxication upon consumption. Ethanol is produced by fermentation, a process by which yeast converts sugar (glucose) to alcohol and carbon dioxide. There are three main groups of alcoholic beverages: beer, wine, and spirits. Beer is produced from barley, hops, water, and live yeast. Wine is produced by fermentation of grapes. Spirits are alcoholic beverages with the greatest percentage of ethanol; they require a distillation step following fermentation. The distillation step enables the ethanol content in an alcoholic beverage to be concentrated and greater than that in beer or wine.

Alcohol use is embedded in many cultures and is perceived as socially acceptable by a majority of people in North American. About 70% of U.S. adults drink alcohol, at least occasionally, and most do so in a responsible fashion. However, 25% of U.S. adults report having alcohol-related problems or have behaviors that put them at risk for developing problems (National Institute on Alcohol Abuse and Alcoholism, 2005). This translates into a very ,large number of people for whom alcohol poses a problem. Human consumption of alcohol has been shown to have both deleterious and

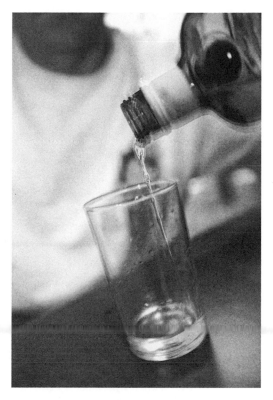

Alcoholic beverages. The alcohol content of beverages varies considerably. In general, health educators consider "one drink" to be the equivalent of 5 fluid ounces of wine, 12 fluid ounces of beer, or 1.5 fluid ounces of liquor. (PhotoDisc, Inc.)

positive effects. The World Health Organization (WHO) estimates that harmful use and abuse of alcohol leads to roughly 2.5 million deaths per year (WHO, 2014).

Cultural History of Alcohol

Alcohol is present in all cultures in some manifestation. Evidence of the earliest preparations of alcoholic beverages can be traced back to 7000 BCE to 6600 BCE in ancient Chinese civilizations (Gately, 2008). Other evidence of the presence of alcohol in ancient cultures is found in the artifacts of people from the Fertile Crescent from around 5400 BCE to 5000 BCE. The artifacts portray people cultivating plants for alcohol production (Gately, 2008). Alcohol production spread from the Fertile Crescent to northern Europe, with evidence found in Scotland of crops grown to produce beer in 3800 BCE (Gately, 2008). Similar evidence of alcohol and its production has been found in Mayan, Indian, Asian, and African ancient cultures. All of

---

Strategies for Reducing Alcohol Intake

The National Institute on Alcohol and Alcohol Abuse (NIAAA) offers excellent information on its website, "Rethinking Drinking," for people who wish to assess their drinking behavior. Some excerpts are included below. The complete online information provides helpful links for measuring and keeping track of drinks, and a downloadable booklet. The NIAAA also suggests that, if people wish to reduce their drinking but have not been able to do so after two or three months, they should consider quitting drinking, getting professional help, or both. Suggested strategies include the following.

- Keep track—Start a list and note each drink before consuming it. This can help slow down a person's drinking, when needed.
- Count and measure—Know the standard drink sizes so that drinks can be counted accurately. Measure drinks when drinking at home.
- Set goals—Decide how many days a week to drink and how many drinks to have, and include some days of no alcohol consumption. Low-risk drinking for alcohol disorders can be as many as 14 drinks per week for men, and 7 drinks per week for women.
- Pace and space—When drinking, pace oneself; sip slowly. Have no more than one standard alcoholic beverage or cocktail per hour. Use "drink spacers"; alternate drinks, and between every alcoholic drink have a non-alcoholic beverage, such as water, soda, or juice.
- Include food—Don't drink on an empty stomach; food helps slow the alcohol absorption.
- Find alternatives—Fill free time by developing new, healthy activities, hobbies, and relationships, or renewing ones that have been missed. Find healthy ways to manage moods or to be comfortable in social situations without drinking alcohol.
- Avoid "triggers." Decide what triggers drinking and plan how to avoid the triggers.
- Plan to handle urges—Remember all the reasons for changing drinking behavior, and even plan to ride out the urges and let them pass.
- Know your "no." Have a polite and convincing "no thanks" ready. The more frequent the hesitation, the more often a person will succumb to drinking.

National Institutes of Health. National Institute for Alcoholism and Alcohol Abuse. (December 21, 2014). *Rethinking drinking*. Retrieved from http://rethinkingdrinking.niaaa.nih.gov/Strategies/TipsToTry.asp

---

these cultures seemed to recognize and use alcohol as a pleasurable or relaxing substance, but they used alcohol for religious reasons as well.

Modern-Day Social and Cultural Aspects of Alcohol

In most modern-day societies, alcohol is viewed as a pleasurable substance or drug rather than a nutrient or a necessary substance. Alcohol frequently is served in social situations of adults and teenagers. Most countries around the world have a legal drinking age of 18; however in the United States, the legal drinking age is 21.

Advocates of lowering the drinking age in the United States believe that lowering the drinking age would decrease harmful, secretive drinking behaviors in adolescents. It has been demonstrated, however, that teenagers across the world engage in harmful drinking patterns, regardless of whether the legal drinking age is 18 years of age or 21 years of age (Grube, 2005). Among teenagers, binge drinking is predominant, as opposed to moderate or safe drinking. Binge drinking is defined as consuming five or more alcoholic beverages in one sitting. It accounts for the three leading causes of death for adolescents aged 12–20, which include unintentional injury, homicide, and suicide (Miller, Naimi, Brewer, & Jones, 2007). Although binge drinking is common in adolescents and young adults, it also is prevalent in older adults. According to the CDC, 70% of all binge drinking episodes can be attributed to adults who are 26 years of age or older, and more than half of the alcohol consumed by adults is via binge drinking (CDC, 2012). Although most adults drink moderately, binge drinking tends to account for a large part of the drinking culture in most societies.

Effects on the Body

Blood Alcohol Concentration

When consumed, ethyl alcohol absorption starts in the stomach and continues in the small intestine. From the small intestine alcohol moves into the blood and travels directly to the liver where only 10% to 20%, of the alcohol in the blood can be broken down at one time. The remaining alcohol circulates in the blood stream until it eventually can be broken down by the liver. It can take roughly 2 hours for one drink to be fully metabolized. The measurement of intoxication therefore can be quantified by blood alcohol content or concentration, known as BAC, which is defined as the percentage of alcohol in one's blood. Research has shown that cognitive function becomes increasingly impaired as BAC rises. At a BAC of 0.05% (5% blood concentration of alcohol), the frontal lobe is defined as sedated and reasoning and judgment become impaired. At 0.10% BAC, the areas of the brain devoted to speech and vision become impaired, resulting in slurred speech and impaired coordination. At 0.30% the drinker experiences stupor and confusion. At a BAC ranging from 0.40% to 0.60% the drinker can suffer from unconsciousness and cardiac or respiratory failure (Insel, Ross, McMahon & Bernstein, 2014).

The speed of alcohol absorption into the body depends on a number of factors, such as the contents of the stomach before drinking an alcoholic beverage, the size of the person drinking, and the sex of the person drinking. On average, women appear to be more susceptible to the effects of alcohol. This partly is due to differences in size and body composition; women are generally smaller than men with a greater percentage of body fat for a given size. Alcohol diffuses primarily into lean tissue. This means that a given amount of alcohol tends to be more concentrated in the lean body mass of women.

The differences in the rate of alcohol metabolism also appear to differ between the sexes. Women's stomachs produce lesser amounts of a key enzyme responsible for breaking down alcohol—alcohol dehydrogenase. Thus, women's bodies generally break down alcohol more slowly, so blood alcohol levels remain high for longer periods. These observations help explain why women develop alcohol-related disorders at lower alcohol intakes than those of men. Larger body sizes also are equipped with larger livers that can metabolize alcohol more effectively. Food also slows the absorption rate of alcohol by the stomach and the small intestine by minimizing contact between alcohol and the permeable lining of the stomach and small intestine. Other factors such as sugar content and aeration of alcohol in a carbonated beverage make alcohol more readily absorbable, thus increasing its effect on the consumer.

Alcohol Metabolization

After alcohol is ingested, enzymes begin metabolizing alcohol in the stomach and small intestine. Alcohol and its byproducts are absorbed in the small intestine and carried to the liver via the portal vein. In the liver, alcohol is converted to acetaldehyde by the enzyme alcohol dehydrogenase. The product of this reaction, acetaldehyde, then is metabolized to acetic acid radicals by acetaldehyde dehydrogenase. The acetic acid from this reaction binds with Coenzyme A to form acetyl-coA using the enzyme acetyl-coA synthetase (HAMS Harm Reduction Network, Inc., 2009). Acetyl-coA then can be used for the energetic needs of the cell. Cytochrome P450, which is highly activated in heavy drinkers, is another enzymatic pathway used to metabolize alcohol in the endoplasmic reticulum of cells (Zakhari, 2006). Catalase is another enzyme in the peroxisomes of cells that metabolizes alcohol and produces hydrogen peroxide in the process. Although there are various pathways to metabolize alcohol, most alcohol is metabolized using the alcohol dehydrogenase and acetaldehyde dehydrogenase mechanism that occurs in the liver.

Alcohol Addiction

Alcohol is considered a drug and can be addicting. Alcoholism is a biological and psychological disorder that is defined by problematic drinking behaviors that include uncontrollable craving and consumption of alcohol. Alcoholism can progress quickly and create severe damage to the health and social well-being of an alcoholic. Alcoholism develops through a myriad of factors including stress, social environment, genetic disposition, and predisposing mental health conditions. Long-term alcohol abuse is detrimental to the physical health of an individual. It causes a variety of disorders including brain damage, psychological disorders, liver disease, and cardiovascular disease, and can lead to systemic organ failure. Alcoholism can be deadly, but many treatment plans have been developed to combat it. Medical professionals can use psychotherapy and drug therapies to help people complete treatment for alcohol withdrawal.

Brain and Behavioral Changes

Alcohol use and abuse can lead to neurological deficits including behavioral changes. Alcohol is a central nervous system (CNS) depressant. Short-term, small-to-moderate consumption of alcohol can cause irritability, aggression, and short-term memory loss. Because alcohol is a CNS depressant, consumption leads to an increase in risk-taking behavior and impaired judgment. Long-term alcohol consumption can lead to decreased concentration, decreased memory ability, and impaired brain development along with many other neurological deficits. Long-term alcohol consumption also can perpetuate many psychological disorders, including depression, anxiety, sleep disorders, bipolar disorder, and substance-abuse disorders. Alcohol particularly affects adolescents and other young people, as the brain is rapidly changing and developing. Studies also have shown that alcohol sensitizes the neurocircuitry of the addiction pathway in adolescents and young adults, making them more prone to alcohol addiction (Guerri & Pascual, 2010).

Alcohol abuse is strongly associated with a plethora of harmful behaviors, including accidental death and injury due to motor vehicle accidents, drowning, burns, and firearm accidents. Alcohol abuse is linked to domestic violence as well as to other forms of violence, including homicide and suicide. Poor decision making under the influence can result in unwanted, unplanned, and unprotected sexual activity and can cause other relationship problems.

Liver Disease

Regular consumption of alcohol is known to cause liver disease. Alcohol contributes to liver disease by infiltrating liver fat, and can cause hepatitis (inflammation of the liver) and cirrhosis (replacement of liver tissue with scar tissue). As alcohol is metabolized, acetaldehyde builds up in the body. Acetaldehyde is a toxin that is considered harmful and promotes liver disease. Liver disease as a result of high levels of alcohol ingestion affects women faster and with use of a smaller amount of alcohol. Roughly 10% to 15% of clinical alcoholics eventually develop liver disease. Alcohol-related fatty liver disease can be fully reversed; however alcohol-induced hepatitis and cirrhosis are not reversible. For alcoholic liver disease that can't be cured; liver transplants are the only treatment option.

In heavy drinkers, the enzymes cytochrome P450 and catalase are highly active. These enzymes contribute to tissue damage. When cytochrome P450 metabolizes ethanol, the following toxic byproducts are produced: Reactive oxygen species (ROS) (free radicals), hydroxyethyl, superoxide anion, and hydroxyl radicals (Zakhari, 2006). When catalase breaks down alcohol, increased levels of hydrogen peroxide occur. The build-up of these toxins leads to the oxidative stress that causes tissue damage associated with liver disease.

Cancers

Alcohol also can lead to liver cancer. The products of the various reactions carried out to metabolize ethanol contribute to the toxic and mutagenic effects of alcohol consumption on the body. The products of alcohol metabolism—acetaldehyde and aldehyde—can alter DNA structure to promote more hepatocyte (liver cell) regeneration. Also, in livers with decreased function due to significant alcohol consumption, hepatocytes regenerate faster than in healthy livers. This could promote dysregulated hepatocyte replication and, therefore, cancer. Acetaldehyde and aldehydes also bind to lysine residues of various cellular proteins and cause them to change and promote tumorigenicity. The ROS produced from cytochrome P450 metabolizing alcohol interact with proteins and DNA, and affect their function and promote tumorigenicity (McKillop & Schrum, 2009).

Alcohol and its metabolites can initiate cancers in other areas of the body as well. Alcohol intake, even at relatively low levels, is associated with increased risk of cancers of the respiratory system; breast cancer; and cancers of the gastrointestinal (GI) tract, including the mouth, esophagus, stomach, colon, and rectum.

Inflammation of the Gastrointestinal Tract and Pancreas

Excessive alcohol intake is the primary cause of esophagitis (inflammation of the esophagus), gastritis (inflammation of the stomach), and pancreatitis (chronic inflammation of the pancreas).

Fetal Alcohol Spectrum Disorders

Scientists have long known that alcohol can be a teratogen, a substance that disrupts fetal development and can cause irreversible damage. Fetal alcohol spectrum disorders include a wide range of physical, behavioral, and cognitive abnormalities that are caused by exposure to alcohol during fetal development. Not all babies exposed in utero to alcohol develop alcohol-related disorders, and scientists continue to look for the biological mechanisms behind alcohol's effects on fetal development. Because researchers have not been able to define a "safe" level of alcohol intake that poses no risk to a developing fetus, pregnant women are strongly encouraged to avoid alcohol.

Positive Effects of Alcohol: Cardioprotective Effects

Many studies have shown that moderate alcohol consumption can be cardioprotective, as moderate alcohol consumption has been linked with a reduced risk for cardiovascular diseases. In particular, red wine consumption has been shown to have cardioprotective qualities. Red wine has antioxidants (flavonoids), which protect the cardiovascular system in many ways. These antioxidants are associated with a decreased concentration of LDL (low-density lipoprotein) cholesterol and an increased concentration of HDL (high-density lipoprotein). These antioxidants also reduce blood clotting and alter lipid profiles after meals. In one study, scientists used a hypercholesterolemic swine model to examine the effects of alcoholic beverages on the heart. Moderate consumption of red wine and vodka was shown to reduce cardiovascular risk by improving collateral-dependent perfusion through various mechanisms (Chu et al., 2012).

Type 2 Diabetes

Alcohol has been shown to decrease the risk of type 2 diabetes in moderate alcohol drinkers. Researchers have shown that some of the reasons alcohol is associated with lowered risk of diabetes is because moderate alcohol consumption increases insulin sensitivity and levels of HDL cholesterol. The anti-inflammatory properties of moderate alcohol consumption also can lead to the protective properties of alcohol against type 2 diabetes. Alcohol consumption at any level greater than moderate consumption, however, increases the risk of type 2 diabetes.

Stress Relief

Moderate amounts of alcohol might provide some relief from stress, because alcohol is a central nervous system (CNS) depressant. Such relief is temporary, however, as the effect of alcohol wears off with time. Although alcohol can be used to relieve stress, being dependent on alcohol for stress relief can lead to addiction. Researchers have found that the results of studies on the relationship between stress relief and alcohol are inconsistent. Experts have come to the consensus, however, that most anti-stress benefits of alcohol are associated with a myriad of other characteristics including family history of alcoholism, environment, types of stress, gender, and personality traits.

Anagha Inguva

Research Issues

According to the World Health Organization (WHO), harmful alcohol use is one of four common risk factors—along with tobacco use, poor diet, and physical inactivity—for the four main groups of noncommunicable diseases: cardiovascular diseases, cancer, chronic lung diseases, and diabetes. Many countries around the world are grappling with the health problems of alcoholism and alcohol abuse. WHO's *Global Status Report on Alcohol and Health* provides more information on this topic.

World Health Organization. (2011). *Action needed to reduce health impact of harmful alcohol use.* Retrieved from http://www.who.int/mediacentre/news/releases/2011/alcohol_20110211/en/index.html

World Health Organization. (2011). *Global status report on alcohol and health.* Retrieved from http://www.who.int/substance_abuse/publications/global_alcohol_report/en/index.html

See Also: Fetal alcohol syndrome and disorders; The French paradox; The liver; Resveratrol.

Further Reading

Centers for Disease Control and Prevention (CDC). (2012). *Fact sheets—binge drinking.* Retrieved from http://www.cdc.gov/alcohol/fact-sheets/binge-drinking.htm

Chu, L. M., Lassaletta, A. D., Robich, M. P., et al. (2012). Effects of red wine and vodka on collateral dependent perfusion and cardiovascular function in hypercholesterolemic swine. *Circulation 126* (11 Supp. 1), S65–72.

Gately, I. (2008*). Drink: A cultural history of alcohol.* New York: Gotham Books.

Grube, J. (2005). *Youth drinking rates and problems: A comparison of European countries and the United States*. U.S. Department of Justice. Retrieved from http://www.udetc.org/documents/CompareDrinkRate.pdf

Guerri, C., & Pascual, M. (2010). Mechanisms involved in the neurotoxic, cognitive, and neurobehavioral effects of alcohol consumption during adolescence. *Alcohol 44* (1), 15–26.

HAMS Harm Reduction Network, Inc. (2009). *How alcohol is metabolized in the human body.* Retrieved from http://hamsnetwork.org/metabolism/

Insel, P., Ross, D., McMahon, K., & Bernstein, M. (2014). *Nutrition.* Burlington, MA: Jones & Bartlett Learning.

McKillop, I., & Schrum, L. (2009). Role of alcohol in liver carcinogenesis. *Seminars in Liver Disease 29* (02), 222–232.

Miller, J. W., Naimi, T. S., Brewer, R. D., & Jones, S. E. (2007). Binge drinking and associated health risk behaviors among high school students. *Pediatrics, 119* (1), 76–85.

National Institute on Alcohol Abuse and Alcoholism (NIAAA). (2005). *Epidemiology of alcohol problems in the United States.* Retrieved from http://pubs.niaaa.nih.gov/publications/Social/Module1Epidemiology/Module1.html

World Health Organization (WHO). (2014). *Management of substance abuse.* Retrieved from http://www.who.int/substance_abuse/facts/en/

Zakhari, S. (2006). *Overview: How is alcohol metabolized by the body?* NIAAA Publications. Retrieved from http://pubs.niaaa.nih.gov/publications/arh294/245-255.htm

Allyl Sulfides (Organosulfurs)

Allyl sulfides (organosulfurs) are organic sulfur-containing phytochemicals (compounds that occur naturally in plants). Allyl sulfides are found in plants belonging to vegetables in the onion and garlic families, including onions, leeks, chives, shallots, and all varieties of garlic. They are known for their pungent odor and possible antitumorigenic properties. Allyl sulfides occur in a variety of classes, the most common of which—allicin—is responsible for the flavor of garlic. The compound is synthesized by the enzyme alliinase which is activated when a garlic bulb is crushed. Garlic has been used over time in traditional Eastern medicine to treat ailments from fungal and bacterial infections to poor digestion and parasites.

The biochemical significance of allyl sulfides in the body is wide ranging. Studies show that the compound helps prevent cancer by blocking the initiation and promotion stages of tumor development. Allyl sulfides modify pathways in charge of cell proliferation, helping to reduce general tumor incidence and suppress tumorigenesis (the creation of new tumors). The main methods by which allyl sulfides block cancerous growth are by inducing apoptosis, or cell death, and by stimulating genes that serve to suppress tumors.

Research shows that garlic preparations featuring allyl sulfides boost the immune system by increasing the presence of natural killer immune cells in the body. Garlic preparations also stimulate digestive enzymes that help remove toxins from the body, and even might be effective in repellents for mosquitoes and other insects. Although allyl sulfide and garlic supplements are widely available, their effectiveness could be tempered through interactions between allyl sulfides and different levels of selenium, vitamin A, and fatty acids. Eating vegetables from the onion and garlic families appears to be associated with more health benefits than consuming dried preparations or supplements.

Patricia M. Cipicchio

See Also: Garlic.

Further Reading

Block, E. (2010). *Garlic and other aliums: The lore and the science.* Cambridge: The Royal Society of Chemistry.

Lavecchia, T., Rea, G., Antonacci, A., & Giardi, M. T. (2013). Healthy and adverse effects of plant-derived functional metabolites: The need of revealing their content and bioactivity in a complex food matrix. *Critical Reviews in Food Science and Nutrition, 53* (2), 198–213. Retrieved from. http.//www.tandfonline.com/doi/full/10.1080/10408398.201 0.520829. doi: 10.1080/10408398.2010.520829.

National Institutes of Health. (2012). *Garlic.* MedlinePlus. Retrieved from http://www .nlm.nih.gov/medlineplus/druginfo/natural/300.html

Norton. K. (2011). *Phytochemicals: 15 health benefits of allyl sulfides.* Health Articles. Retrieved from http://kylenorton.healthblogs.org/2011/09/05/phytochemicals-15-health -benefits-of-allyl-sulfides/

Alpha-Linolenic Acid

Alpha-linolenic acid (ALA) is an essential omega-3 fatty acid, which means that for proper growth and development ALA must be obtained from the diet. This fatty acid contains 18 carbon atoms and 3 carbon-carbon double bonds, and is found in both plant and animal foods. Flaxseed, canola, soy, walnuts, chia seeds, and pumpkin seeds are good sources of alpha-linolenic acid, with flaxseed being the richest. ALA also is found in some dairy foods and red meat, and in cooking oils, medicinal oils, and dietary supplements. Most people consume most of their ALA from soybean oil, as it is found in many different foods such as salad dressings and mayonnaise. ALA deficiencies are rare because people require only a small amount of ALA per day (1.1 to 1.5 grams) (Schardt, 2005).

The two other main types of omega-3 fatty acids are eicosapentaenoic acid (EPA) and docosahexaenoic acid (DHA). These have longer chains and are found in seafood. Omega-3 fatty acids have been associated with a number of health benefits. The human body, however, can convert alpha-linolenic acid into only small amounts of EPA and DHA. The health benefits associated with ALA are not as strongly supported as those of EPA and DHA.

Some evidence suggests that diets with increased ALA help to reduce risk of heart disease and heart attacks. One study showed that over a six-year period, people who had high dietary intakes of ALA had a 59% lower risk of heart attacks, compared to people with the lowest ALA intakes (Therapeutic Research Faculty, 2009). The Nurses Health Study found that women who consumed more dietary ALA had half of the risk of heart disease as those who consumed the least amount (Schardt, 2005). Dietary ALA might slow the buildup of arterial plaque that causes heart disease and reduce the risk of high blood pressure.

Because alpha-linolenic acid can be changed into EPA and DHA, and both are anti-inflammatory, it is thought that ALA also can reduce inflammation. Some preliminary research suggests that diets high in ALA can decrease inflammation and improve lung function in asthma patients (Ehrlich, 2011).

A large epidemiological study found that men who consumed the most ALA in their diet had a greater risk of developing prostate cancer as compared to men consuming the lowest levels of ALA. Other studies, however, have found no risk. A meta-analysis of 16 studies did find a small association between ALA levels in diet, blood, and tissue samples with increased risk of prostate cancer, but attributed this association to publication bias rather than to a negative effect of ALA (Simon, Chen, & Bent, 2009). Nevertheless, such findings suggest that ALA supplements probably should be avoided until research has ruled out the possibility that ALA could increase cancer risk.

People taking anticoagulant medication should check with a health care provider before consuming high amounts of ALA, because ALA can increase the blood-thinning effects of these drugs and raise the risk of bleeding.

Catherine M. Lenz

See Also: Fatty acids.

Further Reading

Ehrlich, S. D. (2011). *Alpha-linolenic acid.* University of Maryland Medical Center. Retrieved from http://www.umm.edu/altmed/articles/alpha-linolenic-000284.htm

Insel, P., Ross, D., McMahon, K., & Bernstein, M. (2013). *Nutrition.* Burlington, MA: Jones & Bartlett Learning.

Schardt, D. (2005, December). *Just the flax.* Nutrition Action Health Letter. Retrieved from http://www.cspinet.org/nah/12_05/flax.pdf

Simon, J. A., Chen, Y.-H., & Bent, S. (2009). The relation of a-linolenic acid to the risk of prostate cancer: A systematic review and meta-analysis. *American Journal of Clinical Nutrition, 89* (5). doi: 10.3945/ajcn.2009.26736E.

Therapeutic Research Faculty. (2009). *Alpha-linolenic acid.* WebMD. Natural Medicines Comprehensive Database. Retrieved from http://www.webmd.com/vitamins-supplements /ingredientmono-1035-ALPHA-LINOLENIC%20ACID.aspx?activeIngredientId=1035

Alpha-Lipoic Acid

Alpha-lipoic acid—also known as lipoic acid and thioctic acid—is an antioxidant that is synthesized by the human body. It is found in every cell and helps the cells convert glucose into energy. It also counteracts the negative effects caused by free radicals in the body. Alpha-lipoic acid is both fat-soluble and water-soluble, which means it can work in all areas of the body. Some research suggests that alpha-lipoic acid might be useful in regenerating and reactivating other antioxidants, such as the vitamins C and E, and thus it could help strengthen the effects of other antioxidants in the body.

Alpha-lipoic acid is found in some foods, such as spinach, broccoli, potato, yam, carrot, beet, yeast, and red meat. After it was first discovered, alpha-lipoic acid was viewed as a vitamin that the body cannot produce, but it later was discovered that the body does synthesize alpha-lipoic acid. The signs of a deficiency for this antioxidant are hard to characterize, because it works with other nutrients in the body. Deficiency symptoms are similar to those of insufficiency of the other antioxidants, such as reduced muscle mass, memory problems, and weakened immune function. There currently is no dietary reference intake for alpha lipoic acid, but it is a popular antioxidant supplement. Dosages of 20 mg to 50 mg per day are generally considered safe but—as with most supplements—long-term safety data are lacking. Some research suggests that high doses of alpha-lipoic acid can cause thiamine or biotin deficiency, and side effects can include headache, muscle cramps, skin rash, and allergic reactions.

Alpha-lipoic acid was discovered in 1937 as a compound in certain bacteria. Its antioxidant functions have been recognized and studied since 1939, and in the 1960s several groups of researchers began to investigate therapeutic applications. Alpha-lipoic acid was observed to work well as a remedy for intake of toxic substances, and physicians prescribed large doses of it to patients diagnosed with mushroom poisoning and heavy-metal poisoning. It was also given to patients with liver cirrhosis and diabetic neuropathy, because it was observed that many of these patients had lower than average levels of alpha-lipoic acid.

Alpha-lipoic acid continues to be prescribed as a treatment for diabetic neuropathy, a painful complication that often is found in people with type 1 diabetes. Diabetic neuropathy is thought to be at least partly a result of oxidative stress, and the ability of alpha-lipoic acid to perform in both water and fat tissue allows it to penetrate all the areas of nerve cells. These treatments use very high doses of alpha-lipoic acid which are administered intravenously with medical supervision. Treatments have proven to be helpful for some patients. Alpha-lipoic acid also has been observed to reduce the blood sugar levels in diabetics. Diabetic patients using alpha-lipoic acid must be monitored to ensure that blood sugar levels do not fall too low.

Additional research investigating other potential therapeutic uses for high doses of alpha-lipoic acid is under way. Some research suggests that alpha-lipoic acid could be helpful in reducing blood sugar levels and improving insulin sensitivity of people who have type 2 diabetes. Other studies aim to establish alpha-lipoic acid's potential ability to treat radiation injury, Alzheimer's disease, cataract formation, and stroke. Studies on the capability of alpha-lipoic acid to lessen some negative side effects of chemotherapy have produced supportive results. Antioxidants, however, also have the potential to reduce the effectiveness of some chemotherapy agents, therefore cancer patients must work with their oncologists to determine whether alpha-lipoic acid supplementation might be useful.

Fei Peng

See Also: Antioxidants; Vitamins.

Further Reading

American Cancer Society. (2008). *Lipoic acid.* Retrieved from: http://www.cancer.org/treatment/treatmentsandsideeffects/complementaryandalternativemedicine/pharmacologicalandbiologicaltreatment/lipoic-acid

EBSCO Publishing. *Lipoic acid.* (2012). NYU Langone Medical Center. Retrieved from http://www.med.nyu.edu/content?ChunkIID=21480

Ehrlich, S. D. (2011). *Alpha-lipoic acid.* University of Maryland Medical Center. Retrieved from http://www.umm.edu/altmed/articles/alpha-lipoic-000285.htm

Weil, A., & Becker, B. (2012). *Alpha-lipoic acid* (ALA). DrWeil.com. Retrieved from http://www.drweil.com/drw/u/ART03051/AlphaLipoic-Acid-ALA.html

Alternative Sweeteners (Sugar Substitutes)

The term "alternative sweetener" refers to a variety of substances that can be used instead of sugar (sucrose) in a range of foods and beverages. Manufacturers choose alternative sweeteners based on whether they are nutritive (have calories and supply energy) or nonnutritive (do not have calories or supply energy), their taste and texture, and their chemical properties. Sugar substitutes in baked goods, for example, must be able to withstand heat, and those used in gum should not promote tooth decay. The names of alternative sweeteners can be confusing, and sometimes even are misleading. Table 1 describes and compares the most common sugar substitutes.

Lisa P. Ritchie

See Also: Agave syrup; Artificial sweeteners; Honey; Stevia; Sugar alcohols.

Table 1. Alternative Sweeteners (Sugar Substitutes)

Name	Description	Examples
Artificial Sweeteners (also called "nonnutritive sweeteners," "high-intensity sweeteners")	Synthetic sugar substitutes are significantly sweeter than sugar. Artificial sweeteners are nonnutritive, and supply few to no calories or carbohydrates per serving.	• Acesulfame potassium (Sunett, Sweet One) • Aspartame (Equal, NutraSweet) • Neotame • Saccharin (SugarTwin, Sweet'n Low) • Sucralose (Splenda)
Sugar Alcohols (also called "artificial sweeteners," "polyols," "nutritive sweeteners")	Sugar alcohols are a group of sweeteners used in processed foods as a lower-calorie substitute for sugar that does not promote tooth decay. On average, they supply 2 calories per gram as compared to 4 calories per gram for sugar. Sugar alcohols can have a laxative effect when eaten in large quantities.	• Erythritol • Hydrogenated starch hydrolysate • Isomalt • Lactitol • Maltitol • Mannitol • Sorbitol • Xylitol
Natural Sweeteners (also called "sugar substitutes," "nutritive sweeteners")	"Natural sweetener" is a general term for sweeteners that contain no added colors, flavors, or other food additives. In the United States, the FDA does not have guidelines for "natural" products. In Canada, "natural" foods must meet standards specifying that they have been minimally processed. The sweeteners provide energy and are chemically similar to sugar, but they have different textures and flavors as compared to table sugar.	• Agave nectar • Barley malt • Date sugar • Fruit juice concentrate • Honey • Maple syrup • Rice syrup

(continued)

Table 1. Continued

Name	Description	Examples
Novel Sweeteners (sweeteners that fit into a variety of categories)	These sweeteners are "novel" because they are new to the market. They do not fit neatly into any of the other categories. Stevia, for example, comes from a plant and many consider it a natural, nonnutritive sweetener; however, only its highly refined form is approved as a food additive in Canada and in the United States. Tagatose also occurs naturally, but is manufactured from lactose. Although it is low in carbohydrates, it is not considered sugar free.	• Stevia extracts (Pure Via, Truvia), also called "Rebaudioside A," "Reb-A," and "rebiana" • Tagatose (Naturlose) • Trehalose

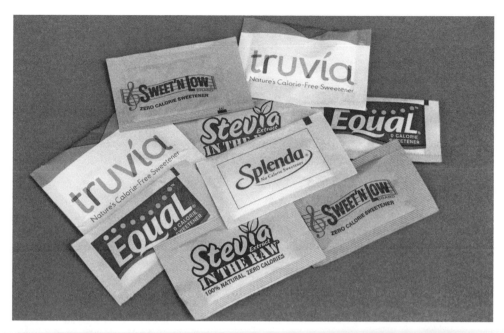

Alternative sweeteners. Consumers often choose alternative sweeteners, such as those pictured here, in order to reduce their intake of sugar and calories. (iStockphoto.com)

Further Reading

Chang, K. (2012, June 11). Choosing a sugar substitute. *The New York Times*. Retrieved from http://well.blogs.nytimes.com/2012/06/11/which-sweetener-should-you-choose/?ref=health

Mayo Clinic Staff. (2012, October 9). *Nutrition and healthy eating: Artificial sweeteners and other sugar substitutes*. Retrieved from http://www.mayoclinic.com/health/artificial-sweeteners/MY00073

Alzheimer's Disease and Nutrition

Alzheimer's disease (AD) is an irreversible, progressive brain disease that accounts for 50% to 60% of all cases of dementia and is estimated to affect 35.6 million people worldwide (WHO & Alzheimer's Disease International, 2012). Dementia is characterized by cognitive decline, reduced daily activities, and neurophysiological abnormalities. Patients with AD progressively worsen until recalling memories and responding to their environment become difficult to impossible tasks. The majority of people who suffer from the disease are 65 years of age and older; however, there are rare cases of early onset AD due to a genetic vulnerability that presents in patients who are between 30 and 50 years old.

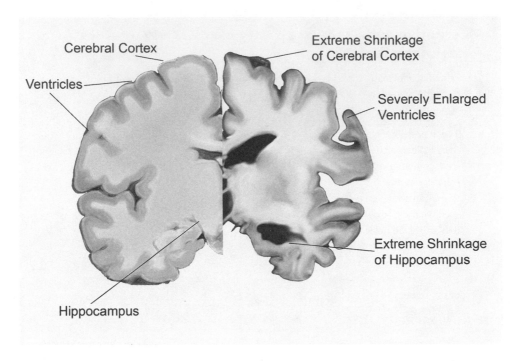

Comparison of a brain before and after development of Alzheimer's disease. Loss of neuron number and function occurs in many areas. (National Institutes of Health/National Institute on Aging)

Although little is known about how the disease begins, it is likely that damage to the brain starts more than a decade before the symptoms appear. The brain is composed of a network of billions of neurons and neuronal connections. In Alzheimer's disease, abnormal protein deposits—specifically intercellular beta-amyloid plaques and intracellular tau tangles—cause neurons to communicate and transmit signals less efficiently. These abnormal protein deposits cause an immune response leading to brain inflammation when cells such as astroglia and microglia—neuronal homologs of pathogen-eating macrophages—gather to destroy the plaques as the tangles initiate cell death. Although at first this might seem beneficial to the brain, AD causes chronic inflammation that stresses and kills nearby healthy cells in addition to the diseased cells. These cells include the astroglia and microglia that die and aggregate at the beta-amyloid plaques due to beta-amyloid's adhesive qualities. Over time, the neurons fail to function properly and fail to communicate, ultimately causing cell death. The damage eventually spreads to an important brain structure—the hippocampus. The hippocampus is vital in memory consolidation, memory recall, and spatial recognition. As a result, the first symptoms to appear are problems in memory and recognition. By the final stages of Alzheimer's, neuronal apoptosis (cell death) is widespread, and the brain tissue has shrunk significantly. Thus, in end-stage AD, patients lose the ability to communicate, sense spatial orientation, and care for themselves.

Alternative and Complementary Health Therapies for Alzheimer's Disease

The following information on the use of complementary and alternative therapies—including nutrition therapy—for Alzheimer's disease and dementia is excerpted from the U.S. government National Center for Complementary and Alternative Medicine.

- There presently is no convincing evidence from a large body of research demonstrating that a dietary supplement can prevent worsening of cognitive impairment associated with dementia or Alzheimer's disease, including the use of ginkgo, omega-3 fatty acids/fish oil, vitamins B and E, Asian ginseng, grape seed extract, and curcumin. Additional research on some of these supplements is under way.
- Preliminary studies of some mind and body practices such as music therapy suggest that they might be helpful for some of the symptoms related to dementia, such as agitation and depression.
- Mindfulness-based stress-reduction programs might be helpful in reducing stress among caregivers of patients with dementia. Studies suggest that a mindfulness-based stress-reduction program is more helpful for improving mental health than is attending an education and support program or just taking time off from providing care.
- Complementary health approaches shouldn't be used as a reason to postpone seeing a health care provider about memory loss. There are treatable conditions, such as depression; adverse reactions to medications; and thyroid, liver, or kidney problems, which all can impair memory.
- Some complementary health approaches and supplements can interact with medications and also can have serious side effects. Talk to a health care provider before adding dietary supplements or other complementary health approaches.

National Center for Complementary and Alternative Medicine (NCCAM). (2014). *5 things to know about complementary health practices for cognitive function, dementia, and Alzheimer's disease.* Retrieved from http://nccam.nih.gov/health/tips/alzheimers

Interestingly, the disease is named after a German psychiatrist and neuropathologist, Dr. Alois Alzheimer, who in the early 1900s cared for a patient with rapidly declining and severe dementia. The patient's symptoms included memory loss, language problems, and erratic behavior (NIH, 2013). The autopsy of the diseased brain revealed cellular changes in the nervous tissue which caused a loss of neuronal connections. These cellular changes later were identified as neurofibrillary tangles and plaques, which are hallmark characteristics of Alzheimer's disease.

Disease Risk Factors

Scientists have not yet determined the causes of Alzheimer's disease; however it is likely that the causes include a mixture of genetic, environmental, and lifestyle factors. Those who have a first-degree relative with Alzheimer's are more likely to develop the disease. The risk increases if more than one family member has been diagnosed. Research has found that there are several genes that increase the risk of having Alzheimer's. The gene that has the strongest link to late onset Alzheimer's is APOE-e4, one of the four common forms of the apolipoprotein E gene. Each individual inherits some form of the APOE gene, and those who have inherited one copy of APOE-e4 have increased risk of developing AD. Those who inherit two copies of the variant 4 gene have an even greater risk of developing the disease; however, the existence of the variant four genes does not guarantee that the person will develop AD. Scientists have estimated that APOE-e4 is implicated in 20% to 25% of Alzheimer's cases (Alzheimer's Association, 2013).

One of the greatest mysteries of Alzheimer's disease remains unsolved: Why does the risk increase with age? Although the disease is not a normal part of growing older, after age 65 the risk of developing Alzheimer's doubles every five years. After age 85, the risk of developing the disease is about 50% (Alzheimer's Association, 2013). Research on how brain function changes with age has begun to illuminate how age-related changes can harm neurons and contribute to the neurological damage observed in Alzheimer's. Normal age-related changes in the brain include neuroinflammation and production of free radicals—both of which contribute to cell death and brain atrophy.

Treatment and Prevention

Medication

Currently there is no cure for Alzheimer's disease. Those who develop Alzheimer's usually are prescribed FDA-approved medication. There are two ways in which AD medication functions. One way is to inhibit cholinesterase, an enzyme that breaks down the memory neurotransmitter acetylcholine. The medication works by inhibiting the activity of cholinesterase, thus slowing the disease progression, as the memory loss experienced is associated with deficiencies in acetylcholine. The second method is medication that regulates the activity of glutamate, which is involved in learning and memory, through an NMDA receptor antagonist. The NMDA, N-methyl-D-aspartate receptor is a glutamate receptor that predominantly is involved in sending excitatory signals in the brain to help form memories. Thus the agonist triggers the NMDA receptor and increases memory-forming activities. The antagonist drugs protect neurons against excess glutamate that is released by cells damaged by Alzheimer's causing excitotoxicity in the brain. Additionally, antagonist drugs target NMDA receptors, because they can become over-activated and trigger an excess of Ca^{2+} ions to enter neuronal cells, thus activating a series of intracellular processes that promote cell death (Alzheimer's Association, 2013).

Lifestyle and Cardiovascular Health

Lifestyle contributes to the development of AD. It has been observed that risk increases with conditions that damage the heart and blood vessels including hypertension, heart disease, stroke, diabetes, and high cholesterol. Autopsy results show that 80% of individuals with Alzheimer's also had some type of cardiovascular disease. In fact, autopsy studies suggest that the hallmarks of Alzheimer's disease—the plaques and tangles—might be present in the brain without causing symptoms unless the brain also shows evidence of vascular disease (Alzheimer's Association, 2013). The brain is nourished by the heart; with each heartbeat, 20% to 25% of the body's blood is carried to the brain to receive oxygen and nutrients. Thus, conditions disrupting blood flow to the brain lead to nerve damage.

Experts believe that controlling cardiovascular risk factors might be the best approach to protect brain health. A heart-healthy lifestyle includes regular exercise. In fact, some research has suggested exercise might directly benefit brain cells as a result of increased blood and oxygen flow. Strong evidence suggests exercise actually protects the brain from AD, due to the proven benefits to the cardiovascular system. Conversely, cardiovascular risk factors also appear to increase AD risk. For example, a long-term study of 1,500 adults found that those who were obese in middle age were twice as likely to develop Alzheimer's, and those who also had high cholesterol and hypertension were six times as likely to develop the disease (Alzheimer's Association, 2013).

Nutrition: Heart-Healthy Diet

A heart-healthy diet is a balanced diet that includes a variety of foods such as vegetables, fruits, whole grains, low-fat dairy products, and lean protein. Nutritionists suggest eating dark-skinned fruits and vegetables, such as kale, eggplants, blueberries, and plums, because these foods have high levels of antioxidants and polyphenols to protect the brain from free radicals and oxidative damage. Metal ions are known to catalyze production of free radicals and induce dementia. Several studies have suggested that metals such as lead, iron, aluminum, copper, and zinc are involved in Alzheimer's pathogenesis. Although specific metal chelators—molecules that bind to metal ions—have been tested in Alzheimer's disease therapy, there has been little success. This is thought to be due to late administration of the chelators after extensive brain damage already has occurred. It therefore is thought that regular consumption of dietary polyphenols, which are known to chelate metals, could prove to be protective against AD (Ramesh, Rao, Prakasam, Sambamurti, & Rao, 2010).

Some studies have suggested associations between an atherogenic blood lipid profile and AD. Diets that are high in added sugars and processed fats are thought to be associated with a poor cholesterol profile. This consists of an increase in low-density lipoproteins (bad cholesterol) and a decrease in high-density lipoproteins (good cholesterol). Experts believe that cholesterol plays a role in AD because cholesterol acts in both the production and aggregation of amyloid beta in the brain. However, HDL (good cholesterol) also has been shown to protect brain cells. Thus, to promote brain health, experts suggest reducing the intake of sugar-sweetened food and beverages, and foods that have added fats and sugars.

Additionally, evidence suggests a relationship between type 2 diabetes and Alzheimer's disease. Type 2 diabetes is characterized by high blood glucose levels and a blunted response of cell membrane receptors to insulin. Of those people with type 2 diabetes, 70% develop Alzheimer's disease (Weller, 2013). Research suggests that the underlying mechanism is the disruption of an essential enzyme that typically rids the brain of amyloid plaques—a hallmark of Alzheimer's pathology. In general, high sugar intake appears to be risk factor for AD, even for people who do not have diabetes.

Nutrition: Omega-3 Fatty Acids

Studies have noted that the consumption of fish is associated with a reduced risk of developing Alzheimer's (Morris, 2009). Long-chain omega-3 fatty acids are found almost exclusively in fish such as salmon, tuna, and mackerel. Docosahexaenoic acid (DHA), a type of omega-3 fatty acid, makes up key structures in the brain, including the neuronal membranes and the phospholipids contained in the cerebral cortex. Animal studies with DHA supplements showed enhanced control of neuronal membrane excitability, marked membrane transmission, and decreased oxidative stress in the brain. In the Framingham Study, those patients who were free of dementia and were being treated with high DHA levels (median age of 76 years) had a significant 47% reduction in the risk of developing dementia in the subsequent nine years (Schaefer et al., 2006). There is consistent evidence across all studies that omega-3 fatty acids and fish can help reduce the risk of Alzheimer's. More studies presently are examining the effect of fish oil supplements on progressive cognitive impairment and on the risk of Alzheimer's disease.

Nutrition: Micronutrients

Some studies suggest that high intake of specific vitamins is associated with a reduced risk of developing Alzheimer's; however reports are inconsistent. Limited evidence suggests that low folic acid concentrations in the blood can increase AD risk. Elevated levels of plasma homocysteine are associated with increased risk for the development of dementia and Alzheimer's disease (and cardiovascular disease); this risk factor is modifiable because plasma homocysteine levels can be reduced by folic acid consumption. Epidemiological studies suggest that vitamin E and vitamin C might help reduce inflammation and oxidative stress in the brain (Alzheimer's Research Center, 2013). Additionally, vitamin D deficiency is common among the elderly, but it has been found that increased serum concentrations of vitamin D are associated with reduced risk of AD.

Nutrition: Ketogenic Diet

A specialized diet that is thought to be beneficial to Alzheimer's patients and decrease the risk of developing the disease is the ketogenic diet. The diet consists of high fat intake, adequate protein intake, and low carbohydrate intake. The diet has been used successfully in epileptic patients in countries around the world. More recently the diet is being used for patients with other diseases, including Alzheimer's disease. A high carbohydrate diet is very deleterious—individuals favoring such diets had an 89% greater risk for mild cognitive deficits, as compared to a 44% risk for individuals on a high-fat diet, according to one analysis (Roberts, 2012). It is not known how the ketogenic diet influences brain activity in epilepsy and AD. The low blood sugar levels achieved with a ketogenic diet are thought to be beneficial, but other explanations for altered brain function also are being explored.

Nutrition: Reducing Brain Inflammation

Oxidative stress and inflammation accompany AD pathogenesis. The process of glycation—or the addition of a sugar group to a lipid or protein—dramatically increases the production of free radicals and inflammation in the brain (Stetka & Perlmutter, 2014). Amyloid-beta—the protein that comprises amyloid beta plaques found in AD-affected brains—can be glycated and promote free radical production and inflammation. It is not well understood whether oxidative stress and inflammation are a cause or consequence of Alzheimer's disease, but it would seem logical to try to reduce its development. This can be accomplished through diet by avoiding obesity, and omitting the added sugars and fats that can spur inflammation. Consuming foods known to be anti-inflammatory also could be beneficial. For instance, omega-3 fatty acids have been known to help reduce inflammation. Thus, it seems to be helpful to eat foods such as salmon, tuna, and mackerel which are high in omega-3 fatty acids. It is most beneficial if fish are baked or broiled rather than fried or salted. Nuts such as almonds and walnuts also can help fight inflammation because they are rich in fiber, calcium, vitamin E, and omega-3 fatty acids. Nuts also have high levels of antioxidants that can defend against and repair damage caused by inflammation. Spices such as turmeric and ginger have been known to reduce inflammation.

Animal studies have shown that diets supplemented with antioxidants result in heightened learning acquisition and memory. Antioxidants can be found in a wide range of fruits and vegetables, such as beets, tomatoes, raspberries, and blueberries, as well as many other foods, including green tea and chocolate. Studies have shown that vitamin E might play a role in protecting the body from pro-inflammatory molecules known as "cytokines." Both the Chicago Health and Aging Project and the Rotterdam study concluded that a high dietary intake of vitamin E is associated with a lower risk of AD. Vitamin E can be found in dark green vegetables, such as spinach, kale, and broccoli.

Kay O. Kulason and Victoria E. von Saucken

Research Issues

Some researchers have suggested that Alzheimer's disease (AD) is similar to type 2 diabetes, and some even are calling AD "type 3 diabetes." The brain manufactures insulin which signals neurons to take up the glucose they need for their work. If the cells in the brain are overwhelmed with too much insulin—produced in response to high blood sugar—then the insulin receptors in the cell membrane become less sensitive to insulin's presence. If poor insulin sensitivity turns out to be a major mechanism in the development of AD, then a healthful diet and the prevention of obesity will become even more central in public health efforts to prevent or delay the onset of Alzheimer's.

Bittman, M. (2012, September 25). Is Alzheimer's type 3 diabetes? *New York Times*. Retrieved from http://opinionator.blogs.nytimes.com/2012/09/25/bittman-is-alzheimers-type-3-diabetes/?_php=true&_type=blogs&_r=0.

See Also: Antioxidants; Blood sugar regulation; Cardiovascular disease and nutrition; Diabetes, type 2; Insulin.

Further Reading

Alzheimer's Association. (2013). *Alzheimer's disease and dementia*. Retrieved September 28, 2013, from http://www.alz.org/

Alzheimer's Foundation of America—Index. (2013). Retrieved September 28, 2013, from http://www.alzfdn.org/index.htm

Alzheimer's Research Center. (2013). *Alzheimer's prevention*. Retrieved from http://www.alzheimersinfo.org/prevention.html

Crane, P. K., Walker, R., Hubbard. R.A., et al. (2013). Glucose levels and risk of dementia. *New England Journal of Medicine 369*, 540–548.

Morris, M. C. (2009). The role of nutrition in Alzheimer's disease: Epidemiological evidence. *European Journal of Neurology 16* 1–7. doi: 10.1111/j.1468-1331.2009.02735.x

National Institutes of Health (NIH). National Institute on Aging. (2013). *Alzheimer's disease fact sheet—Alzheimer's disease education and referral center*. Retrieved September 28, 2013, from http://www.nia.nih.gov/alzheimers/publication/alzheimers-disease-fact-sheet

Ramesh, B., Rao, T., Prakasam, A., Sambamurti, K., & Rao, K. (2010). Neuronutrition and Alzheimer's disease. *Journal of Alzheimer's Disease 19* (4), 1123–1139.

Roberts, R. O., Roberts, L. A., Geda, Y. E., et al. (2012). Relative intake of macronutrients impacts risk of mild cognitive impairment or dementia. *Journal of Alzheimers Disease 32* 329–339.

Schaefer, E. J., Bongard, V., Beiser, A. S., et al. (2006). Plasma phosphatidylcholine docosahexaenoic acid content and risk of dementia and Alzheimer disease: The Framingham Heart Study. *Archives of Neurology 63,* 1545–1550.

Stetka, B. S., & Perlmutter, D. (2014, January 12). *Dementia: Is gluten the culprit?* Medscape. Retrieved from http://www.medscape.com/viewarticle/819232

Weller, C. (2013). Alzheimer's may be late-stage type 2 diabetes: The relationship between insulin, amyloid plaques, and enzyme destruction. *Medical Daily*. Retrieved from: http://www.medicaldaily.com/alzheimers-may-be-late-stage-type-2-diabetes-relationship-between-insulin-amyloid-plaques-and-enzyme

World Health Organization, & Alzheimer's Disease International. (2012). *Dementia: A public health priority*. World Health Organization. Retrieved from http://www.who.int/mental_health/publications/dementia_report_2012/en/

Amino Acids

Amino acids are organic compounds that serve as the building blocks of proteins. Amino acids are essential to human life, and also are found in all plant and animal cells. Researchers have identified hundreds of amino acids in nature. Of these, there are about 20 amino acids that are proteinogenic, from which every living thing produces a large number of proteins. Proteins are responsible for countless functions and provide structure to numerous tissues.

In terms of human nutrition, amino acids can be divided into three categories: essential, nonessential, and conditionally essential. Essential amino acids are amino acids that the body cannot produce on its own, and must therefore be consumed. Nonessential amino acids are naturally produced by the body, and do not need to be supplied through diet as long as sufficient protein is present in the diet. Conditionally essential amino acids are amino acids that the body normally produces, but which become essential during certain circumstances, such as during illness or when the body does not have the proper enzymes to make them; at such time, these amino acids must be consumed through the diet. Amino acids are categorized in Table 1.

Chemical formulas for 20 amino acids. (Dreamstime.com)

Table 1. Classification of Amino Acids

Essential Amino Acids	Nonessential Amino Acids	Conditionally Essential
Histidine	Alanine	Arginine
Isoleucine	Arginine	Cysteine
Leucine	Asparagine	Glutamine
Lysine	Aspartic Acid	Glycine
Methionine	Cysteine	Proline
Phenylalanine	Glutamic Acid	Tyrosine
Threonine	Glutamine	
Tryptophan	Glycine	
Valine	Proline	
	Serine	
	Tyrosine	

Amino Acid Structure

The basic amino acid structure is composed of a central carbon atom (C) that is linked to a hydrogen atom (H), an amino group (-NH$_2$), a carboxylic acid group (-COOH), and a unique side group commonly designated by the letter "R." The R group is what distinguishes different amino acids, and each amino acid has a unique R group. When two amino acids join to form a protein, they form a peptide bond. A peptide bond occurs when the amino group of one amino acid joins with the carboxyl group of another amino acid and water (H$_2$O) is released. A dipeptide is two amino acids that are joined by a peptide bond. Tripeptides have three amino acids joined by peptide bonds, oligopeptides have 4 to 10 amino acids joined by peptide bonds, and a polypeptide has more than 10 amino acids joined by peptide bonds.

Amino acids often are likened to letters, and proteins are words spelled with those letters. Proteins can be quite large, containing thousands of amino acids. These chains of amino acids bend and coil, forming unique three-dimensional structures with shapes that depend upon the amino acid interactions with one another. The function of a protein molecule often depends upon this three-dimensional shape.

Amino Acid Function

Amino acids serve a considerable number of functions in the human body through the action of proteins. Functions include fluid balance, acid-base balance, structural and mechanical support (muscles, bone, skin, hair), immune response (antibodies), regulation of chemical processes (enzymes), chemical messengers (hormones), and transporters (cell membrane channels and pumps, carriers). Individual amino acids often are precursors to specific neurochemicals. For example, tryptophan is a precursor for the neurotransmitter serotonin.

Amino Acid Digestion and Absorption

Amino acids enter the body in the form of proteins. Once ingested, polypeptide bonds are broken down and the end result is single amino acids. Protein digestion begins in the stomach, where hydrochloric acid (HCl) unfolds the protein's unique structure, increasing surface area and thus making it easier for digestive enzymes to gain access to the amino acid chain. This process is known as protein denaturation. Following denaturation the proenzyme pepsinogen is released, and then is activated by the acidic environment of the stomach; the activated form of pepsinogen is pepsin. Next, pepsin breaks down 10% to 20% of ingested proteins into smaller polypeptide units or single amino acids.

After leaving the stomach, polypeptides and amino acids enter the small intestine, where most digestion takes place. The pancreas and intestinal lining then release proteases—enzymes that further break down peptide groups into ever smaller units—which then are absorbed as single amino acids into the bloodstream. Once absorbed, amino acids are available to the body for the synthesis of cellular proteins. Any proteins that are not digested are excreted in feces.

Amino Acid Pool and Protein Turnover

All cells need single amino acids to build proteins. Cells continually break down and build proteins. When proteins are broken down the amino acids are released into the bloodstream. Free amino acids are found throughout the body and collectively are referred to as the "amino acid pool." Amino acids from the amino acid pool are used whenever the body needs amino acids for synthesis of proteins.

The body is skilled at reusing amino acids. This recycling of amino acids is called "protein turnover." Protein turnover helps the body meet its amino acids needs. The body synthesizes about 300 grams of protein each day; about 200 grams of this protein comes from protein turnover (Insel, Ross, McMahon, & Bernstein, 2014). When dietary protein intake is too low to meet the body's needs for amino acids, protein breakdown increases to supply the amino acid pool. This can result in the breakdown of essential body tissues, such as muscles.

Protein Quality

Foods which contain all the essential amino acids are referred to as "complete" or "high-quality" proteins. Those foods that lack one or more essential amino acid are referred to as "incomplete" or "low-quality" proteins. Consuming a balanced and varied diet ensures that all the essential amino acids are present.

Amino Acids and Diet

Amino acids are found in every food group, and it is not difficult to achieve an adequate intake of amino acids with a varied diet. Foods highest in protein include most animal-derived products such as meats, fish, poultry, eggs, and dairy products.

Legumes, nuts, and grains also contain protein. Combining plant sources of protein enables people to ensure they have an adequate intake of all essential amino acids. Combining grains and legumes, for example, provides all essential amino acids. Many health authorities advise including a wide variety of protein foods in a diet, limiting the consumption of certain proteins such as red meat—which has been associated with health risks—and increasing intake of seafood and plant proteins.

Amino Acid Supplements

Many amino acid and protein supplements are marketed and sold to athletes with the promise of enhancing endurance and muscle strength. Amino acids can come from either food or supplements. Protein supplements marketed to athletes often feature whey protein, which is high in the branched-chain amino acids leucine, isoleucine, and valine. "Branched chain" refers to the R group structure. These amino acids might be helpful for recovery from strenuous exercise. Some studies suggest that muscle cell injury and recovery time can be lessened with consumption of these amino acids near the time of exercise.

Amino acids also are given as supplements to people with certain diseases and the elderly, when they either are unable to produce particular amino acids or simply lack adequate protein sources in their diet. Studies suggest that daily essential amino acid supplementation improves the quality of life, symptoms of depression, muscle function, and nutrition of institutionalized elderly patients (Rondanelli et al., 2011).

Paula Sophia Seixas Rocha

See Also: Digestion and the digestive system; Protein; Vegetarian and vegan diets; Whey protein.

Further Reading

Acids in protein? (n.d.). Chem4kids.com. Retrieved from http://www.chem4kids.com /files/bio_aminoacid.html

American Dietetic Association; Dieticians of Canada; American College of Sports Medicine, Rodriguez, N. R., Di Marco, N. M., & Langley, S. (2009). American College of Sports Medicine position stand. Nutrition and athletic performance. *Medicine and Science in Sports and Exercise 41* (3), 709–731. doi: 10.1249/MSS.0b013e31890eb86.

Insel, P. M., Ross, D., McMahon, K., & Bernstein, M. (2014). *Nutrition.* Burlington, MA: Jones & Bartlett Learning.

Rondanelli, M., Opizzi, A., Antoniello, N., Boschi, F., Iadarola, P., Pasini, E., & Dioguardi, F. S. (2011). Effect of essential amino acid supplementation on quality of life, amino acid profile and strength in institutionalized elderly patients. *Clinical Nutrition 30* (5), 571–577. doi:10.1016/j.clnu.2011.04.005.

Therapeutic Research Faculty. (2009). *Branched-chain amino acids.* WebMD. Natural Medicines Comprehensive Database. Retrieved from http://www.webmd.com/vitamins-supplements/ingredientmono-1005-BRANCHED-CHAIN%20AMINO%20ACIDS.as px?activeIngredientId=1005&activeIngredientName=BRANCHED-CHAIN%20 AMINO%20ACIDS

Anthocyanins

Anthocyanins are powerful antioxidants found in plants and provide pigmentation to flowers, fruits, and some leaves. Responsible for providing the vibrant reds, blues, and purples prominent in berry plants like bilberry, strawberry, blueberry, and black currant, these water-soluble substances are critical for attracting animals for pollination and seed dispersal. Anthocyanins also impart color to red onions, red cabbage, black beans, grapes, nectarines, and pomegranates. There are more than 500 different types of anthocyanins, differentiated by the nature and positioning of their attached sugar molecules.

The biological interactions that incorporate anthocyanins are complex, making their actions difficult to study in the human body. Not only is it difficult to track their metabolic breakdown after ingestion, but anthocyanins never act independently and are readily oxidized and degraded. They exist as isolated molecules as well as in highly concentrated groups called "anthocyanic vacuolar inclusions," that could intensify their antioxidant properties. Although the release of reactive oxygen species (ROS) is a normal byproduct of cellular metabolism, abnormally high amounts alter the structure of cell membranes and are indicative of disease. The ability of anthocyanins to scavenge ROS makes them effective in reducing the risk of cardiovascular disease by reducing oxidative stress that can lead to ischemia, high blood pressure, and inflammation (Wallace, 2011). Anthocyanins also serve to regulate various signaling pathways whose dysfunction can contribute to the development of cardiovascular disease (CVD).

Anthocyanins are thought to sharpen visual acuity by enhancing the regeneration of rhodopsin, a pigment found in photoreceptor cells of the eye that helps to detect light. Preliminary research with anthocyanin compounds in vitro suggest possible anti-cancer effects, although it is unclear whether this research will develop into therapeutic applications. Bilberry extract supplements have become popular for people experiencing eye strain and those concerned with eye health. These supplements seem to be safe at doses of 25 mg to 50 mg. No other evidence currently provides strong support for taking anthocyanin supplements. Consuming plenty of anthocyanin-rich fruits and vegetables appears to be the best option for maximizing the protective effects of these helpful phytochemicals.

Patricia M. Cipicchio

See Also: Antioxidants; Phytochemicals.

Further Reading

Basu, A., Rhone, M., & Lyons, T. J. (2010). Berries: Emerging impact on cardiovascular health. *Nutrition Reviews 68* (3), 168–177. doi: 10.1111/j.1753-4887.2010.00273.x.

Wallace, T. C. (2011). Anthocyanins in cardiovascular disease. *Advances in Nutrition 2* (1), 1–7.

Wong, C. (2011). *The scoop on anthocyanins*. About.com Alternative Medicine. Retrieved from http://altmedicine.about.com/od/herbsupplementguide/a/The-Scoop-On -Anthocyanins.htm

Antioxidants

Antioxidants are compounds that neutralize chemicals known as "free radicals." Free radicals are molecules that have a single electron, making the molecules highly reactive as they "look" for another electron to complete the incomplete valence. In cells, free radicals can take electrons from other molecules, including those in important structures such as DNA and cell membranes. By donating electrons to stabilize free radicals, antioxidants in the human body help to prevent or delay some types of cell damage.

Some antioxidants are natural and others are man-made. Antioxidants are found in foods such as fruits, vegetables, and whole grains. Antioxidants such as carotenoids, lutein, lycopene, vitamin C, and vitamin E can help healthy cells from being damaged by free radicals (Academy of Nutrition and Dietetics [AND], 2014). Although there is extensive research supporting the idea that a diet with high intake of fruits and vegetables lowers the risk of many chronic diseases, it is difficult to pinpoint how certain antioxidants might be directly responsible for the lower risks of specific diseases. Furthermore, individuals who consume a large amount of fruits and vegetables often also engage in overall healthier lifestyles, which might account for the lower risks of diseases (NIH, 2014b).

Free Radicals and Antioxidants

Free radicals come from a variety of sources. Individuals can be exposed to free radicals via the environment from sources such as cigarette smoke, air pollution, and sunlight (NIH, 2014b). Free radicals also are produced in the body during normal oxidative metabolism, the process by which energy is produced in the mitochondria from oxygen and the fuel precursors carbohydrates, proteins, and fat. When the human body converts food into energy, unstable molecules are formed as part of the natural process of breaking down food. Free radicals trigger cell damage, which can lead to oxidative stress. Some research shows that oxidative stress is partly responsible for diseases such as cancer, cardiovascular diseases, diabetes, Alzheimer's disease, Parkinson's disease, cataracts, and age-related macular degeneration (NIH, 2014b). Antioxidants counter the damage by counteracting the oxidative stress.

Fruits and Vegetables Rich in Antioxidants

Carotenoids

There are approximately 600 carotenoids in foods, and beta-carotene, lycopene, and lutein are three types that are known to reduce damage from free radicals. Foods high in carotenoids decrease risk of prostate cancer; cancers of the mouth, pharynx, esophagus, stomach, colon, and rectum; and decrease risk of macular degeneration. Good food sources with high concentrations of carotenoids are tomatoes, carrots, spinach, brussels sprouts, sweet potatoes, winter squash, and broccoli.

Vitamin E

Vitamin E is associated with reduced risk of cancer, heart disease, and cataracts. Good food sources of vitamin E are vegetable oils, salad dressings, margarine, wheat germ, whole grain products, seeds, nuts, and peanut butter.

Vitamin C

Vitamin C helps protect against infection and damage to body cells and bruising. Additionally, Vitamin C is essential for collagen production, and for the absorption of iron and folate in the digestive tract. Good food sources of vitamin C are oranges, grapefruits, tangerines, strawberries, sweet peppers, tomatoes, broccoli, and potatoes.

Consuming Antioxidants in Foods

The best way to increase intake of dietary antioxidants is to consume a wide variety of fruits, vegetables, whole grains, nuts, seeds, and plant oils. Foods that are packed with antioxidants and can be consumed as a meal or snack include: peanut butter on whole wheat toast with a fruit salad; baked potato with olive oil topped with broccoli, tomatoes, and carrots; and a spinach salad with sweet peppers, carrots, tomatoes, nuts, seeds with extra virgin olive oil as dressing. One way to consume a nutrient-dense diet is to "eat a rainbow" as part of every meal, by filling half of a plate with a mixture of fruits and vegetables (Fruits and Veggies More Matters [FVMM], 2014). Eating a rainbow every day means consuming red, dark green, yellow, blue, purple, white, and orange fruits and vegetables.

Dietary Supplements

Antioxidants also are available in the form of dietary supplements. Consuming natural antioxidants in fruits and vegetables as part of a normal diet is healthful; taking high-dose supplements of antioxidants might not be safe. Antioxidant supplements can have negative interactions with some medications, so it is important to contact the prescribing health care provider when planning to add antioxidant supplements to a regimen. People taking anticoagulant (blood-thinning) drugs, for example, who also are taking high doses of vitamin E supplements could be at risk for bleeding (NIH, 2014b). Smokers who take high doses of beta-carotene could increase their risk of lung cancer. Taking high doses of vitamin E might increase the risk of prostate cancer and of hemorrhagic stroke.

Susana Leong

See Also: Dietary supplements; Phytochemicals.

Further Reading

Academy of Nutrition and Dietetics. (2014). *What are antioxidants?* Retrieved from www .eatright.org/public/content.aspx?id=6792

Fruits and Veggies More Matters. (2014). *Eat a colorful variety every day.* Retrieved from www.fruitsandveggiesmorematters.org/eat-a-colorful-variety-of-fruits-and-vegetables

National Institutes of Health (NIH). (2014a, February). *Antioxidants.* MedlinePlus. Retrieved from www.nlm.nih.gov/medlineplus/antioxidants.html

National Institutes of Health (NIH). (2014b, January). *Antioxidants and health: An Introduction.* National Center for Complementary and Alternative Medicine. Retrieved from www.nccam.nih.gov/health/antioxidants/introduction.htm

NutritionData. (2014). *Nutrition facts, calories in food, labels, nutritional information and analysis.* Retrieved from http://nutritiondata.self.com

U.S. Department of Agriculture. (2014, February). *Vitamins and minerals: Food nutrition information center.* Retrieved from http://fnic.nal.usda.gov/food-composition/individual -macronutrients-phytonutrients-vitamins-minerals/vitamins-minerals

Appetite

Appetite refers to the psychological desire to eat. It is influenced by a variety of factors, including internal signals and cues from the environment. Sensory perceptions, as well as social and emotional triggers and expectations, all impact what and how people eat. Although there are physiological components to how appetite is experienced, there are a greater number of environmental and psychological influences.

It is important to note that appetite is not the same as hunger. Although hunger is the physiological *need* to eat, appetite describes the psychological *desire* for food. Appetite can cause a craving for a particular food even when hunger is absent. Conversely, appetite can be suppressed due to various emotional or medical reasons even though the body is hungry and in need of nutrients. This is an important topic for many reasons. Appetite—arguably even more than hunger—dictates what a person eats, how much a person eats, as well as when and why a person eats. Eating too little or too much, or eating foods that are not healthy simply because they taste or look good can affect a person's health. Psychological influences on appetite can negatively impact a normally healthy lifestyle.

Although occasionally straying from healthful foods and portion sizes is not harmful, in the long term such eating habits can contribute to many health problems, including obesity, type 2 diabetes, hypertension, and liver disease. Furthermore, discovering how to physiologically control or suppress appetite might be helpful in the prevention and treatment of obesity and obesity-related health problems.

Physiological Factors

A variety of neurochemicals work together to influence appetite. The influences of neuropeptide-Y (NPY) have been researched extensively, it appears to work by increasing feelings of hunger and as an appetite stimulator. Ghrelin, produced in the stomach, and leptin, produced in fat cells, are largely responsible for the rise and fall of NPY, and therefore the increase and decrease of appetite. Although

---

Prescription Medications for Appetite Suppression

Several prescription medications for the treatment of obesity work as appetite suppressants; they help people eat less, but they also can cause problems. The Weight-control Information Network's online information should be consulted for information on how these drugs work and their potential side effects. The medications discussed include the following:

- Lorcaserin (sold as "Belviq")
- Phentermine-topiramate (sold as "Qsymia"); phentermine (sold as "Adipex-P," "Oby-Cap," "Suprenza," "T-Diet," and "Zantryl")
- Benzphetamine (sold as "Didrex")
- Diethylpropion (sold as "Tenuate" and "Tenuate Dospan")
- Phendimetrazine (sold as "Adipost," "Bontril PDM," "Bontril Slow Release," and "Melfiat")

Among these types of drugs phentermine is the one used most often in the United States.

Weight-control Information Network (WIN). (2013). *Prescription medications for the treatment of obesity.* National Institute of Diabetes and Digestive and Kidney Diseases. Retrieved from http://win.niddk.nih. gov/publications/prescription.htm

---

ghrelin promotes hunger by stimulating NPY, rising before a meal and falling afterward, leptin quells hunger by inhibiting NPY, suppressing appetite after a meal.

A release of NPY has been shown to increase food intake in both animal and human studies. Neuropeptide-Y is released in states of starvation or food deprivation, as well as when confronted with psychologically desirable foods. The former is to be expected. When the body is in a state of hunger, it is not surprising that appetite would be signaled. The release of neuropeptide-Y when confronted with psychologically desirable foods affects food intake, and this has clear and dangerous implications for those who are overweight or obese—appetite can be stimulated even when the body is satiated and does not need food. This could lead individuals to develop a habit of overeating, because the eating environment or the person's emotional or social states encourage constant and generous consumption.

Leptin release has been correlated with weight loss as it suppresses appetite. Low leptin levels, whether resulting from decreasing fat stores or abnormal leptin function, are correlated with subjective perceptions of hunger and appetite. Individuals with persistently low leptin levels have been reported to experience incessant feelings of hunger. People who are obese appear to develop leptin resistance; the body does not respond appropriately to the presence of leptin. Leptin resistance is associated with increased appetite and hunger.

Sensory Perception

Sensory perceptions of food can influence mood and appetite before and after meals, and significantly impact an individual's weight. The presentation, taste, smell, and texture of food all influence food intake. These factors often can cause individuals to consume far greater amounts of food than their hunger dictates, and also are likely to determine what types of food individuals choose.

Portion size has a very interesting effect on consumption. Multiple studies have shown that the amount of food people tend to eat increases with larger portion sizes. The bigger the portion or the size of a plate, the more food a person tends to consume. This has strong implications in today's world, where portion sizes now are larger than ever. The current eating environment in the United States promotes over consumption by producing inexpensive food in large quantities. Increasing portion sizes have been revealed to correspond with increasing rates of obesity.

Psychological Factors

Emotional states can work to increase or decrease appetite. Although some people are prone to having increased appetites when experiencing negative emotions, other people lose their appetites—particularly when prompted to feel sad. Many people use eating to cope with negative emotions. When food is utilized to deal with issues such as low self-esteem or depression, disordered eating habits commonly develop. An increased appetite in response to a negative mood appears to be a learned behavior, in which a person learns to associate improvements in mood with food consumption. This mood improvement could result from activation of the pleasure centers of the brain, as well as altered neurochemical levels in other areas of the central nervous system. Negative emotions eventually trigger an increase in appetite and then an increase in eating behavior, which reduces negative emotions.

Generally, eating habits established due to long-term exposure to stressors are not positive. They do not aid in the maintenance of a healthy lifestyle. In an interesting study of college women, researchers found that more than 80% of participants' appetites were noticeably different when stressed, and of the 80% of subjects who reported having healthy diets, 66% failed to make healthy choices when experiencing stress (Kandiah, Yake, Jones, & Meyer, 2006). Stress is likely to negatively impact health, as it encourages individuals to under- or overeat, and to eat unhealthy foods that lack a variety of nutrients.

Social and Environmental Factors

Social factors can influence appetite. When eating with friends or relatives, individuals might feel comfortable and eat only as much as they need. Other times, social environments provide a distraction from one's sense of satiety (the feeling of having had enough to eat), and people can continue to experience an appetite and the drive to continue eating, even though they are full. Social factors could create feelings of stress that influence appetite.

Cultural influences also shape a person's appetite. As children grow up they create associations with particular foods. The presence of comfort foods or foods associated with special occasions can stimulate appetite. Similarly, foods regarded as unpleasant can decrease appetite.

The eating environment could influence appetite. A calm and relaxing environment generally is conducive to a healthy appetite, allowing individuals to experience the drive to eat as pleasant, and eating as being pleasurable. Conversely, a noisy, stressful environment could interfere with appetite signals, decreasing or increasing appetite depending upon how an individual responds to stress. The presence of tasty food can increase appetite even though one has had enough to eat. Seeing the dessert menu, for example, can stimulate appetite even after having just finished a large meal. Obesity experts claim that most areas of North America are "obesogenic environments," in that the environments stimulate appetite and push individuals toward overeating, while limiting opportunities for physical activity.

Appetite Stimulants and Suppressants

Various illnesses and medical conditions can cause a decreased appetite even when the body is hungry and in need of food. A loss of appetite is called anorexia. Many cancer treatments interfere with appetite, for example, causing cancer anorexia. A decreased appetite often is seen with illness, and can result in unintentional weight loss. People experiencing unintentional weight loss and a decreased appetite should consult their health care providers to rule out an underlying illness. Older adults often experience a decreased appetite, especially if their senses of taste and smell become less sharp.

Medications that stimulate appetite are known as orexigenics. One example is a drug that is a synthetic version of marijuana. This drug can stimulate appetite and relieve pain.

Understanding how appetite works in the body and in the mind can be useful in offering treatment to obese individuals. Appetite suppressant medication, however, has not yet proved to be very helpful for the long-term treatment of obesity. These medications suppress appetite in the short term, but appetite eventually returns to normal. Medications also have several negative side effects. People should not take these medications for more than a few months, at which time eating returns to normal and weight lost weight often is regained.

Cassandra C. Greene

Research Issues

A variety of magazine and newspaper articles encourage individuals to exercise to suppress appetite and lose weight. Exercise has been shown to influence appetite short term, especially in overweight individuals. High-intensity workouts such as interval training appear to have a stronger appetite-reducing effect than that of more moderate activity levels. High-intensity exercise can result in longer elevations of blood glucose levels and lower blood concentrations of hunger hormones (Reynolds, 2013a). Theoretically, a regular exercise schedule could suppress appetite continuously and decrease the occurrence of overeating or eating between meals. Most studies on exercise and appetite have been short term, however. Little to no evidence suggests that the effect of exercise on appetite actually leads to significant weight loss.

See Also: Hunger, biology of; Mindful eating; Obesity, causes.

Further Reading

Kandiah, J., Yake, M., Jones, J., & Meyer, M. (2006). Stress influences appetite and comfort food preferences in college women. *Nutrition Research 26* (3), 118–123.

Reynolds, G. (2013a, September 11). How exercise can help us eat less. *New York Times.* Retrieved from http://well.blogs.nytimes.com/2013/09/11/how-exercise-can-help-us -eat-less/

Reynolds, G. (2013b, January 17). The appetite workout. *New York Times.* Retrieved from http://well.blogs.nytimes.com/2013/01/17/the-appetite-workout/

Therapeutic Research Faculty. *Prescription weight loss drugs.* (2013). WebMD. Natural Medicines Comprehensive Database. Retrieved from http://www.webmd.com/diet /guide/weight-loss-prescription-weight-loss-medicine

Vorvick, L. J. (2012). *Appetite—decreased.* MedlinePlus. Retrieved from http://www.nlm .nih.gov/medlineplus/ency/article/003121.htm

Arginine

Arginine, also known as L-arginine, is a semi-essential amino acid involved in protein metabolism and the synthesis of urea and creatine within the body. The body also converts arginine into nitric oxide (NO), which acts as an important vasodilator that causes blood vessels to open wider to increase blood flow. Arginine is considered a semi-essential amino acid because the body normally is able to make it in sufficient amounts. This amino acid, however, could be required to be supplied by diet or supplementation in some physiological conditions, such as malnutrition, excessive ammonia production, burns, infections, peritoneal dialysis, urea synthesis disorders, and sepsis. Deficiencies can result in symptoms including constipation, alopecia, skin problems, slow-healing wounds, and fat buildup in the liver. This amino acid occurs naturally in meats, dairy products, many nuts, legumes, and whole grains such as buckwheat, barley, and brown rice.

Arginine was first isolated from a lupin seedling extract in 1886 by Ernst Schulze, a Swiss chemist. In 1998, the Nobel Prize in physiology was awarded to Robert Furchgott, Louis Ignarro, and Ferid Murad for their discoveries concerning NO as a signaling molecule. Because NO is created from arginine, the pharmaceutical and nutraceutical fields began marketing arginine as a dietary supplement. Because it stimulates the body to make proteins, arginine often is marketed to athletes. Additionally, many athletes look to vasodilation to increase blood flow and the delivery of nutrients and oxygen to exercising muscles, thus stimulating protein synthesis and decreasing recovery time. Current research, however, suggests that physiological concentrations of arginine in healthy individuals are enough to saturate the enzymes responsible for making NO, and concludes that arginine supplementation does not cause an increase in enzymatic activity or NO production (Alvares, Conte-Junior, Silva, & Paschoalin, 2012).

Although arginine supplementation might not be beneficial for healthy individuals, several potentially helpful medical applications are under investigation. Arginine supplementation has been shown to aid patients with urea-synthesis deficiencies—which cause a buildup of dangerous nitrogen in the body—by helping to shift the way nitrogen is processed and aid in its elimination. Early evidence from several studies also suggests that arginine supplementation in patients with coronary artery disease and angina can help increase blood flow to the heart and arteries via the NO pathway. Arginine supplementation could aid other circulatory disorders, including erectile dysfunction and intermittent claudication (poor blood flow) in the legs. Studies also show that arginine can aid in wound healing, and when given with hydroxymethylbutyrate (HMB) and glutamine it can slow muscle wasting in certain disease states, such as AIDS.

The supplemental usage of arginine is limited by its absorption rates and bioavailablity within the body. When consumed, it is converted to L-citrulline or L-ornithine by the liver. After conversion, it can enter the bloodstream and be absorbed by peripheral tissue. Due to poor intestinal uptake of arginine during normal conditions, citrulline supplements might be prescribed instead. During disease conditions intestinal uptake of arginine can increase. There is no standard or well-established dosage recommended for arginine. Research studies commonly use two to three grams administered orally two to three times daily.

It is important to consult a health care provider before starting arginine supplementation due to its unwanted interactions with many medications, herbs, and other dietary supplements. Side effects of arginine supplementation include low blood pressure, stomach cramps, and nausea. Although often prescribed for people with congestive heart failure and chest pain, those who already have suffered a heart attack should not take arginine, as it can increase risk of death in some groups of heart patients. Arginine supplementation also can aggravate herpes symptoms in people with this virus. People with asthma should be wary of taking this supplement, as should people taking prescription medicine to control blood sugar levels.

Chelby J. Wakefield

See Also: Amino acids.

Further Reading

Alvares, T., Conte-Junior, C., Silva, J. T., & Paschoalin, V. M. F. (2012). Acute L-Arginine supplementation does not increase nitric oxide production in healthy subjects. *Nutrition & Metabolism*, *9*, 54. Retrieved from http://www.nutritionandmetabolism.com/content/9/1/54

Examine.com. (2012). *Arginine*. Retrieved from http://examine.com/supplements/Arginine/

Mayo Clinic. (2012). *Arginine*. www.mayoclinic.com/health/l-arginine/NS_patient-arginine.

National Institutes of Health (NIH). (2012). *L-Arginine*. MedlinePlus. March 21, 2012. http://www.nlm.nih.gov/medlineplus/druginfo/natural/875.html

Wax, B., Kavazis, A. N., Webb, H. E., & Brown, S. P. (2012). Acute L-arginine alpha keto-glutarate supplementation fails to improve muscular performance in resistance trained and untrained men. *Journal of the International Society of Sports Nutrition* 9, 17. doi:10.1186/1550-2783-9-17.

Wong, C. (2013). L-Arginine: What should I know about it? *About.com: Alternative Medicine*. Retrieved from http://altmedicine.about.com/cs/herbsvitaminsad/a/Arginine.htm

Arsenic

Arsenic is a naturally occurring element that exists in the environment in both organic and inorganic forms. It is found in soil, rocks, water, and air, and can be released during erosion, forest fires, volcanic activity, and through human acts such as mining. Arsenic is considered an essential nutrient, with daily intake ranging from about 12 mcg to 40 mcg. The function of arsenic in human health is not clear, although animal evidence suggests it might be involved in the metabolic pathways of the amino acid methionine.

Arsenic is an odorless and tasteless class 1 carcinogen, or cancer-causing agent. In small amounts arsenic has been used to combat a variety of ailments as far back as Hippocrates (460 BCE–370 BCE), who employed arsenic sulfate to treat ulcers. In 1909, German scientist Paul Ehrlich discovered an arsenic-based cure for syphilis known as "Salvarsan," which in the 1940s was replaced by penicillin. The harmful health effects of arsenic have largely eliminated its application in contemporary medicine, aside from its use in isolated cancer treatments. It is commonly used in industry to strengthen alloys and is most often found in pesticides and treated wood products.

Because the element dissolves easily in groundwater, it also is found in food—especially fish, poultry, rice, and starchy vegetables. Food products usually contain organic arsenic, which currently is considered less harmful by the Food and Drug Administration, as opposed to inorganic arsenic which can be fatal (FDA, 2011). Total arsenic presence in bottled and public drinking water is restricted to 10 ppb by the Environmental Protection Agency, which also is considering standards for other beverages such as apple juice. In 2011, consumers in the United States became alarmed when arsenic levels greater than 10 ppb were found in samples of apple juice and grape juice, according to *Consumer Reports*, an expert, independent nonprofit organization whose goal is to educate consumers about products in the marketplace (Consumer Reports, 2012). The FDA countered stating that its own testing did not find high arsenic levels in juices, but consumers remain concerned. Especially worrisome is children's arsenic intake, because many children in the United States drink relatively large amounts of apple juice. In 2012, higher than expected levels of arsenic were found—this time by the FDA and several other groups—in many samples of rice from around the world (FDA, 2012). Arsenic levels in rice products, including rice milk, rice baby cereal, and rice cakes also were found to be greater than expected.

Arsenic toxicity is highly variable between individuals and is thought to be affected by nutrition. In rats, the element has been shown to interfere with absorption of copper in the body. Vitamins C and E might help relieve oxidative stress caused by arsenic. Prolonged exposure to arsenic can lead to many types of cancer, particularly of the lung, skin, and bladder. Exposure also can cause skin lesions, anemia, diabetes, and neurological problems (CDC, 2009). Acute effects include headaches, gastrointestinal distress, convulsions, and hair loss. Its lethal dose in adults is estimated to be 70 mg to 200 mg.

Patricia M. Cipicchio

Research Issues

The FDA, USDA, Consumer Reports, and other organizations are continuing to monitor arsenic levels in the food supply. Their websites contain interesting information about their monitoring processes and their findings, as well as advice for concerned consumers.

See Also: U.S. Food and Drug Administration.

Further Reading

Center for Disease Control (CDC): Agency for Toxic Substances and Disease Registry. (2009, October 1). *Case studies in environmental medicine: Arsenic toxicity.*

Consumer Reports. (2012, January). Arsenic in your juice? How much is too much? Federal limits don't exist. *Consumer Reports Magazine.* Retrieved January 12, 2013, from http://www.consumerreports.org/cro/consumer-reports-magazine-january-2012/arsenic-in-your-juice/index.htm

Food and Drug Administration (FDA). (2011, December 6). *Questions and answers: Apple juice and arsenic.* Retrieved January 12, 2013, from http://www.fda.gov/Food/ResourcesForYou/Consumers/ucm271595.htm

Food and Drug Administration (FDA). (2012, September 19). FDA looks for answers on arsenic in rice. Retrieved January 12, 2013, from http://www.fda.gov/forconsumers/consumerupdates/ucm319827.htm

Arthritis and Nutrition

Arthritis refers to a group of diseases that involve painful inflammation and stiffness of the musculoskeletal system, especially the joints. It is the leading cause of disability in adults in the United States (CDC, 2011). The word "arthritis" comes from the Greek word "arthron," meaning "joint," and the Latin term "itis," meaning "inflammation." There are more than 100 different types of arthritis, and they vary in prevalence from common to rare. In the United States, as many as 50 million adults (22%) have been doctor-diagnosed with arthritis, with

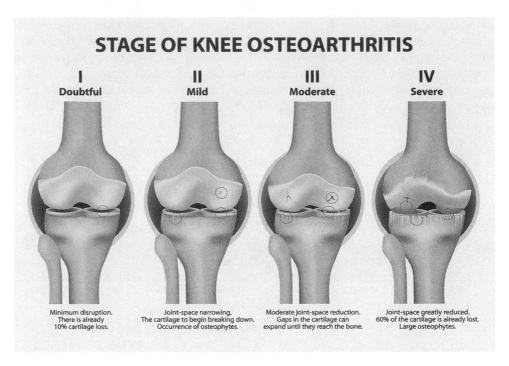

STAGE OF KNEE OSTEOARTHRITIS

I	II	III	IV
Doubtful	Mild	Moderate	Severe

| Minimum disruption. There is already 10% cartilage loss. | Joint-space narrowing. The cartilage to begin breaking down. Occurrence of osteophytes. | Moderate joint-space reduction. Gaps in the cartilage can expand until they reach the bone. | Joint-space greatly reduced. 60% of the cartilage is already lost. Large osteophytes. |

Stages of knee osteoarthritis. (iStockPhoto.com)

the condition being the second most frequent reason for consulting a doctor (CDC, 2011). The most common forms of arthritis are osteoarthritis (OA) and rheumatoid arthritis (RA). Nutrition does not seem to play a major role in the causation of arthritis. Nutrition is, however, an important component of arthritis management, along with other lifestyle-change recommendations and appropriate medications.

Osteoarthritis

Osteoarthritis or "degenerative arthritis" is characterized by the breakdown of cartilage in a joint, often caused by trauma or overuse. It eventually leads to abnormal bone changes and the failure of the joint's mobility. Cartilage is a flexible connective tissue that protects joints, helping to maintain stability and flexibility. Cartilage does not contain blood vessels, which helps to explain why the rate of cartilage growth and repair is relatively slow. Osteoarthritis also might affect the synovium—a fluid-filled sac that surrounds the joint and provides nutrients and oxygen to the joint components. The surrounding muscle and tendons also can be involved.

In the early stages of OA, the cartilage becomes swollen and loses elasticity, which results in the formation of tiny cracks within cartilage tissue that hinder joint function and leave the cartilage vulnerable to further damage. The fragmentation of the cartilage surface can lead to remodeling of the bone and invasion by blood vessels. Inflammation also commonly occurs in the synovium, causing pain and swelling, and can exacerbate cartilage deterioration. Osteoarthritis is not a systemic disease, and only occurs in those joints with deterioration, most commonly affecting the joints of the spine, knee, hand, foot, and hip.

Rheumatoid Arthritis

Rheumatoid arthritis is a chronic, systemic, inflammatory autoimmune disorder affecting the synovium, and leading to joint damage and bone destruction. The disease begins in the small joints, such as the hands and feet, and extends to larger joints. In RA, the immune system attacks the tissues that line joints, including cartilage. The inflamed synovium proliferates across the joint and becomes heavily infiltrated with inflammatory cells. The invading synovium also produces enzymes that decrease cartilage integrity and stimulate bone erosion. Additionally, the surrounding soft tissue becomes inflamed, and new blood vessel growth occurs. Together with the invasion of cartilage and bone into the joint surface, this leads to deformity and progressive physical disability. Intestinal inflammation, abnormal gut microflora, and lipid abnormalities, including insulin resistance correlated to inflammation, also are associated with RA.

Epidemiology

Osteoarthritis is a much more common disease than is rheumatoid arthritis. The number of people affected by arthritis is large with a wide-ranging impact on society. Approximately 1 in 3 people with arthritis (31%) between the ages of 18 and 64 report work limitations due to arthritis, and arthritis is strongly associated with major depression (CDC, 2011). Worldwide, approximately 9.6% of men and 18.0% of women have OA, and about 0.3% to 1% of people have RA (WHO, 2013). Rheumatoid arthritis has a relatively lower prevalence in poorer countries (WHO, 2013). Both OA and RA are more prevalent in women; it has been noted that 24.3% of women and 18.3% of men in the United States have been diagnosed with arthritis; the prevalence increases with age and is higher among women than men in every age group (CDC, 2011).

Although premature mortality is quite low in people with arthritic diseases, the morbidity associated with the disease can be very high, varying greatly among individuals. Joint stiffness and pain are the most prominent symptoms, and arthritis often causes reduced mobility and a lower level of physical activity that result in some degree of physical disability (CDC, 2011). This morbidity related to arthritis also comes as an economic cost to both the individual and to society. Arthritis is among the most common reasons for working days lost, amounting to a huge economic impact worldwide. In 2003, the total cost attributed to arthritis and other rheumatic conditions in the United States was 128 billion dollars, up from 86.2 billion dollars in 1997 (CDC, 2011).

History

Arthritis was one of the first diseases to be clinically recognized, having been described by ancient Egyptian medical texts and Greek scholars. The symptoms of the disease were also referred to in an Ayurvedic medical text. Ayurvedic medicine is a form of Hindu traditional medicine that is native to the Indian subcontinent, 123 CE (Stetka & Wel, 2013). Early Greek scholars, including Hippocrates (~460–357 BCE), and later medieval Europeans ascribed joint maladies to the "flux" of congested humors, in which bad humors were thought to drip into affected joints. Archeological remains also give evidence of arthritis's long past, extending to dinosaurs, Neanderthals, and early humans (Stetka & Wel 2013).

Symptoms and Diagnosis

General signs and symptoms of arthritis include swelling in one or more joints, stiffness around joints that lasts for at least an hour in the morning, constant or recurring pain or tenderness in a joint, difficulty in moving joint, and warmth or redness around joint (CDC, 2011). A general physician or rheumatologist often will review a patient's medical history and order lab tests, including blood and urine tests and imaging tests such as x-rays or MRIs, to make a diagnosis (CDC, 2011). Both OA and RA can be classified according to severity using criteria set out by the American College of Rheumatology.

Osteoarthritis can manifest in different ways, but it is usually diagnosed when health care providers note a loss of cartilage within synovial joints, associated with loss of bone mass and the thickening of the joint capsule. (The joint capsule is the thin, fibrous sac that surrounds the joint and that contains lubricating fluid.) Rheumatoid arthritis usually is diagnosed when patients have arthritis of at least one joint area and achieve a certain "score" that is based on the American College of Rheumatology's criteria. These criteria include location and number of involved joints; symptom duration; severity of RA symptoms such as swelling or deformity; and positive blood results for serum rheumatoid factor.

Causes and Risk Factors

Osteoarthritis sometimes is brought about by another disease or condition. This includes trauma or repetitive use, infectious diseases, or other inflammatory diseases, such as gout. Gout is a complex form of arthritis that occurs when either the kidney does not excrete enough uric acid or the body produces too much, and, consequently, uric acid crystals can accumulate in joints. The accumulation of crystals results in inflammation, swelling, and severe attacks of pain. Obesity is another common contributor to OA, as excess adipose tissue increases systemic inflammation and can put added stress on damaged joints, particularly the knees and hips.

Rheumatoid arthritis appears to be caused by the interaction between many genetic and environmental factors. Genetic susceptibility can be seen in twin and family studies that have shown an increase in the risk of developing RA among relatives. Certain shared alleles, called "rheumatoid epitopes," could help predict disease severity and outcome. Rheumatoid arthritis seems to peak in the fifth decade of life, and socioeconomic status seems to affect the outcome of—rather than cause of—the disease; lower socioeconomic status is linked with a worse prognosis. Smoking and dietary choices also are likely to affect the risk of developing RA and also the outcome of the disease. People in geographic zones that eat a Mediterranean diet, including a lifelong consumption of fish, olive oil, and cooked vegetables, have lower rates of RA occurrence and severity.

Treatment

Arthritis treatment recommendations vary greatly from lifestyle changes to prescription medicine therapies, and depend on type and severity of arthritis and the individual. Because arthritis has no cure, the goals of treatment are to reduce pain, limit joint damage, maximize function, and maintain or improve the quality of life. Treatment usually consists of a combination of medication and nonpharmacologic therapies, such as physical therapy, occupational therapy, patient education, and weight loss (for people who are overweight).

There are many medications on the market to help in the management of arthritis, including analgesics, nonsteroidal anti-inflammatory drugs (NSAIDs), disease-modifying antirheumatic drugs (DMARDs), biologic response modifiers, and corticosteroids (CDC, 2011). These medications aim to reduce pain and decrease inflammation, often by slowing or blocking the immune system—which can leave the patient susceptible to other health problems (CDC, 2011). Other suggested practices include exercise, proper diet, rest and relaxation, surgery (in some cases), and heat/cold therapies (CDC, 2011).

Nutrition

People with arthritis are at risk for nutritional deficiencies. One reason could be that inflammation is associated with the production of cytokines, the activators of immune cells that increase resting metabolic rate and protein breakdown. Medications also can cause conditions that are associated with decreased appetite, such as peptic ulcers or gastritis. People with arthritis who experience significant disability frequently have difficulty shopping for groceries and preparing nutritious meals.

For people with arthritis, a proper diet means eating a variety of foods that balance caloric intake and physical activity, choosing a diet with plenty of vegetables and fruits, and choosing foods low in synthetic trans fats, added sugars, and alcohol. Following a healthy diet nurtures a healthy weight and improves overall health, which might be important in managing arthritis and its symptoms. Additionally, foods with anti-inflammatory properties might help reduce the inflammation associated with both OA and RA. Some of the dietary components and eating patterns that have been investigated as possible factors in the management of OA and RA include the following.

Omega-3 Fatty Acids and Gamma Linolenic Acid

Omega-3 fatty acids play a role in modifying the inflammation process and the regulation of pain, decreasing cytokine activity and cartilage breakdown. It has also been suggested that omega-3 levels are inversely correlated with cardiovascular disease, which is seen in many patients with RA; are associated with lower risk of developing the disease; and can work alongside other medications, such as NSAIDs, to decrease inflammation (Stamp et al., 2005). Omega-3 fatty acids can be found in oily fish (e.g., salmon, tuna, mackerel), some vegetables (including soybeans, tofu, kale, collard greens, and winter squash), and walnuts, flaxseed, and pecans (Nelson & Zeratsky, 2013).

Gamma linolenic acid (GLA) is a fatty acid precursor to anti-inflammatory compounds made by the body. Gamma linolenic acid is found in evening primrose oil, borage oil, and black currant oil supplements. Preliminary research has shown that GLA supplements might help reduce arthritis symptoms.

Antioxidants and Vitamins

Eating foods rich in antioxidants could decrease the oxidation that leads to increased cell and tissue damage in inflammatory arthritis. Antioxidants such as vitamin C, vitamin E, selenium, carotene, lycopene, and flavonoids slow the process of oxidation and remove free radicals. Colorful vegetables and fruits are rich in antioxidants: leafy greens including spinach and kale, beets, blueberries, and cranberries. Beans, nuts, green tea, red wine, dark chocolate, and certain spices such as cinnamon, ginger, and turmeric also are rich in antioxidants. Vitamin D also could exert anti-inflammatory effects. Probiotic foods and supplements could help to address the intestinal inflammation present with RA.

Supplements and Herbs

Although it always is better to consume needed nutrients from whole foods, diet supplementation can be beneficial for arthritis treatment. Some recommended supplements include fish oil (which contains high levels of omega-3 fatty acids), antioxidant supplements, and some herbal supplements (NCCAM, 2013). Although the use of herbal supplements is quite controversial, some of the recommended types are thunder god vine (side effects could outweigh anti-inflammatory benefits), bosweillia, ginger, rosemary, and green tea (NCCAM, 2013; Weil, 2013). Glucosamine and glucosamine chondroitin supplements might help reduce pain in people with moderate to severe arthritis pain, but appear to be less effective for those with milder pain.

Specialty Diets

Some research suggests that vegetarian and vegan diets could improve clinical symptoms of arthritis, as could many low-fat diets that aim to reduce animal product consumption. As noted, another beneficial eating plan suggested is the Mediterranean diet. Other research suggests that dietary lectins—found in carbohydrates such as rice, potato, and wheat products—increase permeability and bacterial overgrowth in the gut that could lead to increased production of immune cells. People with arthritis might find that replacing some dietary lectins with fruits and vegetables helps reduce arthritis symptoms.

Controversial Diets

Little research supports the notion that elimination diets, fasting, and "miracle" food diets are safe and effective ways to reduce inflammation. There is little scientific evidence to show that cutting out a specific food, or relying on one as a cure, are effective treatment options. Fasting, although associated with reduced inflammation in the short term, can lead to dehydration and serious nutritional deficiencies and is not recommended as a viable long-term treatment option.

Micaela A. Young

Research Issues

Research continues to investigate possible foods and supplements that may help to treat both osteoarthritis and rheumatoid arthritis. The website of the Arthritis Foundation (http://www.arthritistoday.org/arthritis-treatment/natural-and-alternative-treatments/supplements-and-herbs/supplement-guide/), lists additional foods and supplements that one day could become established as helpful arthritis remedies.

See Also: Antioxidants; Inflammation; Marine omega-3 fatty acids.

Further Reading

Centers for Disease Control and Prevention (CDC). (2011). *Arthritis.* Retrieved from http://www.cdc.gov/arthritis/index.htm

National Center for Complementary and Alternative Medicine (NCCAM). (2013, July). Rheumatoid Arthritis and Complementary Approaches. Retrieved from http://nccam.nih.gov/health/RA/getthefacts.htm

Nelson, J., & Zeratsky, K. (2013, March 16). *Does diet have a role in rheumatoid arthritis?* Retrieved from http://www.mayoclinic.com/health/diet-and-rheumatoid-arthritis/MY02387

Stamp, L., James, M., & Cleland, L. (2005). Diet and rheumatoid arthritis: A review of the literature. *Seminars in Arthritis and Rheumatism 35,* 77–94.

Stetka, B., & Wei, N. (2013, March 22). Arthritis, then and now. *Medscape.* Retrieved from http://www.medscape.com/viewarticle/780895

Weil, A. (2013, September 28). *Osteoarthritis.* Retrieved from http://www.drweil.com/drw/u/ART00662/osteoarthritis-treatment.html

World Health Organization. (2013). *Chronic rheumatic conditions*. Retrieved from http://www.who.int/chp/topics/rheumatic/en/

Artificial Sweeteners

Artificial sweeteners are used in a variety of products in place of sucrose (sugar). They also are called "high-intensity sweeteners" and "nonnutritive sweeteners" (NNS) because they are many times sweeter than sucrose and can be used in miniscule amounts, providing few (if any) calories. Unlike sugar, they do not promote tooth decay. Artificial sweeteners can be found in diet soda, yogurt, chewing gum, and many other processed foods; they also commonly are tabletop sweeteners, and some can be used in home cooking.

Artificial sweeteners are regulated as food additives in the United States by the U.S. Federal Drug Administration (FDA) and in Canada by Health Canada. These regulatory agencies set acceptable daily intake (ADI) values that represent the maximum amount considered safe to consume daily over a lifetime. Acceptable daily intake values generally are calculated to be 100 times less than the smallest amount that might be harmful to health. For example, the ADI of aspartame is 50 milligrams per kilogram of body weight. For an average adult, this is roughly equivalent to consuming 16 12-ounce diet sodas daily (Insel, Ross, McMahon, & Bernstein, 2013). Despite these regulations, controversy over the safety of artificial sweeteners abounds. For each sweetener some studies confirm safe usage and other studies suggest alarming risks. (See "Research Issues" for more information on the debate.)

A similar debate ensues over the health benefits of artificial sweeteners. Many people use artificial, or nonnutritive, sweeteners and products containing them to help cut sugar and calories from their diet. Both the American Heart Association and the American Diabetes Association support the use of NNS as one way to combat obesity and its resulting complications (Strawbridge, 2012). Yet both institutions also caution that NNS should be consumed in moderation as part of a nutritious diet. This is particularly true for children and pregnant women—NNS, although considered safe, should not be consumed in place of the nutritious foods necessary for growth and development.

The debate centers on studies that have shown a connection between consumption of NNS and weight gain (Strawbridge, 2012). One explanation for this is that people who consume a diet product subsequently allow themselves to eat more food. The reasoning is, "I am drinking diet soda, so I can have the fries," or "These are reduced-calorie cookies, so I can eat the whole box." The result is more caloric intake rather than less. Another hypothesis is that NNS might change the way people experience food. The intensity of the artificial sweetness could cause naturally sweet foods to seem less sweet, and therefore less appealing. This could be compounded by a lack of satiety from foods and beverages containing NNS—although they taste sweet they do not satisfy, which can increase cravings for more sweets.

It could be decades before research confirms purported benefits or dangers of artificial sweeteners. Meanwhile, they are consumed around the world in a wide variety of products, and research and development into new sweeteners is ongoing. Following are descriptions of the artificial sweeteners currently approved for use in the United States and Canada.

Saccharin

Saccharin is more commonly known by the brand name Sweet'N Low. It is 300 times sweeter than sucrose. Saccharin is the oldest of the artificial sweeteners, but its long life has not been without controversy. A white crystalline derivative of a coal-tar compound, it was discovered in 1879 when a chemist forgot to wash his hands before dinner, and his food then tasted remarkably sweet. By the early 1880s, saccharin was being marketed as a nonnutritive sweetener, and it was used not only to sweeten foods and drinks, but also as an all-purpose panacea (Hicks, 2010). The controversy surrounding saccharin began around the end of the 19th century, as Americans began demanding more government oversight of the food industry. Despite several attempts to ban the substance (on the grounds that it was a coal-tar derivative and therefore must not be safe for humans), its popularity persisted— helped in part by the strong backing of President Theodore Roosevelt, who took a saccharin pill daily (Hicks, 2010). During WWI and WWII, it received widespread use as an inexpensive sugar substitute.

In 1958, a mixture of saccharin and another artificial sweetener, cyclamate, was introduced as the pink-packeted sugar replacer, Sweet'N Low, which became a diner staple. The diet soft drink, "Tab"—introduced by Coca-Cola in 1963—propelled saccharin's popularity even further. In 1968, however, researchers found a connection between cyclamate and bladder cancer in rats. A study conducted in 1970 found the same connection between saccharin and bladder cancer in rats. As a result of these findings, cyclamate was banned, and saccharin was required to display the following warning label: "Use of this product may be hazardous to your health. This product contains saccharin, which has been determined to cause cancer in laboratory animals" (National Cancer Institute, 2009). Research continued, both on the effects of saccharin and in the development of artificial sweeteners that could replace it. (Aspartame hit the markets in the early 1980s, followed shortly thereafter by acesulfame potassium, both with research supporting their safety.) Ultimately, researchers concluded that the mechanism causing bladder cancer in rats did not exist in humans, and saccharin's reputation was largely exonerated. In 2000, the warning labels were removed from products in the United States, and saccharin was taken off the U.S. National Toxicology Program's list of substances reasonably anticipated to cause cancer in humans. Canada is considering relisting saccharin as a safe food additive (Health Canada, 2010). Neither country has re-approved cyclamate as a food additive, although it is available for direct purchase in Canada and has a warning label.

Aspartame

Aspartame is known more commonly by the names "Nutrasweet" and "Equal." It consists of a combination of two amino acids, phenylalanine and aspartic acid.

Because aspartame is a protein, the body can digest and absorb it, so it does provide calories. It is 200 times sweeter than sugar and is used in miniscule amounts to sweeten foods, however, so the calories contributed are few. It was approved by the FDA for use in some foods in 1981 and for use in beverages in 1983 (Insel et al., 2013). Products with aspartame must carry a warning label for people that have phenylketonuria, which is a rare genetic disorder that prevents the breakdown of the phenylalanine. Some people report adverse reactions to aspartame, including dizziness, headaches, nausea, and seizures, but research has not confirmed any connection.

Acesulfame K (Acesulfame Potassium)

Acesulfame K is commercially available under the name "Sunette" and is 200 times sweeter than sugar. It has been approved in the United States since 1988 and in Canada since 1994. The human body cannot digest it, therefore it provides no energy. It is heat stable and can be used in baked goods, but it has a strong after-taste, so it is frequently used in combination with other artificial sweeteners.

Sucralose

Sucralose, also known by the brand name "Splenda," has been approved for use in Canada since 1992 and in the United States since 1998. Sucralose is manufactured by replacing three hydrogen-oxygen groups on the sugar molecule with three chlorine atoms; the process creates a nonnutritive compound that is 600 times sweeter than sugar. It is heat stable, so it creates products with long shelf lives, and it can be used in home cooking.

Neotame

Neotame is derived from the same amino acids used to make aspartame, but it is significantly sweeter—7,000 to 13,000 times sweeter than sugar. Neotame is safe for individuals who have phenylketonuria. Neotame is approved for use in the United States and Canada; but as one of the newer sweeteners, it is not yet associated with any brand names and is just beginning to be used in products, frequently in combination with other sweeteners.

Novel Sweeteners

The sweeteners tagatose, trehalose, and refined stevia (this excludes whole leaf and crude stevia) recently have been determined to be "generally recognized as safe" (GRAS) by the FDA. The GRAS status means that enough research on the additive has been completed for it to be used for its intended purposes without regulation. Of these three, only stevia is approved for use in Canada.

Lisa P. Ritchie and Jennifer C. Hsieh

Research Issues

If you type the sentence "Are artificial sweeteners safe?" into an online search engine, you will find thousands of websites, research studies, and opinion pieces arguing for or against the use of these synthetic sweeteners. Some claims are backed by scientific evidence, and others are backed by hearsay and misinformation. Clearly, the debate over the use and safety of artificial sweeteners is complex.

See Also: Alternative sweeteners (sugar substitutes); Food additives; Stevia; Sugar alcohols.

Further Reading

Health Canada. (2010, March 25). *Food and nutrition: Sugar substitutes.* Retrieved from http://www.hc-sc.gc.ca/fn-an/securit/addit/sweeten-edulcor/index-eng.php

Hicks, J. (2010). The pursuit of sweet: A history of saccharin. *Chemical Heritage Magazine.* Retrieved from http://www.chemheritage.org/discover/media/magazine/articles/28-1-the-pursuit-of-sweet.aspx?page=1

Insel, P., Ross, D., McMahon, K., & Bernstein, M. (2013). *Nutrition.* Sudbury, MA: Jones & Bartlett.

National Cancer Institute. (2009, August 5). *Artificial sweeteners and cancer.* Retrieved from http://www.cancer.gov/cancertopics/factsheet/Risk/artificial-sweeteners

Strawbridge, H. (2012, July 16). *Artificial sweeteners: Sugar free, but at what cost?* http://www.health.harvard.edu/blog/artificial-sweeteners-sugar-free-but-at-what-cost-201207165030

Astaxanthin

Astaxanthin is a powerful antioxidant in the carotenoid family. Astaxanthin is a reddish pigment, and contributes to the coloration found in some plants, algae, and bacteria. In the presence of high levels of ultraviolet (UV) light, the algae *Haematococcus pluvialis* produces large amounts of astaxanthin, possibly for protection from UV damage. Astaxanthin also is incorporated into the flesh of animals that consume foods with this pigment, including salmon, trout, lobster, and krill. Astaxanthin is responsible for the pink feathers of flamingos. At birth, flamingoes are white; their feathers become pink as the flamingoes consume red algae and shrimp. Although research suggests that astaxanthin has the potential to confer several health benefits in humans, at present the research is preliminary.

Charles Weedon, an organic chemistry professor, discovered astaxanthin in 1970 when using magnetic resonance spectroscopy to study carotenoid pigments. In 1987, the U.S. Food and Drug Administration approved the use of astaxanthin as an additive in the agriculture and aquaculture industries to enhance the color of farmed meat and fish, and in 1999 it became an approved dietary supplement. One serving of Atlantic salmon has approximately 1 mg of astaxanthin per serving, and Pacific salmon contains 4 mg to 5 mg.

Astaxanthin acts as an antioxidant, and appears to reduce the oxidation of fats in vivo. Oxidation of low-density lipoprotein cholesterol in the bloodstream appears to accelerate the process of artery disease, therefore researchers are investigating whether astaxanthin might slow this oxidative process. Researchers also hope that astaxanthin's antioxidant effects might reduce levels of inflammation. Preliminary investigations in vitro and in animal models suggest this might be the case. A few studies in humans have found that supplementation with astaxanthin did reduce markers of oxidative stress (Fassett & Coombs, 2012). Researchers also are studying astaxanthin's potentional to protect the eye from UV damage, possibly preventing the formation of cataracts and slowing macular degeneration. There currently is no evidence that these effects occur in humans, however. Astaxanthin has been found to reduce hypertension in rats genetically altered to develop hypertension, but not in normotensive rats.

Astaxanthin supplements appear to be relatively safe, although long-term data are not available. Astaxanthin is not recommended for women who are pregnant or nursing. Therapeutic dosages used in research generally have ranged between 4mg and 10 mg daily.

Jennifer Najera

See Also: Antioxidants.

Further Reading

EBSCO CAM Review Board. (2012). *Astaxanthin*. Retrieved from http://healthlibrary .epnet.com/GetContent.aspx?token=e0498803-7f62-4563-8d47-5fe33da65dd4&chunk iid=160132

Fassett, R. G., & Coombes, J. S. (2012). Astaxanthin in cardiovascular health and disease. *Molecules, 17* (2), 2030–2048. doi: 10.3390/molecules17022030

Kidd, P. (2011). Astaxanthin, cell membrane nutrient with diverse clinical benefits and anti-aging potential. *Alternative Medicine Reviews 16* (4), 355–364.

The Atkins Diet

The Atkins Diet, named after cardiologist Dr. Robert C. Atkins, is a nutrition-based weight-loss regime that focuses on carbohydrate restriction as a means to increase the use of fat for energy, and decrease stored body fat. The premise of the diet is that weight gain is produced by excess carbohydrate intake which causes a rise in insulin. The increase in insulin stimulates the uptake and storage of glucose and other nutrients—primarily as triglycerides—contributing to an increase in body fat levels. The Atkins Diet involves eliminating or drastically reducing carbohydrate consumption to reduce insulin levels and to drive the body to burn fat as fuel, producing substantial weight loss.

Many people who adhere to the diet lose weight and often experience associated health benefits, including improved blood sugar regulation and blood lipid levels, reduced blood pressure, and fewer markers of systemic inflammation. Critics argue that the diet is difficult to follow and is not associated with long-term weight-loss maintenance. Some people on the diet experience an increase in blood lipid levels. The diet's low fiber content increases risk for constipation. The high protein intake also might increase the risk of kidney stones and of bone mineral loss.

The dietary regime is organized into four phases, Induction (Kick-Start), Ongoing Weight Loss (Balancing), Pre-Maintenance (Fine-Tuning), and Lifetime Maintenance. The dieter determines the start point and duration of the phases; however, the plan offers suggestions based on degree of obesity, target weight, and individual dietary restrictions. During the Induction phase carbohydrate intake is limited to 20 g per day, 12 g to 15 g of which are expected to come from non-starchy vegetables. This value is increased throughout

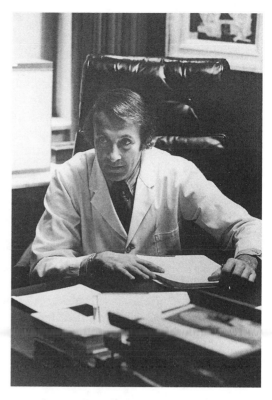

Dr. Robert C. Atkins was the creator of the Atkins diet and best-selling author of *Dr. Atkins' New Diet Revolution* (2002). Although nutritionists originally regarded the Atkins diet as too high in fat, newer research suggests the diet might not be as harmful as once believed, at least over a short period of time. (Time & Life Pictures/Getty Images)

the phases to an individualized amount that is as much as 90 g to 120 g per day. (As a point of reference, the U.S. Dietary Reference Intake is at least 130 g of carbohydrates per day.) The structured diet, listing only the allowed foods for each phase, is often referenced as the Atkins Nutritional Approach (ANA). Exercise is suggested but not required, increased water intake is encouraged to offset the diuretic effect of the diet, and vitamin supplementation is encouraged to replace lost nutrients.

Although Robert C. Atkins is credited with the popularity of carbohydrate-restrictive meal plans, he did not invent low-carbohydrate diets. This credit is attributed to Dr. Alfred W. Pennington, whose extensive research on the impact of animal protein consumption on weight loss was published in the early 1950s. After adopting Pennington's diet for himself, cardiologist Atkins became a medical consultant helping patients reach an ideal weight with his low-carbohydrate diet plan.

Gaining popularity, Atkins was featured on "The Tonight Show" and various magazines before publishing *Dr. Atkins' Diet Revolution* in 1972 (Martin, 2003). After its initial period of popularity, the cardiologist's diet plan became less popular during the 1990s, with the widespread promotion of the health benefits associated with low-fat diets. The diet regained popularity in the early 2000s along with similar low-carbohydrate and high-protein diets including The Zone and The South Beach Diet. In addition to several subsequent diet books, Atkins International markets frozen meals, prepackaged snacks, and shakes throughout the United States. Atkins International also maintains a mobile app, free progress trackers, and an online forum community.

People who adhere to the Atkins Diet generally lose weight, and the diet has been found to be at least as effective as other weight-loss diets in the short term (Shai et al., 2008). People who lose weight on the Atkins Diet often experience health benefits. Unanticipated due to the liberal consumption high-fat meats and dairy thus elevating dietary saturated fat, several studies of the diet have found some reduced cardiovascular risk factors including reduced serum triglycerides, improved HDL cholesterol, and reduced levels of systemic inflammation (Gogebaken et al., 2011). Similar improvements, however, are experienced by people who lose weight by following other types of diets.

During the first phase of the Atkins Diet, dieters achieve a state of ketosis. Ketosis refers to a metabolic state in which the body is producing higher than normal levels of compounds called ketones. The body increases its manufacture of ketones when its supply of carbohydrate is low. Many organs of the body can manufacture energy from ketones. Interestingly, a ketogenic diet has been shown to be very effective in reducing the frequency of seizures in people with epilepsy; and a modified Atkins Diet now is promoted as an accessible way to help people with epilepsy to achieve ketosis (Kossoff, Cervenka, Henry, Haney, & Turner, 2013). The Atkins Diet claims to promote weight loss without hunger. Followers of the diet usually do experience low levels of hunger because of their high protein intake and because they enter a state of ketosis.

Critics of the diet argue that the rapid weight loss often achieved during the induction phase is a result of water loss, or diuresis, and not an increase in adipose metabolism. Carbohydrate-restrictive diets trigger the mobilization of glycogen, depleting the body's storage along with the 2 g to 3 g of water bound to each gram of glycogen. Substantial weight loss in the subsequent phases has been attributed to decreased caloric intake due to limited food options, circulating ketones acting as an appetite suppressant, and a satiation effect of increased protein consumption.

On the grounds that most studies have evaluated the diet for a short period and have used a small sample size, medical professionals fairly conclusively agree that the long-term safety and efficacy of the Atkins Diet remain in question. Reducing dietary glycemic load through avoidance of processed carbohydrates has become an established recommendation for reducing risk for obesity, heart disease, type 2 diabetes, and hypertension; and the Atkins Diet does promote this practice. Some researchers question the wisdom of a high protein intake, however, which increases stress on the kidneys and also might accelerate bone mineral loss (Huggett et al., 2012).

An interesting meta-analysis that examined data from a number of studies on low-carbohydrate diets found that low-carbohydrate diets actually were associated with increased rates of premature death from all causes except from cardiovascular disease (Noto, Goto, Tsujimoto, & Noda, 2013). The meta-analysis included only eight studies, therefore these results are considered preliminary. The researchers have speculated that the low intake of fruits, vegetables, and fiber could explain the greater mortality rates.

Allison R. Ferreira and Barbara A. Brehm

Research Issues

A great deal of research supports the notion that a high intake of fruits and vegetables is associated with positive health outcomes. Using the Atkins diet website (http://www.atkins.com/Program/Overview.aspx), try to construct a list of five to nine fruit and vegetable servings. How many grams of carbohydrates are contained in the foods listed? Imagine trying to consume only 20 grams of carbohydrate per day. Can you find five servings of vegetables that would provide 20 or fewer grams of carbohydrate?

See Also: Ketosis and ketogenic diets; Obesity, treatment.

Further Reading

Atkins Nutritionals. (2014*). The program: Overview.* Low Carb Diet Program and Weight Loss. Retrieved from http://www.atkins.com/Program/Overview.aspx

Gogebaken, O., Kohl, A., Osterhoff, et al. (2011). Effects of weight loss and long-term weight maintenance with diets varying in protein and glycemic index and cardiovascular risk factors; the Diet, Obesity, and Genes (DiOGenes) study: A randomized, controlled trial. *Circulation 124*, 2829–2838.

Huggett, C., Gannon, R. H. T., Truby, H., Hiscutt, R., Lambert, H., Fraser, W. D., & Lanham-New, S. A. (2012). An assessment of the Atkins Diet on skeletal health in contrast to diets rich in alkaline-forming fruits and vegetables. *Proceedings of the Nutrition Society 71* (OCE3), E221.

Kossoff, E. H., Cervenka, M. C., Henry, B. J., Haney, C. A., & Turner, Z. (2013). A decade of the modified Atkins Diet (2003–2013): Results, insights, and future directions. *Epilepsy & Behavior 29* (3), 437–442.

Martin, D. (2003, April 18). Dr. Robert C. Atkins, author of controversial but best-selling diet books, is dead at 72. *New York Times*, pp. 1–2.

Mayo Clinic Staff. (2011). *Atkins Diet: What's behind the claims?* MayoClinic.com. Retrieved from http://www.mayoclinic.com/health/atkins-diet/MY00648

Noto, H., Goto, A., Tsujimoto, T., & Noda, M. (2013). Low-carbohydrate diets and all-cause mortality: A systematic meta-analysis of observational studies. *PLOS One*. January 25, 2013. DOI: 10.1371/journal.pone.0055030.

Shai, I., Brickner, D., Sarusi, B., et al. (2008). Weight loss with a low-carbohydrate, Mediterranean, or low-fat diet. *New England Journal of Medicine 359* (3), 229–241.

Attention-Deficit Hyperactivity Disorder and Nutrition

Attention-Deficit Hyperactivity Disorder (ADHD) is a neurodevelopmental disorder characterized by inattention, distractibility, hyperactivity, and impulsivity. The *Diagnostic and Statistical Manual of Mental Disorders* (DSM-5) is the handbook used to diagnose mental disorders, and it classifies ADHD with several diagnostic criteria. These criteria include at least six symptoms of inattention and/or hyperactivity and impulsivity, lasting for a period of at least six months; onset of the majority of symptoms before age 12; symptoms present themselves in at least two different settings (i.e., home, work, school, social situations); symptoms have a direct impact on social, academic, or occupational functioning or development; and symptoms cannot be better explained by another mental disorder. Individuals with ADHD can present as predominantly inattentive, predominantly hyperactive and impulsive, or a combination of both.

Attention-Deficit Hyperactivity Disorder often is treated with various forms of psychotherapy and psychiatric medications. Stimulants such as Ritalin, Concerta, Focalin, and Adderall regularly are prescribed to adults and children age six years and older. Although these drugs have proven to be effective in those with ADHD, they also can result in serious side effects such as heart palpitations, decreased appetite and weight loss, tics or disordered movements, anxiety, and insomnia. Due to the controversy concerning the over-prescription of stimulants, recent research has explored the relationship between nutrition and ADHD to determine whether dietary factors might help prevent or treat ADHD.

Symptoms of ADHD

Inattention

- Difficulty staying on task
- Easily distracted
- Frequent careless errors
- Difficulty paying attention
- Difficulty organizing activities (i.e., time management, meeting deadlines)
- Frequently loses or misplaces possessions
- Does not seem to listen during conversation
- Difficulty following instructions

Hyperactivity-Impulsivity

- Difficulty remaining seated
- Inability to sit still
- Difficulty waiting one's turn (in activities and/or conversations)

- Blurting out answers before questions have been completed
- Excessive talking
- Difficulty adapting to new situations

Prevalence

- Affects an estimated 11% of children ages 4 to 17 in the United States (CDC, 2013).
- Although most individuals are diagnosed during childhood, ADHD can be diagnosed at any age. Approximately 4.1% of adults ages 18 to 44 in the United States are diagnosed each year (ADHD, 2008).
- The rate of ADHD diagnoses in boys is double the rate for girls (CDC, 2013).
- Girls are more likely to be diagnosed with predominantly inattentive type, and boys are more likely to have a combined-type diagnosis.
- Diagnoses in the United States increased from 7.8% in 2003 to 11% in 2011 (CDC, 2013).

Nutrition and ADHD

Overall, there are mixed conclusions regarding nutrition and ADHD. Some experts claim that artificial food colorings and preservatives are to blame, others believe that symptoms could be due to nutritional deficiencies. Still other experts think that hyperactivity and attention issues can be avoided by eating a healthy, balanced diet. One recent study compared ADHD symptoms in individuals who followed a typical "Western diet" (i.e., processed meats, high-fat dairy products, soft drinks) versus those who adhered to a healthier dietary pattern (i.e., whole grains, fruit, vegetables, legumes, fish) (Howard et al., 2011). ADHD symptoms were markedly diminished in those people adhering to a healthy diet.

Many critics deem ADHD nutritional studies to be unreliable. Dr. Feingold's research (discussed below) has been widely criticized for its lack of double-blind studies and control groups, invalid diagnoses, subjective responses, and small sample sizes. Many studies rely on observational data from teachers and parents, which can drastically impact results. Further, most scientists looking at food colorings fail to study additives individually, making it difficult to identify the true cause of any correlational effect. Finally, ADHD diets could result in several nutritional deficiencies. This can be particularly dangerous for children and individuals with outstanding medical issues.

Nevertheless, many caregivers try dietary manipulations to determine whether such changes might be helpful for children with ADHD. There appear to be several dietary factors that could affect ADHD. Artificial food colorings as well as vitamin and mineral deficiencies might contribute to the duration and intensity of ADHD symptoms. Dietary regimens have been designed specifically for the treatment of ADHD. Many studies have shown a positive relationship between diet and ADHD.

Table 1. Artificial Food Colors

Artificial Food Color	Common Name	Foods
Blue No. 1	Brilliant blue	Baked goods, ice cream, cereals, candy, beverages
Blue No. 2	Indigotine	Candy, beverages
Green No. 3	Fast green	Candy, gelatin, beverages
Red No. 3	Erythrosine	Baked goods, candy, cereals, popsicles
Red No. 40	Allura red	Beverages, candy, pastries, sausages, cereals, gelatin
Yellow No. 5	Tartrazine	Candy, chips, ice cream, pickles, cereals, baked goods
Yellow No. 6	Sunset yellow	Jam, candy, sausages, baked goods, beverages, gelatin
Citrus Red No. 2	Citrus red	Added to skins of some Florida oranges
Orange B		Sausage casings

Source: Created from data in Stevens et al. (2011).

Artificial Food Colorings

There are nine synthetic food dyes currently approved by the U.S. Food and Drug Administration.

Food colorings are added to foods to reduce color loss due to changes in light, air, or temperature; to correct natural variations and changes in color; to make food more appealing; and to enhance natural colors. Many medications (both prescription and over-the-counter drugs) also contain artificial food colorings. Although both natural and artificial dyes can be used, the food industry usually relies on synthetic dyes because they are more efficient, stable, and cost effective. Some experts claim as much as 8% of children with ADHD could have symptoms attributed to artificial food colors, and that 30% might improve with dietary changes (Nigg, Lewis, Edinger, & Falk, 2012). Authors also paired food colorings with the preservative sodium benzoate, however, thus complicating their conclusions. Some research suggests correlation between tartrazine and behavioral problems in children, including increased irritability, restlessness, impulsivity, and sleep disturbances. The possible link between food colorings and ADHD has served as a reference for various ADHD diets.

Diets

In 1973, Dr. Benjamin Feingold suggested a link between hypersensitivity or intolerance to certain foods and hyperactivity in children. He proposed a diet free of natural salicylates and artificial flavors that he called the "Kaiser Permanente Diet," or "K-P Diet." By 1977, Dr. Feingold claimed that 60% to 70% of his pediatric patients had improved. Critics, however, argued that his work was premature and lacked structure. Nevertheless, scientists have used Feingold's work as a basis for their own research studies, as well as for diets that followed.

Table 2. Special Diets That Have Been Tried for ADHD

Diet	How It Works	Avoid
Feingold's Kaiser-Permanente or K-P Diet	Elimination of artificial food colorings, foods containing natural salicylates, and certain preservatives.	All artificial colors and flavors; preservatives BHA (butylated hydroxyanisole), BHT (butylated hydroxytoluene), TBHQ (tertiary butylhydroquinone), and sodium benzoate; and foods with natural salicylates (almonds, apples, apricots, berries, currants, grapes, nectarines, oranges, peaches, plums, tangerines, cucumbers, green peppers, tomatoes, cloves, chili powder, coffee, and tea).
Elimination diet	Elimination of foods for a maximum of 2 weeks, and gradually reintroducing them until the potential triggers are found.	All artificial colors, flavors, and preservatives; chocolate; wheat, rye, barley; eggs; processed meats; citrus fruits; legumes; peanuts
Ketogenic diet	High in fat, low in carbohydrates.	Grains, high-carbohydrate fruits and vegetables, processed foods.
Low-sugar diet	A decrease of glucose in the brain appears to slow EEG rhythms. Many parents believe this to have an effect on their child's hyperactive behavior. Further research is needed, however, to confirm the correlation between sugar and symptoms of ADHD.	Refined carbohydrates, such as sugar, honey, flour, maple syrup, corn syrup, and fruit juice.

Nutrients and Dietary Supplements

Several nutrients have been studied in relation to the prevention and treatment of ADHD. Those best studied include the following.

- Polyunsaturated Fatty Acids (PUFAs)—Omega-3 and omega-6 fatty acids are known to play an important role in cognitive and behavioral functioning. One study found a significant decrease in ADHD symptoms in children assigned to omega-3 and omega-6 supplementation versus placebo (Richardson & Montgomery, 2005). Further research has shown significant variability in results, however, depending on the type of fatty acid used, method of administration, dosage, duration of study, and response measures.
- Zinc—Low serum zinc has been reported in children with ADHD. Zinc promotes dopamine metabolism and functioning involved in ADHD. Serum supplementation has been correlated with increased levels of attention, as well as an increased response to d-amphetamine (Millichap & Yee, 2012).
- Iron—Iron deficiency has been associated with cognitive and learning disorders. Iron helps to regulate the dopaminergic system. Although research is

limited, lower levels of iron have been correlated with more severe ADHD symptoms and cognitive deficits. One study found supplementation to be effective in treating children with ADHD, especially those with the inattentive subtype (Soto-Insuga et al., 2013).

- Magnesium—Low levels of magnesium have been found in children with ADHD. Magnesium is important for several nerve and brain functions, and has been associated with nervous and muscular excitability. Deficiencies in magnesium might be correlated with increased hyperactivity, inattention, insomnia, and distractibility.

Although many studies suggest a nutritional correlation with ADHD, results remain inconclusive. Larger sample sizes, greater age ranges, and long-term follow-up studies are needed to test the validity of these claims.

Nicole D. Teitelbaum

See Also: "Brain foods"; Depression and nutrition; Ketosis and ketogenic diets; Marine omega-3 fatty acids.

Further Reading

ADHD In-Depth Report. (2008). *New York Times*. Retrieved February 8, 2014, from http://www.nytimes.com/health/guides/disease/attention-deficit-hyperactivity-disorder-adhd/print.html

American Psychiatric Association. (2013). *Diagnostic and statistical manual of mental disorders* (5th ed.) (DSM-5). Arlington, VA: American Psychiatric Association.

Centers for Disease Control and Prevention (CDC). (2013). *Attention-deficit/hyperactivity disorder (ADHD): Data and statistics*. Retrieved from http://www.cdc.gov/ncbddd/adhd/data.html

Howard, A. L., Robinson, M., Smith, G. J., Ambrosini, G. L., Piek, J. P., & Oddy, W. H. (2011). ADHD is associated with a "Western" dietary pattern in adolescents. *Journal of Attention Disorders, 15* (5), 403–411.

Millichap, J. G., & Yee, M. M. (2012). The diet factor in attention-deficit/hyperactivity disorder. *Pediatrics, 129*, 1–8.

Nigg, J. T., Lewis, K., Edinger, T., & Falk, M. (2012). Meta-analysis of attention-deficit/hyperactivity disorder or attention-deficit/hyperactivity disorder symptoms, restriction diet, and synthetic food color additives. *Journal of the American Academy of Child & Adolescent Psychiatry, 51* (1), 86–97.

Richardson, A. J., & Montgomery, P. (2005). The Oxford-Durham study: A randomized, controlled trial of dietary supplementation with fatty acids in children with developmental coordination disorder. *Pediatrics 115* (5), 1360–1366. doi:10.1542/peds.2004-2164.

Soto-Insuga, V., Calleja, M. L., Prados, M., Castano, C., Losada, R., & Ruiz-Falco, M. L. (2013). Role of iron in the treatment of attention deficit-hyperactivity disorder. *Anales De Pediatria, 79* (4), 230–235.

Stevens, L. J., Kuczek, T., Burgess, J., Hurt, E., & Arnold, L. (2011). Dietary sensitivities and ADHD symptoms: Thirty-five years of research. *Clinical Pediatrics, 50* (4), 279–293.

Autism and Nutrition

Autism is a neurodevelopmental disorder affecting 1 in 110 children in the United States. This disorder is more common in males and is characterized by impaired social interactions, poor communication skills, gastrointestinal problems, and repetitive behaviors. Children having autism present symptoms by three years of age. Scientists do not yet know what causes autism, but they have proposed some potential risk factors, including genetic vulnerability, reduced gut microbiota, infection, altered immune response, and nutrition. Autistic children are known to have poor diet quality due to their unusual eating patterns and behaviors (Privett, 2013). Data from a comprehensive meta-analysis indicate that children with autism have significantly more feeding problems than do their peers (Sharp et al., 2013). Because many autistic children are found to have food aversions and sensitivities along with behavioral issues, parents and caregivers sometimes turn to dietary interventions hoping to reduce the children's symptoms.

Researchers at Marcus Autism Center at Emory University School of Medicine found that children with autism have inadequate nutrition more often than those unaffected (Autism Speaks, 2013). Those affected by autism might not obtain adequate intake of all nutrients, which theoretically could lead to neurochemical imbalances that in turn could influence behavior. Chronic eating problems have been associated with social difficulties and reduced academic performance. Nutrition is implicated as a potential area for the prevention and treatment of autism. Areas of study have included maternal nutrition during key developmental stages, the impact of dietary supplements on children with autism, and creating special diets for children with autism.

Maternal Nutrition

It is suspected that maternal nutrition might be involved in the onset of autism. Past studies have focused on prenatal vitamins high in folic acid and other B vitamins in relation to autism risk. One research group found that women who took prenatal vitamins three months before conception and in the first month of pregnancy had a 40% lower risk of their child developing autism (Schmidt et al., 2012). Additionally, the children of mothers who took folic acid supplements before or during their first trimester were found to have fewer behavioral problems at 18 months of age, and have social competence and reduced hyperactivity when older than 18 months. This could be because folic acid and other vitamins are crucial for neurodevelopment.

Polyunsaturated fatty acids (PUFAs) have been studied in relationship to autism because they play a critical role in normal brain development. Several studies have shown that arachidonic acid (AA), eicosapentaenoic acid (EPA), and docosahexanoic acid (DHA) are needed for brain growth and memory formation and consolidation. This implies that a maternal PUFA deficiency could contribute to the characteristic behavioral symptoms of children with autism. Polyunsaturated fatty acids are recognized to alter levels of brain-derived neurotropic factors

(BDNFs) that regulate neurogenesis and affect learning and memory. Polyunsaturated fatty acids are precursors to anti-inflammatory lipids that are required for protecting neurons from oxidative stress, which is why some researchers suggest that maternal supplements should include adequate levels of PUFAs. Studies have revealed that children of mothers who had a high intake of PUFAs—such as omega-3 fatty acids—before and during pregnancy had a lesser risk of developing autism as compared to children of mothers with the lowest PUFA intakes (Lyall, Schmidt, & Hertz-Picciotto, 2014).

Vitamin D deficiency has been proposed as a risk factor for autism because vitamin D is important in neurodevelopmental processes, such as neuronal differentiation and metabolism of neurotropic factors (Lyall, Schmidt, & Hertz-Picciotto, 2014). Maternal vitamin D deficiency has been associated with impaired language development in offspring between the ages of 5 years old and 10 years old. Autism has been linked with a mechanism involving both serotonin and vitamin D. Vitamin D regulates the production of the neurotransmitter serotonin in the brain. Maternal vitamin D deficiency results in the overproduction of serotonin. The overproduction of serotonin hinders the metabolic pathway in which vitamin D stimulates the production of a family of T cells that prevent maternal autoantibodies from attacking the fetal brain and causing severe damage (Patrick & Ames, 2014). Supplementation of vitamin D is affordable and could reduce a child's risk of developing autism.

Dietary Supplements

Vitamins (especially A, B6/B12, C, and D) and minerals (especially magnesium, calcium, and zinc) have been suggested to improve symptoms associated with autism. Several studies have found reduced intake of several vitamins and minerals in children with autism as compared to neurotypical children of similar age. In an Autism Research Institute (ARI) survey parents reported that putting their children on supplements improved their children's behaviors. Improvements were noted for vitamin B12 (72% better), vitamin B6 (51% better), and zinc (54% better) (Adams, 2013). Analyzing vitamin D serum levels showed significantly lower measurements for children with autism than for those unaffected (Meguid, Hashish, Anwar, & Sidhom, 2010).

In a large double-blind study, a balanced multivitamin/mineral supplement regimen led to significant improvements for children with autism in their expressive language, tantrumming, hyperactivity, and other behavioral symptoms (Adams et al., 2011). Additionally, there were marked improvements in the children's metabolic processes, which included methylation, sulfation, and oxidative stress. Researchers have hypothesized that a portion of autistic children have inefficient vitamin B metabolism and reduced methylation capacity (Schmidt et al., 2012). Therefore, micronutrient supplementation could help boost deficient metabolic processes in individuals with autism. Interestingly, pharmaceutical treatments were compared to micronutrient supplementation, and it was found that supplements were either comparable to or more effective than pharmaceutical treatments in terms of children with autism positively increasing their scores on clinical scales, such as the Childhood Autism Rating Scale and Childhood Psychiatric Rating Scale (Mehl-Madrona, Leung, Kennedy, Paul, & Kaplan 2010).

In terms of fish and fish oil supplements, there are both studies supporting and negating that they reduce behavioral symptoms. An open-label study of 30 autistic children, for instance, noted that fish oil supplements resulted in improved levels of fatty acids and two-thirds of the cohort had improved behavioral symptoms (Meguid, Atta, Gouda, & Khalil, 2008). Other studies have found no statistical significance of fish oil supplements for reducing hyperactivity and other behavioral problems (Amminger, Berger, Schäfer, Klier, Friedrich, & Feucht, 2006).

Special Diets

The gluten-free, casein-free (GFCF) diet is widely implemented by parents of children with autism (Hurwitz, 2013). Despite its popularity, there is limited evidence supporting drastic change in autistic children on the GFCF diet. The GFCF diet is an elimination diet where the person does not eat anything containing gluten, such as wheat products, or casein, a protein found in dairy products such as milk and yogurt. The diet has the potential to improve an autistic child's functioning and gastrointestinal symptoms, which is why parents try this nutrition regimen. One study noted that 27% of parents have their affected child on a special diet—such as the GFCF diet—at a given time but, overall, half of the cohort had tried a special diet for their child at one time or another (Hurwitz, 2013). Studies claim that the GFCF diet is accessible and can be implemented alongside pharmacological treatment. This special diet is driven by the Opioid-Excess Theory of autism that describes how gluten and casein are not properly digested in the gastrointestinal tract by autistic children. One study found that, in their cohort, 37% of children with autism have abnormal intestinal permeability compared to controls (Kral, Eriksen, Souders, & Pinto-Martin, 2013). Once absorbed, it has been observed that gluten and casein proteins transform into opioid peptides that leak into the bloodstream and cross the brain's blood-brain barrier; this has become known as "the leaky gut hypothesis" (Hurwitz, 2013). In the brain, these opioid peptides behave as real opioids by attaching to the opioid neuroreceptors. The theory describes how opioid receptor binding negatively impacts neurotransmission causing maladaptive behaviors and increasing symptoms associated with autism.

The ideology of the GFCF diet is to remove all gluten and casein from the child's diet to stop the progression of excess opioids in the brain. Studies have reported mixed effectiveness of the GFCF diet in terms of behavioral and developmental effects. In three of the studies of a larger meta-analysis, researchers found no support for the diet as there were no significant improvements in the children's language, attention, and activity level (Hurwitz, 2013). An ARI survey, however, found that 69% of parents rated their children as having improved on the GFCF diet as compared to 28% reporting no change (Adams, 2013). Further research has been conducted, reporting 81% of children with autism improving significantly on the GFCF diet by the third month; large improvements were made in eye contact, mutism or inability to speak, learning skills, hyperactivity, and panic attacks (Cade et al., 2000). Many health care providers recommend that parents try the GFCF diet because trying it is the only way to determine whether the diet will help the particular individual. Other special diets have been proposed for children with autism, but the GFCF diet has by far the most support of parents and the most studies conducted by researchers.

Victoria E. von Saucken

See Also: Marine omega-3 fatty acids.

Further Reading

Adams, J. B. (2013). Summary of dietary, nutritional, and medical treatments for autism—based on over 150 published research studies. *Autism Research Institute.* Retrieved from http://www.generationrescue.org/assets/Published-Science/James-Adams-Summary-of-dietary-nutritional-and-medical-treatment-for-ASD.pdf

Adams, J. B., Tapan, A., McDonough-Means, S., et al. (2011). Effect of a vitamin/mineral supplement on children with autism. *BMC Pediatrics, 11,* 111.

Amminger, Berger, G. E., Schäfer, M. R., Klier, C., Friedrich, M. H., & Feucht, M. (2007). Omega-3 fatty acids supplementation in children with autism: A double blind randomized, placebo-controlled pilot study. *Biological Psychiatry, 61* (4), 551–553.

Autism Speaks. (2013, February 7). *Nutrition and autism.* Retrieved from http://www.autismspeaks.org/science/science-news/nutrition-and-autism

Cade, R., Privette, M., Fregly, M., Rowland, N., Sun, Z., Zele, V., Wagemaker, H., & Edelstein, C. (2000). Autism and schizophrenia: Intestinal disorders. *Nutritional Neuroscience, 3,* 57–72.

Hurwitz, J. (2013). The Gluten-free, Casein-free diet and autism: Limited return on family investment. *Journal of Early Intervention, 35.* doi: 10.1177/1053815113484807

Kral, T. V., Eriksen, W. T., Souders, M. C., & Pinto-Martin, J. A. (2013). Eating behaviors, diet quality, and gastrointestinal symptoms in children with autism spectrum disorders: A brief review. *Journal of Pediatric Nursing, 28*(6), 548–556.

Lyall, K., Schmidt, R. J., & Hertz-Picciotto, I. (2014). Maternal lifestyle and environmental risk factors for autism spectrum disorders. *International Journal of Epidemiology 43*(2), 443–464. doi: 10.1093/ije/dyt282

Meguid, N. A., Atta, H. M., Gouda, A. S., & Khalil, R. O. (2008). Role of polyunsaturated fatty acids in the management of Egyptian children with autism. *Clinical Biochemistry, 41,* 1044–1048.

Meguid, N. A., Hashish, A. F., Anwar, M., & Sidhom, G. (2010). Reduced serum levels of 25 hydroxy and 1,25-dihydroxy vitamin D in Egyptian children with autism. *Journal of Alternative and Complementary Medicine, 16,* 641–645.

Mehl-Madrona, L., Leung, B., Kennedy, C., Paul, S., & Kaplan, B. J. (2010). Micronutrients versus standard medication management in autism: A naturalistic case-control study. *Journal Child and Adolescent Psychopharmacology, 20* (2), 95–103.

Patrick, R. P. & Ames, B. N. (2014). Vitamin D hormone regulates serotonin synthesis. Part 1: Relevance for autism. *The FASEB Journal.* doi: 10.1096/fj.13-246546

Privett, D. (2013). Autism Spectrum Disorder—Research suggests good nutrition may manage symptoms. *Today's Dietitian, 15*(1), 46. Retrieved from http://www.todaysdietitian.com/newarchives/010713p46.shtml

Schmidt, R. J., Hansen, R. L., Hartiala, J., et al. (2012). Prenatal vitamins, one-carbon metabolism gene variants, and risk for autism. *Epidemiology, 22* (4), 476–485. doi: 10.1097/EDE.0b013e31821d0e30

Sharp, G. S., Berry, R. C., McCracken, C., et al. (2013). Feeding problems and nutrient intake in children with autism spectrum disorders: A meta-analysis and comprehensive review of the literature. *Journal of Autism and Developmental Disorders, 43* (9), 2159–2173. doi: 10.1007/s10803-013-1771-5

B

Bariatric Surgery

Bariatric surgery refers to surgical procedures performed for the purpose of reducing body weight in people who are obese. Obesity is a costly health problem associated with several serious chronic health conditions. Many obesity experts think that bariatric surgery is one of the best methods to achieve significant and long-term weight loss and to reduce the negative impact of obesity-related health problems such as type 2 diabetes, hypertension, arthritis, and sleep apnea. Weight-loss surgeries alter the digestive system to facilitate weight loss by physically limiting how much a person can eat, reducing the absorption of calories, or both. Bariatric surgery is suggested for patients in urgent need of decreasing body fat levels and combating physiological problems associated with obesity. It is recommended for those who have exhausted other traditional avenues for weight loss, such as proper diet and exercise. All bariatric surgeries, however, require patients to make permanent changes in eating behaviors to reduce risk of complications, reduce the need for repeat surgeries, and to maintain weight loss.

The National Institutes of Health suggest a list of criteria to evaluate whether a person is a proper candidate for bariatric surgery (National Institutes of Health, 2014). In general, people most likely to benefit from these surgeries and for whom the benefits outweigh the risks include men who are more than 100 pounds overweight and women who are more than 80 pounds overweight, or people who have a BMI exceeding 40. The majority of bariatric surgery patients are severely obese, with average BMI levels exceeding 45 (Padwal et al., 2011). Bariatric surgery also sometimes is recommended for people whose BMI is 30 to 35 or greater and who have obesity-related health problems that will be alleviated by weight loss. It is important for all potential patients to be prepared to commit to positive lifestyle changes following surgery, as the procedure is only the initial step to achieving good health.

Types of Major Bariatric Surgeries

Over time, a variety of bariatric surgeries have been developed. In 1952, Dr. Victor Henrikson of Gothenburg, Sweden, was credited with performing an intestinal resection specifically for the management of obesity. In 1954, A. J. Kremen published the first case report of a jejunoileal bypass (JIB) procedure for

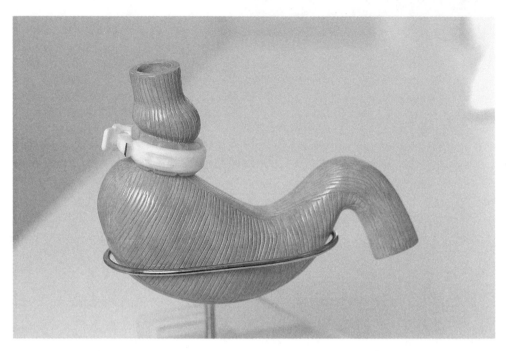

Lap-band placed on a replica stomach. People with the lap-band initially feel full with small volumes of food, and thus reduce their food intake. (iStockPhoto.com)

obesity. This procedure linked the upper and lower parts of the small intestine, thus bypassing the portion of the small intestine between these two points. Despite the effectiveness of JIB, it often was associated with gas-bloat syndrome, electrolyte imbalance, and liver damage. With the introduction of gastric bypass in 1967 as a safer more effective alternative, JIB fell out of favor by the early 1980s.

Current bariatric surgical procedures are classified as either restrictive, malabsorptive, or both. Restrictive procedures leave less room for food intake by physically restricting the stomach size to slow down digestion. The stomach normally holds three to four pints (about one liter), shrinking to just a few ounces post surgery. Food is digested and absorbed normally, however the change in stomach size makes the patient quickly feel full, so the hope is that less food is eaten. Malabsorptive procedures change the way food is digested by rerouting food through the digestive tract, making it harder for the body to absorb calories. Malabsorptive procedures are more invasive. Restrictive procedures generally have fewer complications and lower mortality rates, and the malabsorption procedures lead to greater weight loss. The physician's surgical preference, the patient's health, local hospital circumstances, and new technical developments all influence the choice of which bariatric procedure is best for each individual. The most common procedures are listed below.

- Adjustable gastric banding: Adjustable gastric banding (AGB) restricts food consumption by limiting how much food the stomach can hold. It is the second most common weight loss surgery, following gastric bypass. Adjustable gastric banding—sometimes referred to as the Lap-Band system—involves placing an inflatable silicone ring around the upper portion of the stomach to restrict the amount of food a person can consume. A tube leads from the band to a small port under the patient's skin near the stomach. The physician can manipulate the volume of water injected or withdrawn from the band, which is how the band can be expanded or emptied, similar to inflating or deflating a balloon. When the band is inflated it creates a small pouch where food collects after being swallowed. From within the pouch, food can drain slowly into the rest of the stomach. Gastric banding is considered by many to be the safest and least invasive bariatric surgery.

- Sleeve gastrectomy: Sleeve gastrectomy—also known as vertical sleeve gastrectomy (VSG) or stomach stapling—is another type of restrictive surgery. This type of surgery was introduced in the United States in 2007, and still is considered to be an experimental weight-loss surgery by most insurance companies, so it is much less common than AGB. The procedure surgically reshapes the stomach, leaving much less space for food. Sleeve gastrectomies remove the portion of the stomach responsible for manufacturing ghrelin, the hormone that stimulates hunger, although it is unclear how long this effect lasts. This could help eliminate the physical feeling of hunger in patients. The part of the digestive track where the stomach meets the intestines is left untouched, allowing the stomach to function and empty normally. This surgery sometimes is used in high-risk patients as the first stage of bypass surgery, especially biliopancreatic diversion surgery (described below) for high-risk patients. Many patients lose weight with this surgery alone, however, and avoid further procedures. In other cases, a second surgery occurs within 6 to 18 months after the initial surgery.

- Intragastric balloon surgery: This restrictive procedure inserts an intragastric balloon into the stomach. Once inside the stomach the balloon is inflated. It can remain in the stomach for up to six months. The intragastric balloon has not yet been approved by the U.S. FDA but has been approved in Canada and many other countries.

- Roux-en-Y gastric bypass (RYGB): This bypass surgery is the most common of all bariatric surgeries due to its effectiveness for long-term weight loss. The Roux-en-Y gastric bypass is both a restrictive and a malabsorptive procedure, in which a small stomach is formed, as is done in other restrictive procedures. Additionally, the stomach and small intestine are surgically reconfigured so that food literally bypasses the section of the small intestine that absorbs the majority of calories and nutrients, entering directly into the lower segment of the small intestine. Due to limited nutrient absorption, nutritional supplements are necessary. This procedure is not reversible.

- Biliopancreatic diversion: The biliopancreatic diversion (BPD) procedure also combines restrictive and malabsorptive techniques. Its effect is similar to

Roux-en-Y, but the surgery keeps some stomach function intact after the lower two-thirds of the stomach is removed and attached to the distal segment of the small intestine (the ilium). The BPD procedure generally only is performed on severely obese patients. The BPD usually includes a link from the detached upper portion of the duodenum into the ilium, called the duodenal switch.

When first developed, bariatric surgeries involved open surgical incisions for the surgeon to perform the operation. Currently, about 90% of procedures are performed laparoscopically, requiring several smaller incisions. A laparoscope is a small, tubular instrument with a camera attached; it is inserted through small incisions in the abdomen. Laparoscopy procedures limit the patient's risk for the development of incisional hernias, making it a safer alternative to large-incision surgeries. Surgeons also are developing endoscopic surgical techniques for bariatric surgeries, in which surgery is performed from within the digestive system using very small tools inserted through the patient's mouth.

Eating Post-Surgery

Eating is limited for the initial weeks following weight-loss surgery to allow the stomach and digestive tissues to heal. A liquid diet is mandated for approximately two to three weeks, followed by reintegration of soft foods. Upon the re-entry of solid foods into the diet, the patient will feel full very quickly. Eating must be completed slowly so that foods are thoroughly chewed, so they can pass smoothly through the new opening. Many patients report regurgitating foods during the initial months post-operation due to a lack of room in the stomach. Dry, fibrous foods such as rice, bread, popcorn, and nuts can cause discomfort if not completely chewed.

Effectiveness

Effectiveness rates of bariatric surgeries vary widely. Data on long-term weight-loss maintenance are scarce. Short-term results show weight loss that exceeds the degree of weight loss typically experienced using medications and lifestyle measures only. For the first year following surgery, weight loss is about 30 kg to 50 kg (66 to 110 lbs). Results are higher for RYGB (about 43 kg or 95 lb) than for AGB (about 30 kg or 66 lb) (Osterweil, 2013). Especially intriguing are studies showing that the weight loss experienced with bariatric surgeries has significant health benefits. Patients experiencing significant weight loss have about a 40% lower rate of premature mortality and a 92% lower rate of mortality associated with diabetes (Osterweil, 2013). Data such as these have led to increasing health insurance coverage for bariatric surgeries.

Results vary widely from patient to patient, however. Some people might not lose a significant amount of weight, or even might gain weight post-operation. Achieving maximum results and avoiding regaining weight require permanent lifestyle changes. Regular physical activity and proper nutrition can aid in a patient's weight loss and maintenance. Health indicators are best improved through changing health behaviors, regardless of whether weight is lost. Studies show that many individuals are unable to maintain the weight lost following surgery, thus missing out on long-term benefits.

Risks and Adverse Effects

All surgeries have accompanying risks and weight-loss surgeries are no exception. In fact, surgery becomes riskier as BMI increases. Serious risks associated with the surgeries include excessive blood loss, blood clots, infection, adverse reactions to anesthesia, and leaking of the digestive contents from the digestive system. In rare cases—less than 1 in 1,000 procedures—death can result. Problems that can develop following surgery include a variety of gastrointestinal symptoms such as nausea and vomiting, stomach pain, and gastroesophageal reflex disease. Many patients experience stretching of the esophagus or stomach pouch over time. For AGB surgery, sometimes the gastric band moves or even injures the stomach, which requires an additional surgery. Some patients develop incisional hernias, and the intestines push through the incision site. Gallstones are common with rapid weight loss. Some people experience obstruction of the stomach, small intestine, or bowel; stomach perforation; or ulcers. Patients also can experience dumping syndrome, in which food passes too quickly from the stomach into the small intestine, causing diarrhea, nausea, and weakness. According to the medical literature, AGB procedures generally have the lowest risk of adverse events, approximately 7% (Osterweil, 2013). RYGB procedures have about a 17% risk. The more complicated BPD procedure has adverse complication rates of about 38%.

Malabsorption surgeries require lifelong adherence to dietary supplements, because the malabsorption extends to nutrients as well as calories. Especially problematic are poor absorption of iron, which can lead to iron-deficiency anemia; poor absorption of calcium, which can lead to low bone mineral content and osteoporosis; and low absorption of vitamin B12 with multiple deficiency symptoms.

Approximately one quarter of bariatric surgery patients undergo plastic surgical corrections after significant weight loss has occurred (Klassen et al., 2012). Massive amounts of excess skin and remaining fat tissue can cause hygiene issues and self-esteem problems, and are corrected by plastic-surgery body "lifts." The body's natural ability to retract skin depends on the patient's age and speed of weight loss, and often is exhausted within the first few months following weight loss.

Impact on Psychological Well-Being

Psychosocial benefits of bariatric surgery are related to freedom and lifestyle flexibility following weight loss, such as increased mobility, stamina, and improved self-esteem and body image. Bariatric surgery patients often feel good about taking control of their lives and value their weight loss success. Patients experiencing psychological problems before surgery, however, still might experience these problems following surgery.

A significant proportion of patients who undergo bariatric surgery have binge-eating disorder. Binge eaters are more likely to report psychological disorders, drop out of weight-loss treatment, and regain weight following surgery. Binge eating often is a coping mechanism for stress and can induce potentially dangerous effects post-surgery. In patients, binging on sugary foods or overeating can induce sweating and nausea, involuntary vomiting, or diarrhea. Weight-loss surgery, however, also is viewed as a therapeutic intervention for limiting food consumption and eliminating binge-eating symptoms, therefore promoting psychological improvement.

Allison M. Felix

Research Issues

Should bariatric surgeries be performed on adolescents? Adolescents appear to recover at least as well as adults from the surgeries and experience similar health benefits. Some experts argue that having surgery as early in life as possible will reduce the negative health effects of obesity. Others worry that adolescents might not be psychologically prepared to cope with the demands of surgery and will have more difficulty sticking to the lifestyle changes required by the surgical procedures.

See Also: Digestion and the digestive system; Energy balance; Obesity, causes; Obesity, definition and health effects; Obesity, treatment.

Further Reading

Klassen, A., Cano, S. J., Scott, A., et al. (2012). Satisfaction and quality-of-life issues in body contouring surgery patients: A qualitative study. *Obesity Surgery, 22* (10), 1527–1534. doi: 10.1007/s11695-012-0640-1

Mayo Clinic. (2014). *Tests and procedures: Gastric bypass surgery; definition.* Retrieved November 24, 2014 from http://www.mayoclinic.com/health/gastric-bypass/MY00825

National Institutes of Health. Weight-Control Information Network. (2014, January 24). *Bariatric surgery for severe obesity.* Retrieved from http://win.niddk.nih.gov/publications/gastric.htm

Osterweil, N. (2013). Bariatric surgery reduces mortality in obese diabetic patients. *Internal Medicine News.* Retrieved from http://www.internalmedicinenews.com/news/diabetes-endocrinology-metabolism/single-article/bariatric-surgery-reduces-mortality-in-obese-diabetic-patients/c0d5c01046183b1c9bdcc8e9b8a16a68.html

Padwal, R., Klarenbach, S., Wiebe, N., et al. (2011). Bariatric surgery: A systematic review of the clinical and economic evidence. *Journal of General Internal Medicine, 26* (10), 1183–1194. doi:10.1007/s11606-011-1721-x

Therapeutic Research Faculty. (2014, November 4). *Weight loss surgery: What to expect.* WebMD. Natural Medicines Comprehensive Database. Retrieved from http://www.webmd.com/diet/weight-loss-surgery/slideshow-weight-loss-surgeryϵtty_rm_photo_of_bariatric_surgery_target_area-_.jpg

U.S. National Library of Medicine. (2014, November 13). MedLine Plus. *Weight loss surgery.* Retrieved from http://www.nlm.nih.gov/medlineplus/weightlosssurgery.html

Berberine

Berberine is a bright yellow alkaloid found in the roots, stems, and bark of plants of the *Berberis* species. Some of the common members of this group are goldenseal, Chinese goldthread, Oregon grape, tree turmeric, and barberry. Berberine, traditionally used in Chinese and Ayurvedic medicines, is most widely recognized for its antimicrobial properties. This alkaloid is used clinically to treat bacterial diarrhea, ocular trachoma, and intestinal infections caused by parasites. Preliminary research suggests that berberine also could have anti-inflammatory effects as well as qualities that combat cardiovascular conditions, high cholesterol, type 2 diabetes, and tumors.

Berberine appears to influence bacterial diarrhea caused by organisms such as *Escherichia coli* and *Vibrio cholerae* in a variety of ways. Studies in both animals and humans suggest that berberine acts to decrease the amount of water and electrolytes secreted by the intestines, as well as to slow contractions of intestinal smooth muscle—prolonging the time it takes for substances to pass through. In vitro studies suggest berberine also can act directly on microbes by blocking the ability of the bacteria to bind to the epithelial cells lining the intestinal lumen, which prevents the first step of infection.

Berberine traditionally has been used for its antifungal and antiprotozoal abilities and presently is used to treat intestinal parasites. Experiments have shown that berberine can cause morphological changes; inhibition of growth, multiplication, and respiration; can interfere with nuclear DNA; and can destroy many pathogenic organisms.

Two small clinical studies conducted on humans have suggested that berberine might be effective for the treatment of an eye infection known as ocular trachoma. When berberine chloride was used in eyedrops of patients with this infection—caused by the bacteria *Chlamydia trachomatis*—berberine seemed to enhance protective mechanisms in the host cells that then were able to eliminate the infection (Berberine, 2000).

Berberine appears to have beneficial effects on the cardiovascular system and reduces symptoms of the metabolic syndrome. Berberine sometimes is used in the treatment of heart failure. It seems to prevent harmful arrhythmias by encouraging cardiac contractions and reducing blood pressure. Studies also have shown that this alkaloid can act as a vasodilator. A recent meta-analysis of clinical trials in humans indicates that berberine lowers blood level of total cholesterol and LDL cholesterol and raises HDL cholesterol levels (Dong, Zhao, Zhao, & Lu, 2013). Berberine might help regulate glucose and lipid metabolism. A study in patients with type 2 diabetes mellitus comparing berberine to the diabetes drug metformin over a three-month period found that hemoglobin A_{1c}, fasting blood glucose levels, plasma triglycerides, and insulin resistance all were decreased in patients taking berberine. The results were comparable to the effects of the diabetes drug metformin (Yin, Huili, & Jianping, 2008).

Some research suggests berberine someday could be useful in the prevention or treatment of some cancers. In vitro experiments have demonstrated that

Berberine can inhibit the transcription factor activator protein 1 (AP-1), which normally functions to affect proliferation, differentiation, and programmed cell death. Berberine also might be involved in signal cascades that concern inflammation and the formation of cancer. The alkaloid has also been found to inhibit DNA synthesis in lymphocytes, leading to its anti-inflammatory effects. Berberine is part of a third anti-inflammatory mechanism that inhibits key molecules of the inflammatory process in response to an injury (Singh, Duggal, Kaur, & Singh, 2010). Berberine has been shown to inhibit cyclooxygenase-2 (COX-2) transcription and N-acetyltransferase (NAT) activity in colon and bladder cancers in vitro, giving it anti-tumor qualities. Preliminary studies also suggest that berberine could be helpful for preventing osteoporosis and dementia.

For most clinical uses, 200 mg is taken by mouth two to four times a day. Increased intake can cause GI-tract irritation, low blood pressure, heart damage, and other symptoms. It should not be taken by women who are pregnant because it can cause uterine contractions. Berberine also can cause brain damage in infants, and therefore should not be used by infants or women who are breast-feeding.

Reneé J. Robilliard

See Also: Herbs and herbal medicine.

Further Reading

Berberine. (2000). *Alternative Medicine Review 5* (2), 175–177. Retrieved from http://www.altmedrev.com/publications/5/2/175.pdf

Berberine. (2014) Wellness.com. Retrieved from http://www.wellness.com/reference / herb/berberine

Dong, H., Zhao, Y., Zhao, L., & Lu, F. (2013). The effects of berberine on blood lipids: A systematic review and meta-analysis of randomized controlled trials. *Planta Medica* (March 2013) (epub ahead of print).

Singh, A., Duggal, S., Kaur, N., & Singh, J. (2010) Berberine: Alkaloid with wide spectrum of pharmacological activities. *Journal of Natural Products, 3,* 64–75.

Therapeutic Research Faculty. (2009) WebMD. *Berberine.* Retrieved from http://www.webmd.com/vitamins-supplements/ingredientmono-1126-BERBERINE.aspx?activeIngredientId=1126&activeIngredientName=BERBERINE

Yin, J., Huili, X., & Jianping, Y. (2008). Efficacy of berberine in patients with type 2 diabetes mellitus. *Metabolism Clinical and Experimental, 57,* 712–717. doi: 10.1016/j.metabol.2008.01.013.

Beta-Carotene

Beta-carotene is a member of the carotenoid family, which includes naturally occurring fat-soluble compounds responsible for the red, orange, and yellow pigments found in fruits, vegetables, and some whole grains. Beta-carotene can be found naturally or produced synthetically and is known for its antioxidant properties. It is not itself an essential nutrient but is a source for the essential nutrient, vitamin A. There is some evidence that, taken long-term as a supplement, beta-carotene could have harmful effects, especially in smokers.

Scientist Heinrich Wachenroder coined the term "carotene" in the 19th century, after he crystallized the compound from the carrot root. Carrots now are well known as a major source for beta-carotene. Other foods rich in beta-carotene include pumpkins, mangos, apricots, cantaloupe, sweet potatoes, spinach, kale, and red peppers. (In dark green vegetables, the chlorophyll masks the beta-carotene pigment.) Beta-carotene and other carotenoids are responsible for about 50% of the recommended intake of vitamin A in the North American diet.

Beta-carotene is converted to the essential nutrient, vitamin A, in the small intestine. Vitamin A is an important nutrient in regulating a number of biological functions; and deficiencies of the vitamin can lead to abnormal bone development, problems in the reproductive system, drying of the cornea, and eventually death. To receive adequate vitamin A from beta-carotene, a daily intake of 1,800 mcg (1.8 mg) of beta-carotene is recommended. Daily consumption of five servings of fruits and vegetables generally yields about 6 mg to 8 mg of beta-carotene.

The history of research on beta-carotene supplements provides one of the best cautionary tales regarding the failed promises of dietary supplements. Epidemiological studies conducted in the early 1980s found associations between higher fruit and vegetable consumption and reduced risk of several types of cancer. A high intake of fruits and vegetables was similarly associated with a high intake of beta-carotene. Scientists reasoned that, in diets high in fruits and vegetables, beta-carotene might be the component responsible for reducing cancer risk.

Eager to reap the potential benefits of this association, a number of experimental trials were begun to test this hypothesis. One of the first trials was conducted in Finland, using male smokers as subjects. Researchers thought that the effects of beta-carotene on cancer risk would be especially apparent in this vulnerable population. The experiment, called the Alpha-Tocopherol, Beta-Carotene (ATBC) study followed 29,133 men for 5 to 8 years. When the results were analyzed in 1994, they revealed that subjects receiving the beta-carotene supplement showed a surprising 18% increase in risk of lung cancer (EBSCO, 2012).

In 1996, a similar trial was ended early when subjects receiving beta-carotene showed a 46% greater cancer risk. This study, known as the Beta-Carotene and Retinol Efficacy Trial (CARET) included male subjects who were either current or former smokers, or had been exposed to asbestos. Subsequent studies in women and men, including smokers and nonsmokers, have not found a significant benefit associated with beta-carotene supplements. A high intake of fruits and vegetables still is recommended, and associated with a decreased risk of many types of cancer. Nutrition experts believe that the antioxidant activity of beta-carotene is probably beneficial when beta-carotene is consumed in foods as part of a healthful diet.

Beta-carotene supplements are considered effective in reducing the risk of sunburn in people with the inherited disease erythropoietic protoporphyria (EPP) and might be effective for people who sunburn easily but do not have the disease. High-dose antioxidants might interfere with chemotherapy drugs or radiation therapy. Thus, the decision to take beta-carotene supplements while undergoing cancer treatment should be carefully considered (Mayo Clinic, 2012). Low doses of beta-carotene often are found as a component of multivitamin supplements, to provide all or part of the recommended intake for vitamin A. Because beta-carotene is fat soluble, requiring dietary fat for absorption, beta-carotene in food and supplements is absorbed more effectively when taken with meals containing some fat.

Signs of a toxic level of beta-carotene include dizziness and a (reversible) yellowing of hands and feet. Although beta-carotene likely is safe when taken in limited quantities or for specific medical concerns, supplements are not recommended for general use due to increasing evidence of the dangers of beta-carotene supplementation. Many health authorities (American Heart Association, American Cancer Society, World Cancer Research Institute, and World Health Organization's International Agency for Research on Cancer) recommend getting beta-carotene from food sources until research concludes that supplements are equally as safe and effective.

Eliza N. Cooley

Research Issues

Researchers do not yet understand why beta-carotene supplements are associated with an increased risk of cancer in smokers and people exposed to asbestos. Some experts have suggested that high beta-carotene intake from supplements might inhibit the absorption and utilization of other carotenoids that could be important. Other researchers suggest that, at high doses, some antioxidants can become harmful.

See Also: Antioxidants; Carotenoids; Vitamin A.

Further Reading

EBSCO Complementary and Alternative Medicine (CAM) Review Board. (2012). *Beta-carotene*. Natural and alternative treatments. Retrieved November 25, 2014, from http://healthlibrary.epnet.com/GetContent.aspx?token=e0498803-7f62-4563-8d47-5fe33da65dd4&chunkiid=21547

Mayo Clinic. (2012). *Beta carotene*. Retrieved from http://www.mayoclinic.com/health/beta-carotene/NS_patient-betacarotene

National Institutes of Health. (2011). *Beta-carotene*. Medline Plus. Retrieved from http://www.nlm.nih.gov/medlineplus/druginfo/natural/999.html

National Institutes of Health. National Cancer Institute. (2014, January 16). *Antioxidants and cancer prevention: Fact sheet*. Retrieved from http://www.cancer.gov/cancertopics/factsheet/prevention/antioxidants

Biotin

Biotin is a B vitamin; it also is called vitamin B7, vitamin H, and coenzyme R. Biotin, like all vitamins, is an organic compound that is necessary for normal growth, development, and maintenance of basic functions in the body. Biotin is water soluble, which means that the body does not store it, so it must be consumed regularly. Biotin deficiency is rare because it exists in a variety of foods and only is needed by the body in small amounts (approximately 30 mcg for the average adult) (Ehrlich, 2011). Bacteria that reside in the small and large intestine also synthesize biotin, but it is unknown how much of this the body absorbs. All B vitamins act as coenzymes, or compounds that help enzymes function, and play a critical role in energy metabolism.

Background

A variety of researchers played a role in discovering biotin and its functions, which started with the investigation of a curious condition called, "egg white injury." In 1916, scientist W. G. Bateman discovered that rats consuming a surplus of raw egg whites with an otherwise healthy diet fared poorly, but consumption of cooked egg whites caused no problems. In 1933, another researcher, Margaret Averil Boas, found that rats consuming raw egg whites developed a skin rash. In 1936 German scientists Fritz Kogl and Benno Tonnis isolated a substance in egg that they called "biotin" because of its similarity to substances called "bios" that are needed for yeast growth. A number of other researchers isolated the same substance and gave it other names, including vitamin H and coenzyme R.

In 1942, biotin's structure was confirmed, although for many years its biological functions remained unclear (Ensminger, Ensminger, Konlande, & Robson, 1993). It now is known that biotin is required for many metabolic processes. The reason raw egg white consumption often led to skin rashes and other symptoms is because egg whites contain a substance called avidin. When raw, avidin binds to biotin and prevents its absorption. (Heat denatures avidin, therefore consuming cooked egg whites presents no risk for biotin deficiency.) "Egg white injury" is caused by biotin deficiency.

Role of Biotin in the Body

Biotin is absorbed in the upper part of the small intestine. Once inside a cell, biotin's coenzyme form is activated to assist with fat and carbohydrate metabolism. Biotin promotes the synthesis of fatty acids and glucose by helping to break down amino acids and transfer carbon dioxide to other compounds. Fatty acids and glucose then can be used by the body as fuel for energy.

Biotin Deficiency

Biotin deficiency is rare for people consuming a healthy diet. Instances of deficiency often are connected to conditions or circumstances that make it difficult for individuals to absorb nutrients, such as Crohn's disease, diabetes, long-term intake of antibiotics or antiseizure medication, long-term tube feeding, or as a result of the surgical removal of the stomach. Biotinidase deficiency is a genetic disorder that occurs in approximately 1 in 60,000 newborns. It results in an inability to re-use or recycle biotin, but can be managed with lifelong biotin supplements (U.S. Library of Medicine, 2008). Individuals or animals that consume an excess of raw egg whites (a dozen or more daily over multiple months) also can develop a biotin deficiency (Insel, Ross, McMahon & Bernstein, 2013).

Symptoms of biotin deficiency can include the following.

- Thinning hair
- Glossitis (a bright red, swollen tongue)
- Red, scaly rash around the eyes, nose, and mouth
- Dry eyes
- Muscle pain
- Muscle weakness
- Tingling in the arms and legs
- Fatigue
- Depression

Daily Recommended Intakes

Because biotin deficiency is rare, there is little research on how much biotin individuals should consume. The average intake therefore is determined mathematically from the average intake of infants, which is based on biotin levels in human milk (Insel, Ross, McMahon, Bernstein, 2013). Recommendations are as follows (Ehrlich, 2011).

- Adolescents 14 to 18 years: 25 mcg
- 19 years and older: 30 mcg
- Pregnant women: 30 mcg
- Breast-feeding women: 35 mcg

Food Sources

The food sources containing biotin include liver, salmon, cauliflower, carrots, cereals, bananas, yeast, soy flour, cooked oats, egg yolks, rice bran, milk, soybeans, nuts, wheat, legumes, pork, cheese, avocado, raspberries, and oysters.

Health Benefits of Biotin

Biotin is necessary for proper growth and function of the body. Biotin supplements, however, only are necessary for individuals with proven biotin deficiency. Many biotin supplements are advertised as an effective treatment for a variety of issues, from hair loss and graying hair, to brittle nails and improved blood sugar regulation. None of these claims has been confirmed consistently by research. A study in 2008 showed that a supplement containing both chromium and biotin helped regulate blood sugar levels in people with diabetes. Further research is needed, however, to understand how significant the benefits might be (University of Maryland Medical Center, 2013).

Upper Level Intake and Toxicity

There is no determined Tolerable Upper Intake Level (UL) for biotin. If biotin is overconsumed, then the body removes it through sweat, urine, and feces.

Amari J. Flaherty and Lisa P. Ritchie

See Also: Vitamins.

Further Reading

Ehrlich, S. (2011, June 26). *Vitamin H (Biotin)*. Retrieved from http://umm.edu/health/medical/altmed/supplement/vitamin-h-biotin

Ensminger, A. H., Ensminger, M. E., Konlande, J. E. & Robson, J. R. K. (1993). *Foods and Nutrition Encyclopedia* (2nd ed.). Retrieved from http://books.google.com/books?id=XMA9gYIj-C4C&q=biotin#v=snippet&q=biotin&f=false

Insel, P., Ross, D., McMahon, K., Bernstein, M. (2013). *Nutrition*. Burlington, MA: Jones and Bartlett Learning.

Pantothenic acid and biotin. (2013, February 18). *New York Times*. Retrieved from http://health.nytimes.com/health/guides/nutrition/pantothenic-acid-and-biotin/overview.html

University of Maryland Medical Center. (2013, May 7). *Chromium*. Retrieved from https://umm.edu/health/medical/altmed/supplement/chromium

U.S. National Library of Medicine. (January 2008). Biotinidase deficiency. *Genetics home reference*. Retrieved from http://ghr.nlm.nih.gov/condition/biotinidase-deficiency

Black Cohosh

Black cohosh is a dietary supplement made from the root of the black cohosh plant, which grows naturally in the eastern United States. The plant is a perennial wood-land plant that grows 4 to 8 feet tall and has long white flowers. The scientific names for black cohosh are *Actaea racemosa* and *Cimicifuga racemosa*. It is also known as black snakeroot, bugbane, bugwort, rattleroot, and rattlewood. The herb is often recommended to relieve menopausal symptoms, such as hot flashes, irritability, mood swings, and sleep disturbances.

Nearly 200 years ago, Native Americans used black cohosh root to relieve menstrual cramps, symptoms of menopause, and a multitude of other ailments. In 19th-century America, black cohosh was popular among a group of alternative practitioners. They called it "macrotys" and prescribed it to treat rheumatism, lung conditions, neurological conditions, and conditions that affected women's reproductive organs. In Europe, black cohosh has been used widely to treat premenstrual discomfort, painful menstruation, and menopausal symptoms for more than 40 years.

Black cohosh is most often taken to treat menopausal symptoms, premenstrual symptoms, and menstrual cramps. Germany's regulatory agency for herbal medicine, Commission E, has approved black cohosh for these purposes. Black cohosh is the main ingredient in an over-the-counter German menopausal remedy called Remifemin. Scientific studies regarding the efficacy of black cohosh for the treatment of menopausal symptoms, however, have produced mixed results. Several studies have found black cohosh to be as effective as hormonal treatments, but others have found black cohosh to be no more effective than placebo treatments.

Women with breast cancer often seek help for menopausal symptoms, which are frequent side effects of treatment. Black cohosh has been believed to contain phytoestrogens, including a compound called fukinolic acid, potentially exerting estrogen-like effects in the body. The exact action of the compounds in black cohosh is unclear, however, as studies on possible estrogen-like effects have been contradictory. Additionally, some in vitro studies on human breast cancer cell lines have found black cohosh to inhibit cancer development, and other studies have reported that black cohosh stimulates cancer development. This confusion has led to a general reluctance to recommend the use of black cohosh to women with breast cancer.

Black cohosh can be used in several different forms including capsules, solutions, tablets, tinctures, and powders. The typical suggested dose is 20 mg to 200 mg daily, 1 g to 2 g of dried root powder, or 10 to 60 drops of tincture a day. It also can be made into a tea; however, teas might not be as effective as the standardized extract of black cohosh in relieving menopausal symptoms. Black cohosh can be taken for up to six months and then it should be stopped, as studies demonstrating the safety of long-term use are lacking.

Black cohosh has been associated with some negative side effects, including stomach discomfort, headaches, and weight gain. Rash, nausea, and vomiting also have been reported. Slow heart rate, uterine cramps, dizziness, tremors, joint pain, and light-headedness have been observed with very high doses. In a few cases, liver damage associated with use of black cohosh has been reported. Black cohosh therefore is not recommended for people who consume alcohol regularly or who have liver disorders. It also should not be used by women who are pregnant or breast-feeding.

Alexandra A. Naranjo

See Also: Herbs and herbal medicine; Phytoestrogens.

Further Reading

American Cancer Society. (2011). *Black cohosh*. Retrieved from http://www.cancer.org/treatment/treatmentsandsideeffects/complementaryandalternativemedicine/herbsvitaminsandminerals/black-cohosh

Mayo Clinic. (2011). *Black cohosh (Cimicifuga racemosa [L.] Nutt.)*. Retrieved from http://www.mayoclinic.com/health/black-cohosh/NS_patient-blackcohosh

National Institutes of Health. (2008). *Dietary supplement fact sheet: Black cohosh.* Office of Dietary Supplements. Retrieved from http://ods.od.nih.gov/factsheets /BlackCohosh-HealthProfessional/

Palacio, C., Masri, G., & Mooradian, A. D. (2009). Black cohosh for the management of menopausal symptoms: A systematic review of clinical trials. *Drugs & Aging, 26* (1), 23–36. doi:10.2165/0002512-200926010-00002

University of Maryland Medical Center (UMMC) (2011). *Black cohosh.* Retrieved from http://www.umm.edu/altmed/articles/black-cohosh-000226.htm

Blood Sugar Regulation

The term "blood sugar" refers to blood glucose levels. The body regulates blood glucose levels very carefully because blood glucose is an important source of energy, especially for the central nervous system (CNS). When blood glucose levels fall too low or rise too high, people experience symptoms of CNS dysfunction, including dizziness, disorientation, confusion, unconsciousness, and—in extreme cases—even death.

Blood glucose levels are controlled by two important hormones produced by the pancreas—insulin and glucagon. Specialized cells in the pancreas, called "beta cells," release insulin when blood glucose levels get too high. Insulin binds with receptors on cell membranes that enable cells to take up glucose from the blood, thus reducing blood glucose levels. The cells either use the glucose for energy, if energy is needed, or store it for future use. Liver and muscle cells can convert glucose to glycogen, a type of carbohydrate that quickly can be converted back into glucose as needed. If glycogen stores are full, then the glucose can be converted to triglycerides and stored as fat. Fat is stored in adipose tissue but can also be stored in muscles and in the liver. "Fatty liver" is a harmful condition that can result when energy intake exceeds energy needs over time. (Fatty liver also can develop due to excessive alcohol intake.)

If blood glucose levels fall too low, other specialized cells in the pancreas, called "alpha cells," release the hormone glucagon. Glucagon signals the liver to break down glycogen and release glucose into the bloodstream. As the liver releases glucose into the blood, the blood glucose levels rise to meet the body's immediate energy needs. The liver also can produce glucose from other precursors, such as amino acids; the process is known as "gluconeogenesis."

Another hormone, epinephrine, released by the adrenal glands as part of the stress response—the "fight-or-flight" response—also increases blood sugar level via the same mechanisms as glucagon. The stress hormone cortisol increases blood sugar level by stimulating gluconeogenesis. Adequate blood sugar is essential when responding physically to stress—to fuel muscle contraction, increased heart rate and breathing rate, and the other systems that contribute to fighting or fleeing. Of course, modern-day humans do not always respond to sources of stress by fighting or running away, but blood sugar rises nonetheless as the body prepares to respond to a perceived danger. Drugs that mimic the effects of epinephrine—such as caffeine and nicotine—also raise blood sugar levels.

Blood sugar levels also vary in response to the foods a person consumes, and foods vary in their effect on blood sugar level. Foods with low carbohydrate content contribute little glucose as these foods are digested and absorbed. Foods with high carbohydrate content result in rising blood sugar levels because the glucose is released into the bloodstream. The rate at which a food raises blood sugar levels depends upon the chemical structure of that food. A measurement known as glycemic index represents the speed with which glucose appears in the bloodstream and how high blood sugar levels rise following consumption of a given food. A food with a high glycemic index raises blood sugar levels quickly and to relatively high levels. Foods with lower glycemic indices are digested more slowly, and glucose is released more gradually into the bloodstream. The higher the blood sugar level, the greater the amount of insulin released by the pancreas. High glycemic index foods include white bread, white potatoes, and sugar-sweetened beverages. Low glycemic index foods include those composed primarily of protein and fat, such as eggs, meat, and seafood, and low-starch vegetables such as lettuce, spinach, broccoli, and sweet peppers.

Knowledge of blood glucose regulation enhances understanding of the difficulties presented by conditions that disrupt this process. In people with type 1 diabetes mellitus, the pancreas loses the ability to produce insulin due to the destruction of insulin-producing beta cells. Without insulin, blood glucose levels rise after food consumption as carbohydrates are digested and absorbed, but the glucose is unable to enter the cells. People with type 1 diabetes are able to give themselves insulin. They must time its administration to achieve good control of blood sugar levels. People with type 1 diabetes develop a schedule of insulin administration, meals, and physical activity that tries to mimic nature's intended insulin response, making sure insulin is available when nutrients are being absorbed from meals and that blood sugar does not dip too low during physical activity.

People with type 2 diabetes mellitus usually produce adequate insulin (until later stages of the illness), but the insulin receptors on the cell membranes do not respond well to insulin. People with this condition are said to be insulin resistant, meaning that their insulin receptors "resist" the action of insulin. Although insulin is present in adequate concentrations in the blood, blood glucose remains high because the cell membrane receptors for insulin are not responding and allowing the cells to take up the glucose from the blood. Insulin resistance and type 2 diabetes are often components of the metabolic syndrome usually associated with obesity and low levels of physical activity.

Barbara A. Brehm

Research Issues

How does the body provide optimal glucose levels to muscles during exercise? Scientists do not yet have the full answer to this question. During exercise, great volumes of glucose must be able to enter the exercising muscle cells. Yet, during exercise, insulin levels decline as glucagon and other hormone levels rise to stimulate the liver to release glucose into the bloodstream. How does glucose get into the cells if insulin is not present to stimulate the glucose transporters? The same glucose transporters help cells take up glucose at rest and during exercise; however, signaling molecules other than glucose must be involved in facilitating this process. Interestingly, when muscle is stimulated by insulin, the glucose taken up primarily is stored, and muscle stimulated by exercise oxidizes the glucose to produce energy for muscular contraction, rather than storing it (Wasserman et al., 2011).

See Also: Carbohydrates; Cardiometabolic syndrome; Diabetes, type 1; Diabetes, type 2; Glucose; Glycemic index and glycemic load; Glycogen loading; Hyperglycemia; Hypoglycemia; Insulin.

Further Reading

American Diabetes Association. (2012). Standards of medical care in diabetes—2012. *Diabetes Care, 35* (Supp. 1), S11–S63.

Brehm, B.A. (2014). *Psychology of health and fitness.* Philadelphia: F.A. Davis.

Dugdale, D.C. (2012). *Glucose test—blood.* MedlinePlus. Retrieved from http://www.nlm.nih.gov/medlineplus/ency/article/003482.htm

Sugar homeostasis. (n.d.) *Biology online.* Retrieved from http://www.biology-online.org/4/3_blood_sugar.htm

Therapeutic Research Faculty. (2011). *Blood glucose.* WebMD. Natural Medicines Comprehensive Database. Retrieved from http://diabetes.webmd.com/blood-glucose

Wasserman, D. H., Kang, L., Ayala, J. E., Fueger, P. T., & Lee-Young, R. S. (2011) The physiological regulation of glucose flux into muscle in vivo. *Journal of Experimental Biology, 214* (2), 254–262. doi: 10.1242/jeb.048041.

Body Composition

Body composition refers to an estimate of the proportions of a person's mass that are composed of fat, bone, muscle, and other tissues. Body composition tests used in a nutrition and health context typically divide body mass into fat mass (FM) and everything else, or fat-free mass (FFM). Body composition is interesting because two people who have the same height and weight can look very different and have very different body types. Data from body composition tests can help nutrition professionals make nutrition and weight control recommendations for clients.

How Is Body Composition Measured?

There are many ways to estimate body composition. All are based on the fact that muscle and fat differ in important ways. Each technique uses one of these differences to estimate how much of the body is FM. Some techniques are used primarily in research and medical settings, and others are likely to be available in exercise physiology laboratories and in health and fitness facilities. Techniques used in research and medical settings including the following.

- Hydrometry. Hydrometry methods give an estimate of total body water (TBW). Because fat tissue contains very little water, finding out how much water is in a given body allows researchers to estimate FM and FFM for a given body size. Subjects are given some form of tracer that diffuses into all water compartments. A sample of water, such as saliva, is taken, and TBW extrapolated from the tracer amount in the sample. Hydrometry procedures are expensive and are used primarily for research and medical purposes.
- Dual-energy x-ray absorptiometry. Dual-energy x-ray absorptiometry (DEXA) technology uses two x-ray energies to measure bone density and body composition. It is becoming common for older clients at risk for developing osteoporosis to receive DEXA scans to evaluate and monitor changes in bone density. Dual-energy x-ray absorptiometry technology produces a very accurate estimate of body composition. It currently is used to assess body composition primarily in research settings.
- Medical imaging techniques. Magnetic resonance imaging (MRI) and computed tomography (CT) both are used to assess body tissues and can be used to calculate body composition. MRIs and CT scans also can provide information on the location of adipose tissue stores. These techniques provide good information but are expensive and primarily are used for research on body composition.

Techniques more widely available, and more likely to be used in nutrition and health settings, include the following.

- Hydrostatic or underwater weighing. For this test, a subject sits on a seat underwater. The seat is attached to a scale which measures the person's weight. The heavier a person is in the water, the greater his or her density. Density refers to weight per volume. Two people with the same weight for a given height, or body mass index (BMI), can have different densities. A denser person has more FFM and less fat. By calculating density from water weight, a person's body fat percentage can be estimated. Error can occur with this measure because the density of non-fat tissues, such as bone, varies from person to person; the test calculations, however, rely on an average value. Similarly, percent fat prediction equations take into account the air remaining in the lungs after a complete exhalation. If this volume is estimated and not measured, or if the person has difficulty exhaling and holding the breath underwater, then body-composition estimates will not be as accurate. Underwater weighing tanks most likely are found in research and academic settings, such as in kinesiology department facilities.

- Air displacement. Some instruments estimate body composition from air displacement. The heavier a person is for a given size, the denser the person is. As with underwater weighing, higher density means less fat tissue. Individual variations in tissue density reduce the accuracy of body composition predictions. Air-displacement equipment is most commonly found in research and academic settings.
- Bioelectrical impedance analysis (BIA). Bioelectrical impedance analysis tests are based on the fact that fat conducts electricity more slowly than nonfat tissue, which contains quite a bit of water. BIA equipment sends a weak electrical current through the body. The speed of the current reflects relative fat in the body. BIA measures assume a constant body water content for various tissues, so anything that alters hydration status or causes water retention affects BIA body-composition estimates. Dehydration, premenstrual water retention, elevated muscle glycogen levels, and food in the stomach also can interfere with the accuracy of BIA body composition estimates. BIA equipment is found in many health and fitness facilities. Because equipment is quite portable and easy to use, BIA often is the technology of choice at health fairs.
- Anthropometric measures. Anthropometry means "the measurement of humans," and refers to measures that describe physical characteristics. The anthropometric measures used for estimating body composition include circumferences and skinfolds. Circumference, in this context, refers to the distance around a particular body part, such as the waist, hips, or upper arm. Circumferences are usually taken with a tape measure, and then entered into an equation to predict body fat. Skinfold thickness is measured with calipers at several standard anatomic sites. These measurements then are entered into prediction equations to predict body composition. Circumference and skinfold measures are most accurate when taken by an experienced test administrator; however, body-fat predictions based on these measures often still are inaccurate because the equations that are used are based on population averages and might not apply to a given individual. Some health and nutrition professionals use circumferences and skinfolds as "stand alone" measures. When taken over time they can show changes in and of themselves, without predicting body composition from them. If a person is losing fat, for example, the waist circumference might decrease. Anthropometric measures are the least expensive—but also are the least accurate—means of estimating body composition.

Researchers have a fairly rough idea of the range of body fat percentiles that are normal and healthy for various population groups, although less information is available for ethnic minorities. The healthy range for adult males can be anywhere from 6% to 24%, and for adult women are anywhere from 14% to 34%, depending upon the person's build and body type. Athletes tend to be leaner, although this varies by sport.

The most accurate measures of body composition are not readily available to most people. The most common measures have an error range of at least +/-4 percentage points. This means that if a body composition test—such as a hydrostatic weighing or skinfold test—estimates body composition at 20%, it actually can be somewhere between 16% and 24%. Because body composition changes very slowly, even with weight loss, the most readily available assessment methods lack the precision required to find meaningful change.

When Are Body Composition Tests Helpful?

Body composition tests can be helpful in several situations, including the following.

- A person who has begun exercising more—especially performing more strength training—and is gaining a little scale weight, but appears to be getting more muscular, not fatter. Body composition tests might verify that lean or muscular people are not fat. Their weight gain is healthy muscle gain (not fat gain).
- People who have a normal BMI or weight but lack muscle size and strength. These people could fall into the category of "normal weight obesity," which is associated with the same health risks as obesity. A body composition test might help motivate such people to improve eating and exercise behaviors.
- Athletes attempting to reach a specific weight category or weight minimum might find body composition tests helpful to see if their weight goal is realistic. Coaches and athletic trainers, for example, often monitor high school wrestlers' body composition scores to be sure athletes are not trying to lose too much weight to get into a lower weight category.
- People who have a high BMI (or weight) but appear fairly muscular. A body composition test can help reassure them that they are not overly fat, and that they should not focus on losing weight, unless other obesity-associated health risks indicate that some weight loss would be beneficial.

Body composition tests are most accurate when performed by experienced professionals. If body composition measures are taken over time, then the same test should be used repeatedly and, if possible, the same professional should perform the test each time.

Barbara A. Brehm

Research Issues

When do excess adipose tissue stores become a health risk? Exploring information from the entries in this encyclopedia on adipose tissue, body mass index, and obesity provides a good context for understanding how body composition assessment is useful in clinical settings.

See Also: Adipose tissue; Body mass index; Obesity, definition and health effects.

Further Reading

Brehm, B.A. (2014). *Psychology of health and fitness.* Philadelphia: F. A. Davis.

Esmat, R. (2012). *Measuring and evaluating body composition.* American College of Sports Medicine. Retrieved from http://www.acsm.org/access-public-information/articles/2012/01/12/measuring-and-evaluating-body-composition

McArdle, W. D., Katch, F. I., & Katch, V. L. (2009). *Exercise physiology: Energy, nutrition, and human performance.* Philadelphia: Lippincott, Williams, & Wilkins.

Body Mass Index

Body mass index (BMI) is a measure commonly used to assess weight and obesity, and is calculated from a person's weight and height. Although BMI is not a measure of body composition, it can be a useful indicator of body fat of most people—especially when used in conjunction with other measures, such as waist circumference. Unlike most body composition assessment techniques, BMI is easy to obtain and can help guide individuals and clinicians in their assessment of a person's risk for the development of obesity-related health problems. Body mass index is even more useful as a public health indicator; epidemiologists use BMI to observe population obesity trends. For some individuals, BMI might not be a good indicator of body composition. Body size alone might not reflect body composition, especially for people with an exceptionally great amount of muscle mass, or people with sarcopenic obesity, for whom BMI appears normal but the person has such low muscle mass that "normal" weight is composed of too much body fat.

Body mass index has been used as an assessment tool since the middle of the 19th century. Originally created by Belgian mathematician Adolphe Quetelet, it was called the Quetelet index. It is calculated by dividing a person's weight by the square of his or her height. The formulas provided below are used (CDC, Body Mass Index, 2014).

For metric units of measure:

- BMI = weight (kg) / [height (m)]^2
- Example: Weight = 68 kg, height = 165 cm (1.65 m)
- Calculation: $68 \div (1.65)^2 = 24.98$

For English units of measure:

- BMI = weight (lb) / [height (in)]$^2 \times 703$
- Example: Weight = 150 lbs, height = 5'5" (65")
- Calculation: $[150 \div (65)^2] \times 703 = 24.96$

Online tools are widely used to calculate BMI (CDC, Body Mass Index, 2014). Body mass index charts also are available (*see* table 1).

- To use the table, find the appropriate height in the left-hand column labeled height.
- Move across to a given weight (in pounds).
- The number at the top of the column is the BMI at that height and weight.
- Pounds have been rounded off.

BMI is interpreted for adults 20 years of age and older using the following categories.

- Underweight: BMI below 18.5
- Normal: BMI = 18.5–24.9
- Overweight: BMI = 25–29.9
- Obese: BMI 30.0 and greater

Table 1. Body Mass Index (BMI) Calculation

BMI	19	20	21	22	23	24	25	26	27	28	29	30	31	32	33	34	35
Height (inches)	Body Weight (pounds)																
58	91	96	100	105	110	115	119	124	129	134	138	143	148	153	158	162	167
59	94	99	104	109	114	119	124	128	133	138	143	148	153	158	163	168	173
60	97	102	107	112	118	123	128	133	138	143	148	153	158	163	168	174	179
61	100	106	111	116	122	127	132	137	143	148	153	158	164	169	174	180	185
62	104	109	115	120	126	131	136	142	147	153	158	164	169	175	180	186	191
63	107	113	118	124	130	135	141	146	152	158	163	169	175	180	186	191	197
64	110	116	122	128	134	140	145	151	157	163	169	174	180	186	192	197	204
65	114	120	126	132	138	144	150	156	162	168	174	180	186	192	198	204	210
66	118	124	130	136	142	148	155	161	167	173	179	186	192	198	204	210	216
67	121	127	134	140	146	153	159	166	172	178	185	191	198	204	211	217	223
68	125	131	138	144	151	158	164	171	177	184	190	197	203	210	216	223	230
69	128	135	142	149	155	162	169	176	182	189	196	203	209	216	223	230	236
70	132	139	146	153	160	167	174	181	188	195	202	209	216	222	229	236	243
71	136	143	150	157	165	172	179	186	193	200	208	215	222	229	236	243	250
72	140	147	154	162	169	177	184	191	199	206	213	221	228	235	242	250	258
73	144	151	159	166	174	182	189	197	204	212	219	227	235	242	250	257	265
74	148	155	163	171	179	186	194	202	210	218	225	233	241	249	256	264	272
75	152	160	168	176	184	192	200	208	216	224	232	240	248	256	264	272	279
76	156	164	172	180	189	197	205	213	221	230	238	246	254	263	271	279	287

For BMI greater than 35, see http://www.nhlbi.nih.gov/health/educational/lose_wt/BMI/bmi_tbl2.htm

Source: National Heart, Lung, and Blood Institute. (n.d.) Body Mass Index Table 1. Retrieved from http://www.nhlbi.nih.gov/guidelines/obesity/bmi_tbl.htm

Body mass index is calculated the same way for children and adults, but the BMI of children and adolescents is evaluated in terms of how their BMIs compare to others of their age and gender. Tools for calculating and evaluating the BMI for children and teens can be found on the Centers for Disease Control and Prevention website (CDC, About BMI for children and teens, 2014).

Barbara A. Brehm

See Also: Body composition; Obesity, causes; Obesity, definition and health effects; Obesity, treatment.

Further Reading

Centers for Disease Control and Prevention (CDC). (2014, July 11). *About BMI for children and teens.* Retrieved from http://www.cdc.gov/healthyweight/assessing/bmi/childrens _bmi/about_childrens_bmi.html

Centers for Disease Control and Prevention (CDC). (2014, July 16). *Body mass index.* Retrieved from http://www.cdc.gov/healthyweight/assessing/bmi/Index.html

Boron

Boron is an essential trace mineral vital to plant health and occurs naturally in compounds called borates, which are a variety of salts and minerals found in the earth's crust. In humans, boron appears to participate in a number of important roles. Preliminary research suggests that boron is involved with bone growth as well as regulation of inflammatory and immune-system responses, and probably brain health (Samman, Foster, & Hunter, 2012). Healthy amounts could be involved in steroid-hormone metabolism, might participate in the actions of vitamin D and estrogen, and could assist with the proper absorption of magnesium and calcium (EBSCO, 2012). Boron supplements increasingly are being used by postmenopausal women to promote bone health and mass, although evidence for benefits is preliminary.

In the 1870s, boron became the main ingredient in substances used for preserving meat and dairy foods (Nielsen, 2008). These preservatives proved critical in avoiding food crises during both World War I and II, but fell out of favor by 1950, due to increasing evidence for boron's toxicity in high doses. Boron still is mined for its use in glass and ceramics, as well as is flame retardants, detergents, and soaps.

A key component for cell walls in plants, the element is found in most fruits and vegetables, especially dried fruits such as prunes and raisins. It also is found in other plant foods including nuts and legumes. The boron content of all foods varies with geographical location and soil content. Lack of boron has been found to disrupt the life cycle of frogs, causing atrophy of reproductive organs and death of more than 80% of embryos within the first 96 hours (Nielsen, 2008). Boron deficiency interferes with proper brain function in humans, with subjects exhibiting poor performance on psychomotor tasks involving manual dexterity and eye-hand coordination, as well as on cognitive tests of attention, spatial perception, and short- and long-term memory (Penland, 1998). A few correlational studies suggest that greater intakes of boron could be associated with reduced risk of hormonally sensitive cancers, such as breast and prostate cancers (Samman, Foster, & Hunter, 2012). These studies suggest that further research in this area is warranted. Although no daily recommended intake (DRI) has been set for boron, its intake is considered to be insufficient below 0.4 mg per day, with optimal health effects gained from ingesting about 1 mg per day (Nielsen, 2008). Usual dietary intake is between 0.87 and 1.35 mg per day for adults (Neilsen, 2008). Exposure to excess boron is rare. Symptoms include nausea, poor appetite, weight loss, and decreased sexual activity. The Tolerable Upper Intake Level for boron is 20 mg per day for adults.

Patricia M. Cipicchio

See Also: Minerals.

Further Reading

EBSCO Complementary and Alternative Medicine (CAM) Review Board. (2012). *Boron.* ConsumerLab.com. Retrieved from http://www.consumerlab.com/tnp.asp?chunkiid =21616&docid=/tnp/pg000397

Insel, P., Ross, D., McMahon, K., & Bernstein, M. (2013). *Nutrition.* Burlington, MA: Jones & Bartlett.

Nielsen, F. H. (2008). Is boron nutritionally relevant? *Nutrition Reviews, 66* (4), 183–191.

Penland, J. G. (1998). The importance of boron nutrition for brain and psychological function. *Biological Trace Element Research 66*, 299–317.

Samman, S., Foster, M., & Hunter, D. (2012). The role of boron in human nutrition and metabolism. In *Boron science: New technologies and applications*, N. S. Hosmane (Ed.). Boca Raton, FL: CRC Press.

U.S. Department of Health and Human Services (2010). *Boron toxicology.* Toxicology Profiles: Agency for Toxic Substances and Disease Registry. Retrieved from http://www.atsdr.cdc.gov/toxprofiles/tp26.pdf

Bottled Water

"Bottled water" refers to drinking water that is sold in a variety of containers, including individual serving bottles, quarts, liters, and "carboys" (a large glass or plastic bottle) for water coolers. Bottled water can come from any of several water sources, including springs, aquifers, and even municipal water supplies. The production and marketing of bottled water became popular in North America in the 1980s, and the market has continued to expand as consumers worry about pollution of their local water supplies. As health authorities urge people to consume fewer sugar-sweetened beverages, many individuals are turning to bottled water as a convenient and healthful beverage alternative. Environmental groups have recently become alarmed, however, at the environmental costs of the bottled water industry. Discussions concerning the purchasing of water supplies by private organizations to sell as bottled water have brought questions of water-supply ownership and management into the public eye.

Several types of bottled water are available (FDA, 2010). Mineral water comes from a protected underground source and must contain at least 250 parts per million (ppm) of dissolved minerals, such as calcium and magnesium. Spring water is taken from an underground supply that flows naturally to the surface. Artesian water comes from a confined underground aquifer located below the natural water table. Purified water is tap water or groundwater that has been treated by distillation, deionization, or reverse osmosis.

The debate about whether bottled water is healthier than tap water has been of great significance in recent years, especially as bottled water becomes more pervasive. Bottled water often is thought to be cleaner and taste better than public tap water, but this difference varies depending upon the source and processing of the bottled water, as well as the specific municipal water supply. Bottled water often is claimed to originate from springs, lakes, or mountain streams, and tap water is assumed to come from more local supplies. In reality, some tap water comes from the same places as bottled water, including springs and lakes. Additionally, many types of bottled water actually are forms of filtered tap water. Investigations in 2006–2008 revealed that some bottled waters contained more contaminants than are found in most municipal water supplies. This news prompted many consumers to become more aware of the quality of their tap water and that of their bottled water.

Standards for municipal water are set and enforced in the United States by the Environmental Protection Agency (EPA) and in Canada by Health Canada. Municipal water suppliers must release reports at regular intervals listing contaminants found. Bottled-water products are not required to do this. The production and labeling of bottled water is regulated by the Food and Drug Administration in the United States. In Canada, Health Canada is responsible for the health and safety standards for bottled water, and also helps to regulate labeling policies. The Canadian Food Inspection agency is responsible for setting and enforcing standards for the packaging, labeling, advertising, and production of bottled water. Bottled water and tap water generally have the same safety and the same problems. Consumers therefore should make decisions about what type of water to drink by considering the safety of their home water supply; the cost, taste, and fluoride content of water; and the environmental concerns about the costs of bottled water.

Many consumers have expressed fear about contamination of bottled water by the bottle itself. Evidence suggests that chemicals from the plastic bottle can leak into the water. This is especially likely to occur as the bottles age or are exposed to heat, such as being left in a hot car.

Environmental groups have attempted to educate consumers about the hidden costs of bottled water, including the generation of solid waste, as a majority of bottles end up in landfills rather than recycling facilities. The production of bottled water requires petroleum and water to produce the plastic bottles and transport the product, often for long distances. Additionally, some groups are concerned that the privatization of global water supplies and the diversion of water to produce bottled water for resource-rich countries could leave some communities in resource-poor areas with inadequate water supplies.

Barbara A. Brehm and Catherine E. Tocci

Research Issues

Some schools and workplaces have attempted to reduce use of bottled water by supplying people with reusable containers and urging them to fill containers at home or from drinking fountains. In schools, these efforts often are promoted by student clubs and organizations that focus on environmental awareness and sustainability.

See Also: Water needs, water balance.

Further Reading

Environmental Working Group. (2012). *EWG's bottled water scorecard, 2011*. Retrieved from http://www.ewg.org/research/ewg-bottled-water-scorecard-2011

Health Canada. (2011). *Frequently asked questions about bottled water*. Retrieved from http://www.hc-sc.gc.ca/fn-an/securit/facts-faits/faqs_bottle_water-eau_embouteillee-eng.php

International Bottled Water Association. (n.d.). *Regulation of bottled water*. Retrieved November 26, 2014, from http://www.bottledwater.org/education/regulations

Nelson, J. K. (2012). *Is tap water as safe as bottled water?* Mayo Clinic. Retrieved from http://www.mayoclinic.com/health/tap-water/AN02167

Owen, J. (2006, February 24). Bottled water isn't healthier than tap, report reveals. *National Geographic News*. Retrieved from http://news.nationalgeographic.com/news/2006/02/0224_060224_bottled_water.html

U.S. Food and Drug Administration (FDA). (2010, June 28). *Bottled water everywhere: Keeping it safe*. Retrieved November 26, 2014, from http://www.fda.gov/ForConsumers/ConsumerUpdates/ucm203620.htm?utm_campaign=Google2&utm_source=fdaSearch&utm_medium=website&utm_term=bottled%20water&utm_content=1

"Brain Foods"

The term "brain foods" refers to food that is thought to have a positive influence on brain structure and function. Research suggests that food-derived signaling molecules influence metabolism and synaptic plasticity which reflects positively on cognitive function. Cognition is defined as the mental processes used to gain knowledge and process information through responses such as learning, attention, and memory. Foods that contain omega-3 fatty acids, flavonols and antioxidants, folic acid, and vitamin E show some evidence of contributing to brain health.

Evidence indicates that omega-3 fatty acids, including α-linolenic acid, eicosapentaenoic acid (EPA), and docosahexaenoic acid (DHA), have a significant role in cognition and mental health. Studies have found an increased risk of schizophrenia, depression, and dementia in subjects that have deficiencies in omega-3 fatty acids (Dauncey, 2008). Specifically, high levels of DHA have been found to increase protein-lipid interactions. This results in enhanced cell membrane flexibility because DHA is a key component of neuronal membranes—which translates to increased neuronal activity and better cognitive functioning.

Some studies suggest that, in rodent models, supplementation with DHA could promote greater concentrations of hippocampal brain-derived neurotropic factor (BDNF) and enhanced cognitive function. Brain-derived neurotropic factors alter specific cell signaling pathways in the brain which results in an increase in neurogenesis, learning, and memory. The known pathway where the conversion of α-linolenic acid to EPA to DHA occurs is not efficient. Thus, the required EPA and DHA levels for brain functioning are dependent on dietary intake (i.e., oily fish). Dietary intake, however, is more complicated than just eating foods high in omega-3 fatty acids to enhance cognition; there must be a balance between the intake of foods that are high in both omega-3 and omega-6 fatty acids. Fatty acids in general can affect multiple pathways molecularly in the brain, based upon their binding to receptors in the cell nucleus. In this way, fatty acids can regulate the transcription of various genes important for brain structure and function.

Flavonols are a member of the flavonoid family, a group of compounds found in various fruits, tea, and cocoa (Vauzour, 2012). Studies suggest that flavonol-rich foods improve blood flow in the brain. Optimal blood flow to the brain enhances adult neurogenesis (the creation of new nerve cells) and positively affects cognitive performance. Additionally, flavonols could help to reduce the oxidative damage that the brain experiences due to its high metabolic rate and the vulnerable polyunsaturated fatty acids that comprise neural membranes. The antioxidant lycopene—found in tomatoes and other fruits and vegetables—might help protect the brain against free-radical damage to cells (Lewin, 2014). Several flavonol and flavonoid-based diets have become highly publicized due to the link found between foods high in antioxidants and benefits to neural functioning (Gómez-Pinilla, 2008). For instance, studies examining blueberry supplementation in aged animals showed improved memory and learning (Vauzour, 2012). These results seem to occur in humans, as well. One study found that blueberry juice supplementation for 12 weeks had beneficial effects in humans in terms of improving learning and memory (Joseph, Shukitt-Hale, & Willis, 2009).

Folic acid found in foods such as spinach and orange juice has been shown to be vital to brain structure and function, especially during development (Gómez-Pinilla, 2008). Folate deficiency can result in neurological disorders, such as depression and cognitive deficits. Preliminary studies have indicated that long-term folic acid supplementation can minimize age-related cognitive decline in older adults. Folic acid also is thought to lower homocysteine levels in the blood. Elevated levels of homocysteine could increase the risk of stroke and cognitive impairment (Lewin, 2014).

The micronutrient vitamin E has been shown to correspond to better cognitive functioning (Sorgen, 2014). Foods high in vitamin E include nuts, seeds, and green leafy vegetables. It has been suggested that dietary intake of vitamin E can act as a protective factor against cognitive decline, particularly in the elderly. Vitamin E has been associated with improved mitochondrial activity, which translates to better cognitive function (Gómez-Pinilla, 2008). The mechanisms behind vitamin E are not well understood, but likely relate to antioxidants' effects on ridding the brain of free radicals to protect synaptic membranes from oxidation. Research on use of vitamin E supplements indicates that they sometimes are linked with negative health effects, therefore nutritionists usually advise consumers to obtain adequate vitamin E from food.

Nutritionists also advise that, although research on single nutrients and brain function might seem intriguing, it is unlikely that a single nutrient will be found to exert a strong effect on the brain, given the many nutrients, foods, and lifestyle factors that influence brain development and health. Rather, individuals should strive to consume a healthful diet, including brain foods such as nuts, seeds, oily fish, blueberries and other berries, a variety of vegetables, moderate amounts of tea, and even a little dark chocolate.

Victoria E. von Saucken

See Also: Alzheimer's disease and nutrition; Antioxidants; Attention-Deficit Hyperactivity Disorder and nutrition; Autism and nutrition; Depression and nutrition; Fatty acids; Phytochemicals; Polyphenols.

Further Reading

Dauncey, M. J. (2008). New insights into nutrition and cognitive neuroscience. *Proceedings of the Nutrition Society, 68* (4), 408–415. DOI: http://dx.doi.org/10.1017/S0029665109990188

Gómez-Pinilla, F. (2008). Brain foods: The effects of nutrients on brain function. *National Review of Neuroscience, 9* (7), 568–578.

Joseph, J. A., Shukitt-Hale, B., & Willis, L. M. (2009). Grape juice, berries, and walnuts affect brain aging and behavior. *Journal of Nutrition, 139,* 1813S–1817S.

Lewin, J. (2014). *10 foods to boost your brainpower*. BBC Good Food. Retrieved from: http://www.bbcgoodfood.com/howto/guide/10-foods-boost-your-brainpower

Sorgen, C. (2014). *Eat smart for a healthier brain*. Wed MD. Retrieved from http://www.webmd.com/diet/features/eat-smart-healthier-brain

Vauzour D. (2012). Dietary polyphenols as modulators of brain functions: Biological actions and molecular mechanisms underpinning their beneficial effects. *Oxidative Medicine and Cellular Longevity* 2012, article ID 914273. Retrieved November 26, 2014, from http://dx.doi.org/10.1155/2012/914273

Breast-Feeding

The term "breast-feeding" refers to the practice of nourishing an infant with human milk, generally by allowing the infant to suck on the mother's breast. Breast-feeding practices, however, also can include feeding breast milk to the infant using a bottle. Health organizations, including the World Health Organization, the U.S. Centers for Disease Control and Prevention, and Health Canada, unanimously agree that—with very few exceptions—breast milk is the best source of nutrition for infants. Breast milk provides infants practically all of the nutrients required until they reach six months of age. Although infant-formula producers have tried to replicate the composition of breast milk, they have not yet been able to create the many growth factors, enzymes, antibodies, and other immune-system compounds found in human milk. In addition to its superior nutritional benefits, the act of breast-feeding offers benefits for mothers and contributes to strong emotional bonds between mother and child. Breast-feeding at birth is associated with a number of health benefits for babies, both while children are young and also later in life. Although breast milk is the preferred choice for infants, it is not always an acceptable option for mothers. Many mothers struggle with the physical challenges presented by breast-feeding and find it difficult to balance the demands of lactation and work.

Breast-Milk Nutrition

Breast milk provides almost all of the nutrients that are essential to an infant's growth and development. A combination of fats, cholesterol, proteins, carbohydrates, vitamins, minerals, and other components present in breast milk create the ideal recipe for the health and vitality of infants.

Fats are the primary source of calories in an infant's diet. Infants grow at a rapid rate and therefore require much sustained energy. A diet rich in fat helps promote growth and weight gain. Infants are able to ingest only a certain amount of fluid each day, therefore that fluid must provide an adequate amount of fat. In addition to providing caloric energy, fat plays a role in infant brain development and neural networks. Recent research has focused on the presence of long-chain polyunsaturated acids in human milk, specifically arachidonic acid (AA), and docosahexenoic acid (DHA). These acids are found in the structural lipids of cell membranes and are especially important in the structure of the neurons in the central nervous system, including the brain. The fat content of breast milk varies widely, depending upon the mother's diet. Women who consume strictly vegetarian diets and few marine products can produce lesser amounts of the fatty acids AA and DHA. Breast milk contains enzymes that speed the infants' digestion of fats, thus the fat in breast milk is digested more easily than that in formula.

Breast milk also contains an abundance of cholesterol, which is important in infant brain development. Cholesterol is a primary component in the myelin sheaths located on the axons of the neurons. Myelin sheaths allow for neural impulses to be conducted efficiently.

Human breast milk contains two types of proteins—whey and casein—in a 60:40 ratio. This protein ratio contributes to the digestibility of breast milk and supports the growth of helpful bacteria, such as lactobacillus, in the infant's digestive tract. Lactose (milk sugar) is the primary carbohydrate found in breast milk.

Breast milk contains adequate amounts of all vitamins except for vitamin D. In recent years, pediatricians in North America have recorded several cases of vitamin D deficiency in breast-fed babies. Deficiency is especially likely to develop in babies born in winter months, and in those always protected from the sun by clothing and sunscreen products. For this reason, mothers are advised to give babies a vitamin D supplement and allow babies to be exposed to sunshine, when possible, to stimulate vitamin D production.

Breast milk appears to contain an adequate amount of iron for the first six months of an infant's development. Although the iron content in breast milk is relatively low as compared to formula, the iron in breast milk is absorbed more easily. Iron-containing foods, including iron-fortified foods, should be introduced into a baby's diet by six months of age.

Health Benefits

The first three to five days of an infant's life are the most crucial for breast-feeding. This is because breast milk is at first a sweet, yellow substance known as colostrum, which contains a high concentration of immune cells. The presence of colostrum has been correlated with positive development of an infant's immune system. The protective benefits of breast milk, however, continue throughout the breast-feeding period.

Several substances in breast milk enhance immunity in the baby's gastrointestinal (GI) tract, including the secretory immunoglobulin A (IgA) antibodies. When a mother encounters pathogens, her body manufactures antibodies specific to each one. The antibodies pass into the mother's breast milk and escape breakdown in the baby's GI tract because they are protected by the so-called "secretory" component. Once in the baby's GI tract, the antibodies bind with the targeted infectious agents and prevent them from passing through the lining of the GI tract. This protection is especially important in the earliest days of life, because the infant does not begin to make his or her own secretory IgA until several weeks or months after birth. The secretory IgA antibodies disable pathogens without harming helpful GI tract flora or causing inflammation. This is important because, although inflammation helps fight infection, sometimes the process overwhelms the GI tract. An infant could suffer more from the inflammatory process than from the infection itself when inflammation destroys healthy tissue.

The large quantities of the immune system molecule interleukin-10 found in breast milk also help inhibit inflammation. A substance called "fibronectin" enhances the phagocytic activity of immune cells (called "macrophages"), inhibits inflammation, and helps repair tissues damaged by inflammation. Several other breast-milk molecules help disable harmful microbes. Mucins, certain oligosaccharides (sugar chains), and glycoproteins (carbohydrate–protein compounds) bind to microbes and prevent them from gaining a foothold in the lining of the GI tract. Many of breast milk's immune cells, including T lymphocytes and macrophages, attack invading microbes directly.

Breast-milk compounds also help in other ways. Some decrease the supply of nutrients such as iron and vitamin B12 that harmful bacteria need to survive. A substance called "bifidus factor" promotes the growth of helpful gut flora which crowd out pathogens. Retinoic acids—a group of vitamin A precursors—reduce the ability of viruses to replicate. Some of the hormones and growth factors present in breast milk stimulate the baby's GI tract to mature more quickly, thus making it less vulnerable to dangerous invaders. These immune benefits of breast milk result in fewer GI tract infections, ear infections, and respiratory tract infections for breast-fed babies.

Studies have found that breast-fed babies have reduced rates of childhood asthma and other allergies, lower rates of sudden infant death syndrome (SIDS), and reduced risk for developing type 1 diabetes. Breast-feeding advocates often cite reduced rates of childhood obesity as a positive impact of breast-feeding, which could help to explain why breast-fed babies have lower rates of type 2 diabetes and cardiovascular disease later in life.

Benefits to Mothers

The practice of breast-feeding offers several benefits to mothers. The hormone oxytocin that is released during breast-feeding stimulates the uterus to contract more quickly to its pre-pregnancy size. Oxytocin often is called the "bonding hormone," because it is associated with feelings of pleasure, love, and relaxation, which might help to explain why women who breast-feed have reduced rates of post-partum depression. Women who breast-feed appear to have a lesser risk for breast and ovarian cancers later in life. Because the production of milk in the mammary glands requires a large supply of calcium, research indicates that nursing mothers could lose bone mineral during lactation, although bone density appears to recover once lactation ends.

Breast-Feeding Recommendations

Public health experts and pediatricians in North American universally recommend breast-feeding exclusively for a baby's first six months of life, and continued breast-feeding (in addition to appropriate solid food) for at least the first year. The World Health Organization recommends exclusively breast-feeding for the first six months, with continued breast-feeding for at least the first two years of a child's life. Longer breast-feeding practices are associated with improved infant survival and child health, better maternal health, and reduced health care costs for families and communities.

Contraindications to Breast-Feeding

Mothers infected with HIV or who have untreated tuberculosis are discouraged from breast-feeding in countries where safe infant formula can be obtained. Women taking any medications should check with their health care providers to be sure that breast-feeding is recommended. Many drugs make their way into breast milk and could have harmful effects on an infant.

Prevalence of Breast-Feeding

Until relatively recently in human history, breast-feeding has been the norm for infant nutrition. Mothers carried their infants throughout the day and fed them as needed. Royalty and upper-class women in some cultures hired other lactating mothers, often known as "wet-nurses," to provide their infants with breast milk. The practice of breast-feeding began to decline dramatically in the United States and Canada in the early 1900s, as infant formula and bottles became available. The popularity of breast-feeding began to increase in the 1960s, however, as research establishing the benefits of human milk and breast-feeding developed.

Government surveys estimate that, in the United States, presently about 75% of mothers begin breast-feeding their babies at birth, but less than 50% of mothers are still breast-feeding after 6 months. Many women introduce other sources of nutrition, including formula, and only about 16% of mothers feed their babies only breast milk for 6 months (CDC, 2011). Breast-feeding rates in Canada are higher, with more than 85% of mothers initiating breast-feeding at birth, and about 26% exclusively breast-feeding for at least 6 months (Health Canada, 2012). Factors associated with greater rates of breast-feeding include a higher level of education attained by the mother, greater household income, and a mother who is married rather than unmarried.

Challenges to Breast-Feeding

Despite the evident superiority of breast milk to infant formula, many women still choose not to breast-feed. Some mothers experience physical difficulties with breast-feeding. It can take several days to establish a breast-feeding routine that works for both mothers and babies. Babies initially might have difficulty latching on and drinking enough to support adequate growth and development. Some mothers experience a great deal of physical discomfort when breast-feeding.

Lactation consultants—professionals who specialize in breast-feeding—often can help resolve such issues.

Several social factors can interfere with breast-feeding. Partners and other family members might discourage the practice. Some cultural groups regard breast-feeding as unnecessary or a nuisance. A majority of women in North America today work for pay, and most work environments are not conducive to breast-feeding. Lactating employees must take several breaks during the day to either feed their babies or to pump and refrigerate their milk.

Environmental Impact of Infant-Feeding Practices

Breast-feeding is associated with a lesser environmental impact than that of formula feeding. Lactating mothers must consume more calories to produce milk, therefore their food consumption increases by about 600 calories per day. The environmental impact of this increased food consumption varies with the mother's food choices. The manufacture of formula has a greater impact, as it requires factories, supplies, and fuel. Formula must be placed in containers and shipped, often long distances, requiring more fuel. Plastic bottles, nipples, and other feeding paraphernalia also have environmental costs associated with their production, disposal, and recycling.

Lisa A. Kelley and Barbara A. Brehm

Research Issues

The U.S. Centers for Disease Control and Prevention think that hospitals could do much more to promote breast-feeding practices, especially by providing support to new mothers and their families. Some of their suggestions can be found on the CDC website, listed in the Further Reading section.

See Also: Colostrum; Infant formula; Lactation.

Further Reading

American Academy of Pediatrics. (2012). Policy statement: Breastfeeding and the use of human milk. *Pediatrics 129* (3), e827–e841. doi: 10.1542/peds.2011-3552

Centers for Disease Control and Prevention (CDC). (2011). *Hospital support for breastfeeding.* Retrieved from http://www.cdc.gov/vitalsigns/breastfeeding/

Committee on the Evaluation of the Addition of Ingredients New to Infant formula, Food and Nutrition Board, Institutes of Medicine. (2004). *Infant formula: Evaluating the safety of new ingredients.* National Academies Press. Retrieved from: http://books.nap.edu/catalog.php?record_id=10935

Health Canada. (2012). *Breastfeeding initiation in Canada: Key statistics and graphics (2009–2010).* Retrieved from http://www.hc-sc.gc.ca/fn-an/surveill/nutrition/commun/prenatal/initiation-eng.php

U.S. Department of Health and Human Services, Office on Women's Health. (2010). *Why breastfeeding is important.* Womenshealth.gov. Retrieved from http://womenshealth .gov/breastfeeding/why-breastfeeding-is-important/index.html

World Health Organization (WHO). (2002). *The World Health Organization's infant feeding recommendation.* Retrieved November 26, 2014, from http://www.who.int /nutrition/topics/infantfeeding_recommendation/en/

Brown Adipose Tissue

Brown adipose tissue (BAT), unlike white adipose tissue, is a special type of fat that is associated with positive health benefits. Greater levels of BAT are associated with lower measures of body mass index (BMI), a weight-for-height measure used to estimate obesity. In other words, people with more BAT are less likely to be obese. Once thought to play a negligible role in human physiology, researchers now believe that humans have significant amounts of BAT, and that this fat tissue acts as an endocrine organ, producing neurochemicals that influence processes such as blood glucose regulation and resting metabolic rate.

Brown adipose tissue seems to have been described as early as 1551, but it wasn't until the 1900s that it was recognized as being present in all mammals. Scientists initially were interested in the role BAT plays in generating heat, especially for mammals during their arousal following hibernation. This ability to produce heat plays an essential role in the survival of these mammals, which must function in a cold environment. The heat production by BAT also was recognized as providing a survival advantage for human infants—about 5% of an infant's body mass is BAT. Brown adipose tissue enables infants to generate heat without shivering, a process known as "non-shivering thermogenesis." Once thought to be present in significant amounts only in infants, nuclear imaging techniques have shown that BAT also is present in human adults (Ravussin & Kozak, 2009).

Brown adipose tissue contains a greater density of capillaries and mitochondria (the cellular organelles responsible for energy production) than that of white fat. Although most mitochondria produce adenosine triphosphate (ATP) to fuel metabolic processes, the mitochondria in BAT are "energy inefficient" for ATP production and produce heat from fuel precursors, such as glucose and fats, instead of producing ATP. In addition to keeping people warm, BAT appears to help them get rid of extra calories by "burning them up"—turning them into heat, rather than storing them (Ravussin & Galgani, 2011). Researchers have speculated that the higher levels of BAT in lean individuals as compared with obese individuals could partly explain differences in body composition. Greater levels of BAT might contribute to an increased resting metabolism and the ability to consume a more than average amount of calories without gaining weight.

Research suggests that regular exercise stimulates white adipocytes to become brown adipocytes (Bostrum et al., 2012). During exercise, a cellular messenger made in muscles and dubbed "irisin" (named after the Greek messenger goddess

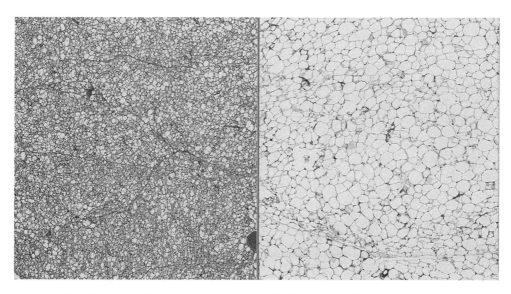

Brown fat's color comes from its greater density of blood vessels. Brown fat is metabolically more active than white fat, expending more calories, and thus, helping to prevent excess body fat. (Vetpathologist/Dreamstime.com)

Iris) is produced. Irisin moves from the muscle to the bloodstream and appears to communicate with white adipose tissue, "telling" it to develop into BAT, especially in the visceral area. Increasing irisin levels in the blood of mice results in an increase in energy expenditure, with no changes in physical activity level or food intake (Bostrum et al., 2012).

Research suggests that BAT might play an important role in blood glucose regulation and energy balance. One interesting study transplanted BAT from healthy mice into mice that had developed pre-diabetes as a result of a high-fat diet (Stanford et al., 2013). After 8 to 12 weeks, the mice receiving the BAT transplant had decreased body weight and fat mass, and improved blood sugar regulation, increasing their insulin response to blood glucose. Brown adipose tissue appears to achieve these results in part because it increases levels of important signaling molecules that improve blood glucose regulation. This effect of BAT could help to explain why regular exercise, by increasing BAT, improves blood glucose regulation.

Barbara A. Brehm

Research Issues

Researchers hope that by understanding the signaling messengers—such as irisin, which is generated by brown adipose tissue—new drugs to treat obesity can be developed. Although availability of these drugs still is a long way off, pharmaceutical treatment of obesity generally has been disappointing, and new strategies are needed.

See Also: Adipose tissue; Energy balance; Obesity, definition and health effects.

Further Reading

Bostrum, P., Wu, J., Jedrychowski, M. P., et al. (2012). A PCG1-alpha-dependent myokine that drives brown-fat-like development of white fat and thermogenesis. *Nature, 481* (7382), 463–468. doi:10.1038/nature10777

Brehm, B. A. (2014). *Psychology of health and fitness*. Philadelphia: F.A. Davis.

DeNoon, D. (2009). *Can brown fat make you thin?* WebMD. Retrieved November 26, 2014, from http://www.webmd.com/diet/news/20090407/can-brown-fat-make-you-thin

Ravussin, E. & Galgani, J. E. (2011). The implication of brown adipose tissue for humans. *Annual Review of Nutrition, 31,* 33–47.

Ravussin, E. & Kozak, L. P. (2009). Have we entered the brown adipose tissue renaissance? *Obesity Reviews 10* (3), 265–268.

Stanford, K. I., Roeland, J. W., Middelbeek, R. J. W., et al. (2013). Brown adipose tissue regulates glucose homeostasis and insulin sensitivity. *Journal of Clinical Investigation, 123* (1), 215–223. doi:10.1172/JCI62308

Wein, H. (2009, April 20). Overlooked "brown fat" tied to obesity. *NIH Research Matters*. Retrieved from http://www.nih.gov/researchmatters/april2009/04202009obesity.htm

C

Caffeine

Caffeine is a bitter substance found in the seeds, leaves, and fruits of certain plants. Beverages made from these plant components also contain caffeine. The most commonly consumed caffeinated beverages are coffee and tea. Caffeine also occurs naturally in chocolate. Caffeine is added to many foods, beverages, dietary supplements, and over-the-counter drugs. It is somewhat addictive, and withdrawal symptoms include headache, fatigue, drowsiness, and irritability.

One of the most-studied drugs in the world, it has been consumed in some form for centuries by people in just about every culture. Research examining the effect of the consumption of caffeine and caffeine-containing beverages on health suggests that, in general, small doses do not appear to do too much harm to most people. Small-to-moderate amounts even can provide beneficial effects for some people. Caffeine does become harmful at higher doses, however, and some people are better off avoiding caffeine altogether.

Caffeine is similar in structure to the neurochemical adenosine, which slows brain activity. By blocking adenosine receptors caffeine blocks adenosine's effects. This explains caffeine's positive psychological effects, such as reducing feelings of fatigue, improving concentration, and enhancing mood. Caffeine's negative psychological effects, including increased anxiety, irritability, nervousness, and insomnia, also are a result of blocking the action of adenosine in the brain.

Considered a sympathomimetic drug, caffeine's effects mimic those of the sympathetic nervous system—the branch of the nervous system that produces the fight-or-flight stress response. This response causes heart rate, blood pressure, and muscle tension to temporarily increase as the body prepares to fight or flee in response to danger. Metabolic rate increases somewhat and appetite can be reduced, which is why many weight-loss products contain caffeine.

Sensitivity to the effects of caffeine varies considerably from person to person. Smokers remove caffeine from their bodies twice as fast as nonsmokers and thus could be less sensitive to caffeine's effects. People who rarely consume caffeine generally are much more sensitive to caffeine's many effects, but people accustomed to caffeine experience less-pronounced reactions.

Most adults appear to self-regulate caffeine consumption fairly well. They learn—perhaps through trial and error—what amount of caffeine helps them feel alert and productive and at what point to stop consuming it before any negative effects develop. Negative side effects, such as stomachache, nausea, nervousness, insomnia, and anxiety, encourage most people to limit caffeine consumption.

Some people, however, develop negative symptoms from very small doses of caffeine and therefore should avoid it entirely. Experiencing any of the effects listed below suggests that one should limit or eliminate caffeine intake.

- Irregular heartbeat: Some people experience an irregular heartbeat when they consume caffeine. Their hearts feel like they are beating much too fast or are "skipping beats."
- Feelings of stress and anxiety: Many people experience feelings of stress and anxiety when they consume caffeine. Adding insult to injury, people also are more likely to overindulge in caffeine when they feel stressed. Yet, because caffeine's effects mimic the stress response, it can leave people feeling even more stressed.
- Insomnia: People who suffer from difficulty sleeping should try reducing or giving up caffeine to see if this solves the problem. Some people find that even when they consume caffeine only in the morning it aggravates sleep problems that night.
- High blood pressure: Blood pressure rises for a fairly short time following caffeine ingestion. Although this rise does not appear to be harmful for most people, those with hypertension might benefit by reducing caffeine intake.
- High intake: High intake of coffee and other caffeinated products has been associated with some health problems, such as increased risk for ovarian and pancreatic cancers. Risks usually are associated with consuming more than five cups of coffee per day (Lueth, Anderson, Harnack, Fulkerson, & Robien, 2008).
- Bone density and osteoporosis: Some studies have suggested a link between caffeine consumption and the risk of osteoporosis in elderly women. This has not been found, however, for younger women who drink just a cup or two of a caffeinated beverage a day (Cooper et al., 2009).
- Reproductive concerns: A high caffeine intake might interfere with fertility, therefore couples having difficulty conceiving should try reducing caffeine. High caffeine consumption during pregnancy is associated with birth defects in laboratory animals, and with miscarriage and low birth weight in humans, therefore only small amounts of caffeine (or none) should be consumed during pregnancy (Patel & Rizzolo, 2012). Caffeine makes its way into breast milk, and nursing mothers who consume caffeine could end up with irritable, fussy babies who have trouble sleeping.
- Ulcers and heartburn: Coffee, not caffeine, increases the production of stomach acids, therefore decaffeinated coffee is not a solution for related problems. People having digestive problems should reduce coffee intake or switch to tea.

Barbara A. Brehm

Research Issues

Many people have suggested that the caffeine content of food, beverages, supplements, and over-the-counter drugs should appear on the label. It is easy to consume caffeine without realizing how much one is ingesting. Caffeine is added to many body-building and sports supplements, for example because it has a slightly ergogenic effect, allowing people to work harder than they work without caffeine. Caffeine also can give users a more positive feeling, and thus make users more likely to consume the supplement again. Caffeine also works to reduce perception of pain, so it is added to many pain-reliever formulations. Tables of caffeine content in familiar foods are available from the Center for Science in the Public Interest (CSPI) (http://www.cspinet.org/new/cafchart.htm), but labeling would further reduce guesswork.

See Also: Chocolate; Coffee; Energy drinks; Tea.

Further Reading

Center for Science in the Public Interest (CSPI). (November 2014). *Caffeine content of food & drugs.* Retrieved from http://www.cspinet.org/new/cafchart.htm

Cooper, C., Atkinson, E. J., Wahner, H. W., et al. (2009). Is caffeine consumption a risk factor for osteoporosis? *Journal of Bone and Mineral Research, 7* (4), 465–471.

Lueth, N. A., Anderson, K. E., Harnack, L. J., Fulkerson, J. A., & Robien, K. (2008). Coffee and caffeine intake and the risk of ovarian cancer. The Iowa Women's Health Study. *Cancer Causes and Control, 19* (10), 1365–1372.

Mayo Clinic Staff. (2014, April 14). *Caffeine: How much is too much?* Retrieved from http://www.mayoclinic.com/health/caffeine/NU00600

Patel, S. & Rizzolo, D. (2012). When the patient asks: Is caffeine safe during pregnancy? *Journal of the American Academy of Physicians Assistants, 25* (5), 69.

Calcium

Calcium is the most abundant mineral found in the human body and plays a key role in a variety of functions. Not only is calcium essential to maintain the structural integrity of bones and teeth, it also is necessary for signaling and enzymatic processes in blood vessels, neurons, and the endocrine system, and plays an important role in muscular contraction. Calcium is found in a variety of foods and dietary supplements and has many health-related effects.

Calcium is an essential nutrient that must be consumed for a person to maintain health. It is absorbed in the body by two different mechanisms. When calcium is consumed, either from a food or supplemental source, it moves through the esophagus and stomach until it reaches the small intestine. In the small intestine, calcium passes into the endothelial lining of the duodenum via active transport. Once inside the cell, the calcium molecule binds to the carrier protein, "calbindin," whose formation is dependent upon vitamin D. Calbindin transports calcium to the basal membrane (where the absorptive cell of the digestive tract communicates with the bloodstream), where calcium is actively pumped out of the cell and into the bloodstream. After entering the bloodstream, calcium is transported throughout the body to perform its many functions. If calcium intake is high, then the mineral also is absorbed in the jejunum and ileum via passive diffusion then passes through the tight junctions and into the bloodstream.

The amount of calcium that is absorbed depends on the calcium source, the amount taken at one time, the person's age, vitamin D availability, and other food components. On average, people absorb about 30% of the calcium they consume. Increased levels of vitamin D allow for more calcium to be absorbed from the gastrointestinal tract. Absorption rate is highest during peak growth times of life, including infancy, puberty, and pregnancy. As people age, their ability to absorb calcium declines. Oxalic acid, which is found in many vegetables, and phytic acid, found in greens, also can reduce the amount of calcium that is absorbed. Two major forms of calcium, citrate and carbonate, are found in most calcium supplements. Calcium carbonate is best absorbed when it is taken with food and calcium citrate can be absorbed with or without food.

Calcium is found in many foods, but is highest in concentration in dairy products such as milk, yogurt, and cheese. It also is found in many vegetables including Chinese cabbage, kale, and broccoli as well as in fish with edible bones. Grains, such as bread, pasta, and cereals naturally have very little calcium in single servings, but because they often are eaten in large quantities they can be a source of calcium. Grains and other foods also commonly are fortified with calcium and therefore can be good sources of the mineral. Many people take calcium citrate or calcium carbonate in the form of dietary supplements.

Excess calcium is stored in bones and teeth, and 99% of the body's calcium can be found in these structures. Blood calcium levels are highly regulated and when calcium levels become too low more is released from the bones into the blood. Throughout life, bones are continuously being remodeled. During times of growth, however, more bone is being built than broken down, therefore it is important to have a sufficient calcium intake. Thus, recommended calcium intake differs with age, sex, and stage of life.

Infants, growing children, and adolescents require significant amounts of calcium to grow strong bones. In the United States and Canada, the Recommended Dietary Allowance (RDA) for calcium suggests that both males and females ages 9 to 18 years old consume 1,300 mg per day, because bone is being formed. During early and middle adulthood bones reach peak bone mass (at ~30 years old), and at this point the rates of building and breakdown are the same. For people ages 19 to 50 years old, the RDA is 1,000 mg per day of calcium. In aging adults and postmenopausal women, more bone is being broken down than is being built. Women older than age 50 and men older than age 70 should consume 1,200 mg of calcium per day. Pregnant and lactating women should try to consume 1,300 mg per day.

Young women with amenorrhea, due either to low caloric intake or too much exercise, have lower calcium absorption (because of reduced estrogen levels), which puts them at risk for inadequate calcium levels. Lactose intolerance and vegan diets, due to a lack of dairy products, also are often found to cause low calcium levels. Not only can calcium deficiency be caused by malabsorption or low intake, it can be due to increased excretion from the body. Calcium excretion in the urine increases when there is high protein and high sodium intake. Excretion also can be affected by some medicines (Office of Dietary Supplements, 2013).

Calcium performs important roles in bone as well as in other tissues. In bones, calcium becomes part of a crystalline structure called hydroxyapatite, which surrounds collagen. Osteoblasts and osteoclasts work to form and dismantle bone, respectively. Calcium is important for bone strength, but can be released into the bloodstream when it is needed in other body tissues and to maintain a constant blood calcium concentration. The process of turning bone into calcium is regulated by vitamin D, parathyroid hormone, and the hormone calcitonin.

When calcium is not being stored in the bones it is aiding in many other functions. In neurons, action potentials travel down axons and trigger a calcium release. This calcium release causes vesicles within the neuron to release neurotransmitter into the synapse, to propagate the nerve signal throughout the body. In muscles, the neurotransmitter acetylcholine is released onto the muscle cells, which leads to downstream calcium release within the muscle fibers. The calcium molecules bind to proteins that are part of the contractile machinery, controlling muscle contraction. Calcium also can bind to the protein calmodulin. The calcium-calmodulin complex plays a part in regulating secretion, cell division, and the movement of cilia. Calcium also is important for blood clotting.

Too much or too little calcium can influence a wide range of health issues. Adequate levels of calcium must be consumed to reach peak bone density by age 30. If not enough calcium is absorbed to replace bone calcium loss, low bone mineral levels and, eventually, osteoporosis can develop. Osteoporosis is a disease of porous and fragile bones that affects more than 10 million adults in the United States, 80% of whom are women (Office of Dietary Supplements, 2013). Studies show that getting adequate calcium might reduce risk of hypertension. Some studies have found that high calcium consumption lowers the risk of colon and renal cancers as well as reducing the risk of nonmalignant colon tumors. Conversely, other research, such as the results of the Women's Health Study, does not show a correlation between calcium levels and colon or rectal cancer. Some studies even suggest that high calcium intake increases the risk of prostate cancer.

Many studies have attempted to elucidate the effect of calcium on cardiovascular disease (CVD). It is thought that by decreasing the intestinal absorption of lipids, relatively high levels of calcium could decrease the risk of CVD. Recent studies found that men who ingested more than 1,000 mg per day of supplemental calcium, however, had a 20% increase in their risk of CVD. Results from the Women's Health Initiative suggest that taking calcium supplements increased the risk of CVD in women, but results from the Women's Health Study found that calcium decreased the risk. Experts agree that, at some level, high intakes of calcium can lead to hypercalcemia, which is high blood calcium. Hypercalcemia can lead to increased blood clotting, calcification of the blood vessels, and stiffening of the arteries, all of which contribute to cardiovascular disease (Xiao et al., 2013). Experts recommend that calcium be obtained from food rather than supplements when possible, as risks appear to be higher with supplements. Additionally, upper limits for calcium have been set at fairly low levels to discourage high consumption of calcium. The U.S. and Canadian recommendations for upper limits of calcium intake are 2,000 mg per day for people older than age 51, 2,500 mg per day for people ages 19 to 50, and 3,000 mg per day for people ages 9 to 18.

Calcium might interact with certain medications. It can reduce the absorption of bisphosphates, fluoroqinolones and tetracycline antibiotics, levothyroxine, phenytoin, and tiludronate disodium. Diuretics also have been found to decrease calcium excretion in the kidneys which increases blood calcium concentration. Glucocorticoids, mineral oil, laxatives, and antacids with magnesium or aluminum can lead to reduced blood calcium levels.

Renée J. Robilliard

Research Issues

Not everyone agrees with the high calcium Daily Recommended Intakes of the United States and Canada. In many countries calcium intake is about 300 mg to 600 mg per day, compared with the recommended 1,000 mg to 1,200 mg per day for Americans, depending on age. Osteoporosis rates are very low in many of these countries, perhaps because citizens get more exercise or sun exposure (Harvard School of Public Health, 2013).

See Also: Cardiovascular disease and nutrition; Female athlete triad; Osteoporosis.

Further Reading

Harvard School of Public Health. (2013). *Calcium and milk: What's best for your bones and health?* Retrieved from http://www.hsph.harvard.edu/nutritionsource/calcium-full-story/

Health Canada. (2012, March 22). *Vitamin D and calcium: Updated dietary reference intakes.* Retrieved from http://www.hc-sc.gc.ca/fn-an/nutrition/vitamin/vita-d-eng.php

National Institutes of Health. Office of Dietary Supplements. (2013). *Calcium. Dietary supplement fact sheet, health professional.* Retrieved from http://ods.od.nih.gov/factsheets/Calcium-HealthProfessional/

USDA National Nutrient Database for Standard Reference, Release 17. *Calcium content of selected foods per common measure, sorted by nutrient content.* Retrieved from http://www.nal.usda.gov/fnic/foodcomp/Data/SR17/wtrank/sr17w301.pdf

Xiao, Q., Murphy, R. A., Houston, D. K., Harris, T. B., Chow, W.-H., & Park, Y. (2013). Dietary and supplemental calcium intake and cardiovascular disease mortality: The National Institutes of Health–AARP Diet and Health Study. *Journal of the American Medical Association Internal Medicine, 173* (7). doi:10.1001/jamainternmed.2013.3283

Calorie

A calorie is a unit of heat energy, and the term comes from the Latin root for heat, "calor." A calorie is the amount of energy needed to raise the temperature of one gram of water by one degree centigrade under standard conditions. Because the heat absorption capacity of water changes with water temperature, water temperature should be defined for calorie definitions. Standard initial water temperature is usually defined as 14.5 degrees C, at 1 atmosphere pressure. In common usage, the term calorie also refers to energy, both the energy contained in food and the energy expended by animals, including humans. On food labels, the term calorie generally refers to a kilocalorie (kcal) (1,000 calories) and is the amount of energy needed to raise the temperature of one kilogram of water by one degree centigrade. Sometimes the term "Calorie" (rendered with an initial capital letter) is used to represent kilocalorie. A calorie is equal to approximately 4.184 joules.

The calorie first came into use as a unit of heat energy in early 19th-century France, when Nicholas Clément introduced the term in a series of lectures on the fuel efficiency of steam engines. Several decades after its first use, the term was translated into English and came to represent the energy needed to raise the temperature of water. The use of calories in relation to human dietary needs was popularized in the United States by W. O. Atwater in 1887, after he used calories in his articles on food and in his tables of food composition (Hargrove, 2007). At the start of the 20th century, the word became further entrenched in common usage in the United States, due in great part to the USDA Farmers' Bulletins food databases. From there, as Americans became increasingly interested in weight management, the word began appearing in articles and books, garnering the interest of non-scientists across the country. The calorie was adopted for use in the nutritional facts panels on U.S. food labels, in contrast to the many other countries that use kilojoules rather than kilocalories in describing food energy content.

Continued use of the calorie in a nutrition context is a practice mostly isolated to the United States and the United Kingdom. Although the calorie predates the joule as a unit of food energy by nearly 60 years, many nations officially transitioned from the use of the calorie to use of the joule in 1954, when the International System of Units (SI) was adopted (Hargrove, 2007). Within the SI system, the unit for energy in any form is the joule (J), which—in direct contrast to the comparatively ambiguous nature of the calorie—corresponds with energy measurements and conversion factors in all other SI-based branches of science (Food and Agriculture Organization of the United Nations, 1971). Regardless of its context within the realm of international scientific standards, however, the calorie remains the primary unit of food energy for hundreds of millions of consumers around the world.

As units of food energy, calories convey how much energy is stored in a food's chemical bonds waiting to be released when the body breaks down those bonds for its own energy. Chemical bond energy is measurable in the form of heat given off during the oxidation of a given substance. The chemical bond energy in a particular food can be determined using a calorimeter. This device functions by completely burning a given food sample in a chamber that is surrounded by a fluid, such as water. The temperature change of the fluid reflects the energy value of the food. Temperature change then can be directly converted into calories. In a similar fashion, calorimetry can measure energy expenditure in people and animals. For example, a person could be placed in a chamber surrounded by water. The heat given off by the person causes an increase in the water temperature, which is measured and converted to calories.

The calorie content of food as measured by calorimetry probably does not exactly match the calories actually captured by people with the processes of digestion, absorption, and metabolism of food (Nelson & Zeratsky, 2013). Nevertheless, calorie counts on food labels still provide a helpful guide for evaluating the relative energy content of foods. In general, carbohydrates and proteins provide 4 kcals per gram; fat provides 9 kcal per gram; and alcohol contains 7 kcal per gram.

Erin K. McDaniel

See Also: Energy balance; Metabolic rate; Metabolism.

Further Reading

Food and Agriculture Organization of the United Nations (1971). *The adoption of joules as units of energy.* Retrieved November 26, 2014, from http://www.fao.org/docrep/meeting/009/ae906e/ae906e17.htm

Hargrove, J. L. (2006). History of the calorie in nutrition. *Journal of Nutrition, 136* (12), 2957–2961. Retrieved from http://jn.nutrition.org/content/136/12/2957.full

Hargrove, J. L. (2007). Does the history of food energy units suggest a solution to "calorie confusion"? *Nutrition Journal, 6* (44). Retrieved from http://www.nutritionj.com/content/6/1/44

Nelson, J., & Zeratsky, K. (2013). *Calories reconsidered: Old assumptions questioned.* Mayoclinic.com. Retrieved from http://www.mayoclinic.com/health/calorie-counts/MY02403

U.S. Department of Agriculture (n.d.). *Calories.* Retrieved from http://www.choosemyplate.gov/weight-management-calories/calories.html

Cancer and Nutrition

Cancer is a class of more than 100 diseases that is characterized by unregulated cell growth. Cancer begins with changes to a cell's genetic material, its DNA, which alter the cell's normal behavior. Rather than growing, dividing, and dying in a typical way, cancer cells do not stop dividing—producing abnormal cells that continue to reproduce. In most types of cancer (the exception is cancers of the blood cells), the abnormal cells accumulate and cause the formation of masses of tissue called "tumors." Malignant (cancerous) tumors eventually can crowd and replace healthy tissue, interfering with organ function. Malignant tumors also can release cells that travel to other parts of the body, via the lymphatic system or bloodstream, in a process called "metastasis," in which the cells invade other organs and cause new tumors. The transformation that produces cancer cells from normal cells involves multiple steps. Only about 5% to 10% of cancers seem to be caused primarily from inherited genetic factors. The rest are believed to be caused by repeated damage to DNA and the cells over time by environmental factors, such as radiation, viruses, and chemicals. Lifestyle behaviors, including smoking, unprotected sexual activity, sun exposure, physical activity, and diet contribute to cancer risk by causing genetic changes or by influencing other factors that help or hinder cancer cell growth and development. In the United States, researchers suggest that about one-third of cancer deaths can be attributed to tobacco use, and another third is linked to poor diet and inadequate physical activity, including obesity and being overweight (Kushi et al., 2012). The causes and risk factors for many cancers, however, are unknown.

The word "cancer" has been traced to Greek physician Hippocrates, who lived around 460 BCE to 370 BCE. In his writings, Hippocrates described several kinds of cancer tumors with the Greek words "carcinos" and "carcinoma," from the Greek word for crab, presumably from the projections reaching out from the tumor body that produced a crab-like shape (ACS, 2014). Another Greek physician, Galen, who lived and worked in the second century CE, used the word "oncos," which means "swelling," to describe the tumors he observed (ACS, 2014). Today, the word "oncologist" refers to a cancer specialist.

Approximately half of all men and one-third of all women in the United States will face a cancer diagnosis at some point during their lives (ACS, What is cancer? 2012). Many cancers are curable, especially if caught early; there are millions of cancer survivors in the United States and around the world. Nevertheless, cancer is a leading cause of death, with 8.2 million deaths worldwide being attributed to cancer in 2012 (WHO, 2014). For men in the United States, the most common cancers that cause death are cancers of the lung and bronchus, prostate, colon and rectum, pancreas, and liver. For women, the leading causes of cancer deaths are cancers of the lung and bronchus, breast, colon and rectum, pancreas, and ovary (ACS, Cancer Facts & Figures 2012, 2012). The many types of cancer differ significantly from one another in terms of causation, risk factors, diagnosis, and treatment. Dietary recommendations for cancer prevention, however, are similar for the types of cancer that appear to be influenced by diet.

Research on cancer and lifestyle behaviors can identify "in the long run, on the average" cancer risks; it cannot explain why any given individual develops cancer. Many people with healthful lifestyles still develop cancer, but others with multiple cancer risk factors never do.

The Processes of Cancer

The development of cancer is a complex, multistep process. It involves changes in a cell's DNA as well as the metabolic pathways in which proteins that influence cellular function are created from the DNA template. It also is influenced by the processes involved with cell division and differentiation. These changes generally occur over a long period, often decades. Food components can influence these processes—both positively and negatively—at every step.

Cancer begins with changes in a cell's genetic material, the DNA that resides in the chromosomes found in the nucleus of the cell. These initial changes are caused by carcinogens, typically chemicals (e.g., asbestos and formaldehyde), microbes (e.g., hepatitis C virus, some strains of human papilloma virus), or radiation (ultraviolet light; x-rays) that alter the DNA. Researchers estimate that cells and their DNA experience hundreds of injuries each day that have the potential to cause the DNA changes that lead to cancer (WCRF/AICR, 2007). Fortunately, very few of these cause harm. Some damage does not influence the genes that lead to cancer. Often, DNA repair mechanisms fix or eliminate damaged sections, including those that might cause cancer; and cells could die before the damage becomes permanently captured in daughter cells. Over time, however, DNA damage can accumulate. Carcinogens and other compounds also can cause cell damage by altering how DNA is translated (or not) into proteins; influencing DNA repair mechanisms; and affecting communication among cells within a tissue.

Cells respond to a wide variety of messenger molecules known as "cytokines," which help to stimulate or suppress cell division and differentiation, and cell death ("apoptosis"). Some compounds (dietary and other) favor the proliferation of potentially cancerous cells over normal cells through a variety of pathways, a process known as "promotion." Estrogens are believed to be promoters for certain types of cancer, for example, because they increase the proliferation of cells in the breast, and over time, increase the risk of some types of breast cancer. Some systemic factors—such as high levels of oxidation and inflammation—favor the development of cancer by setting the stage for more DNA damage and increased levels of growth factors that signal cells to replicate (WCRF/AICR, 2007).

Bioactive substances in the diet—including nutrients and phytochemicals—can enhance or inhibit cancer development via these pathways and processes. Dietary factors also can influence the strength of the immune system, which in some cases attacks cancer cells in the body. Dietary factors can inhibit the process of angiogenesis (the formation of new blood vessels) that, in the context of cancer, provide oxygen and nutrients and remove wastes from growing cancerous tumors.

Cancer and Nutrition

Research suggests that some foods and beverages and their components, as well as overall dietary patterns, are associated with cancer risk. In addition to the foods themselves, agricultural and food-processing practices, along with methods of food preservation and preparation also influence cancer risk (WCRF/AICR, 2007). It has become apparent that excess body fat, which itself is influenced by dietary pattern as well as physical activity, increases cancer risk.

Identifying helpful and harmful foods, food components, and dietary patterns is difficult for a number of reasons. People consume a wide variety of foods each day, and a person's diet also can vary considerably from day to day; thus, simply obtaining accurate food records from people is challenging. Individuals generally consume more than 25,000 bioactive food constituents—including nutrients and phytochemicals—in any given diet, so it is not easy to tease out the influence of a specific compound (WCRF/AICR, 2007). Results obtained in the laboratory with in vitro cell cultures could have little relevance for humans. For example, although beta-carotene slows cancer cell growth in vitro, use of beta-carotene supplements by former smokers is associated with an increased, rather than decreased, risk of lung cancer.

Dietary compounds interact with the digestive system and other constituents from food as food is broken down and absorbed. Too much supplementary vitamin E (which usually is available as d-alpha tocopherol), for example, can block the uptake of the other seven types of vitamin E that occur in the diet, or of other important compounds. After digestion and absorption, potentially helpful nutrients and phytochemicals travel in the bloodstream and are metabolized and stored via various biochemical pathways in the liver, kidney, and other organs—they might never even come into contact with cancerous cells. If they do, they could behave differently in the body than they do in the lab. Animal studies can be helpful, but might not always apply to people. Dietary components probably influence different people in different ways, depending upon their genetics, as demonstrated in the fields of nutrigenomics and nutrigenetics.

To further complicate research on nutrition and cancer, the influence of a given factor upon cancer risk depends upon dose of the nutrient or other phytochemical. Many compounds are ineffective at low doses, helpful at moderate doses, and harmful at high doses. Timing in the life cycle also can shape the influence of particular dietary factors on cancer risk. For example, as compared to adequately fed females, women who experience famine before the age of 10 have a reduced risk of precancerous breast tissue later in life, and women who experience famine after the age of 18 have greater risk (WCRF/AICR, 2007).

The World Cancer Research Fund and the American Institute for Cancer Research administer ongoing reviews of cancer-related research (WCRF/AICR, 2014). In addition to periodic reports, the agencies also strive to keep their database of research current through the Continuous Update Project (WCRF/AICR, 2014). Expert panels release dietary guidelines that reflect their analysis of the research conducted to date. Their recommendations include the following.

- Be as lean as possible within the normal range of body weight. The panel advises that people should avoid excess weight gain at all ages, and especially avoid becoming overweight or obese. Evidence linking cancer risk, including cancer mortality, to excess body fat has grown significantly in recent years. Extra body fat increases level of inflammation throughout the body, and promotes the growth of many types of cancer.

- Be physically active as part of everyday life. Physical activity levels should be appropriate for the individual's health and fitness. Research suggests that public health guidelines for physical activity are a good start, but that more is generally better in terms of reducing cancer risk. Physical activity reduces inflammation and contributes to healthful body fat levels.
- Limit consumption of energy-dense foods and sugary drinks that promote weight gain. To reduce cancer risk, the panel advises replacing foods with little nutrition value with healthful foods, especially vegetables.
- Eat mostly plant foods. Consume at least five servings of non-starchy vegetables and fruits each day. Consuming additional servings—especially of vegetables— is even more beneficial. Relatively unprocessed grains and legumes are preferred over refined products, as consumption of refined starchy foods should be limited. A diet based mostly on plant foods has high levels of many nutrients, phytochemicals, and dietary fiber, which all are linked with reduced cancer risk. Plant-based diets also tend to be low in red and processed meat, and foods made with refined grains and added sugars.
- Limit intake of red meat and avoid processed meat. Red meat refers to beef, pork, lamb, and goat. Processed meats include meats that are salted, smoked, cured, or have preservatives added, and include hot dogs, sausages, salami, pepperoni, ham, and many deli meats. These meats have been linked with increased cancer risk, partly due to the dietary patterns in which they are found, but also because of the cancer-causing chemicals such as nitrosamines that form from red meat components such as carnitine. Polycyclic aromatic hydrocarbons, which are produced in meats cooked at high temperatures, have been shown in human epidemiological studies to increase the risk of cancer. According to a report from the National Cancer Institute (2010) researchers found that "high consumption of well-done, fried, or barbecued meats was associated with increased risks of colorectal, pancreatic, and prostate cancer."
- Avoid or limit alcohol. Alcoholic drinks all increase cancer risk in a dose-related fashion, with no health benefits associated with light or moderate drinking (unlike the relationship between alcohol intake and cardiovascular disease). Even consuming just 1 or 2 drinks per week increases risk of breast cancer, for example. Scientists do not understand exactly how alcohol increases risk, although they know that one of the products of alcohol metabolism—acetaldehyde—is a carcinogen. Alcohol also might increase cancer risk because it can increase a woman's blood estrogen level.
- Avoid salted-preserved, salted, and salty foods. These have been associated with an increased risk of stomach cancers.
- Limit exposure to aflatoxins by avoiding moldy grains and legumes. Aflatoxins are carcinogenic compounds produced by certain species of mold, most common in corn and peanuts.
- Aim to meet nutritional needs through diet alone. Research on dietary supplements is not very supportive using supplements to prevent cancer. Although

evidence for some supplements occasionally suggests beneficial effects, there usually is equal evidence for a given supplement as showing no effect and, in a few cases, as causing harm. The WCRF/ACRI experts acknowledge that dietary supplements can be helpful for some people in certain situations, such as vitamin B12 for vegans. Dietary supplements even might be advised for the prevention of a few cancers. The panel recommends that a person meet with a qualified nutrition expert to determine which supplements might be individually recommended. The panel, however, discourages supplement use on a general basis. Even though supplements might provide a few dietary components, they do not provide the thousands of components that occur naturally in a plant-based whole-foods diet.

Barbara A. Brehm

Research Issues

Why does obesity increase cancer risk? Obesity might contribute to cancer risk in several ways. Scientists are examining certain biochemical pathways that could help to explain this risk. Obesity is associated with insulin and leptin resistance, for example. Chronically elevated blood insulin and leptin levels increase the production of certain growth factors that stimulate cell proliferation, potentially increasing the growth and reproduction of potentially cancerous cells. Enzymes in adipose tissue convert sex hormone precursors to active hormones—including estrogens—in women. Increased estrogen levels are associated with cancers of the breast and uterus. The World Cancer Research Fund/American Institute for Cancer Research report in the Further Reading section provides more information on the biochemical mechanisms associated with a variety of cancer risk factors, including obesity.

See Also: Alcohol; Antioxidants; Beta-carotene; Carnitine; Dietary supplements; Fiber; Food additives; Heterocyclic amines and polycyclic aromatic hydrocarbons; Inflammation; Nutritional genomics; Obesity, definition and health effects; Phytochemicals; Phytoestrogens; Sodium and salt; Vegetarian and vegan diets; Vitamin E.

Further Reading

American Cancer Society (ACS). (2014). *Early history of cancer*. Atlanta: American Cancer Society. Retrieved from http://www.cancer.org/cancer/cancerbasics /thehistoryofcancer/the-history-of-cancer-what-is-cancer

American Cancer Society (ACS). (2012a, January 11). *ACS guidelines for nutrition and physical activity for cancer prevention*. Atlanta: American Cancer Society. Retrieved from http://www.cancer.org/healthy/eathealthygetactive/acsguidelinesonnutritionphysi-calactivityforcancerprevention/acs-guidelines-on-nutrition-and-physical-activity -for-cancer-prevention-guidelines

American Cancer Society (ACS). (2012b). *Cancer facts and figures 2012*. Atlanta: American Cancer Society. Retrieved from http://www.cancer.org/acs/groups/content/ @ epidemiologysurveilance/documents/document/acspc-031941.pdf

American Cancer Society. (2012c, March 21). *What is cancer?* Atlanta: American Cancer Society. Retrieved from: http://www.cancer.org/cancer/cancerbasics/what-is-cancer

Crosta, P., (2013, July 19). What is cancer? *Medical News Today*. Retrieved from: http://www.medicalnewstoday.com/info/cancer-oncology/

Kushi, L. H., Doyle, C., McCullough, M., et al. (2012). American Cancer Society guidelines on nutrition and physical activity for cancer prevention: Reducing the risk of cancer with healthy food choices and physical activity. *CA: A Cancer Journal for Clinicians, 62* (1), 30–67. doi: 10.3322/caac.20140

National Cancer Institute. (2010, October 15). *Chemicals in meat cooked at high temperatures and cancer risk*. Retrieved from http://www.cancer.gov/cancertopics/factsheet /Risk/cooked-meats#r1

World Cancer Research Fund/American Institute for Cancer Research (WCRF/AICR). (2007). *Food, nutrition, physical activity, and the prevention of cancer: A global perspective*. Washington DC: AICR. Retrieved from http://www.dietandcancerreport .org/cancer_resource_center/downloads/Second_Expert_Report_full.pdf

World Cancer Research Fund/American Institute for Cancer Research (WCRF/AICR). (2014, July). Second expert report: Overview. Retrieved from http://www.dietandcancer report.org/expert_report/report_overview.php

World Health Organization (WHO). (2014, February). *Cancer: Fact sheet*. Retrieved from http://www.who.int/mediacentre/factsheets/fs297/en/

Capsaicin

Capsaicin is a chemical compound found in many types of hot peppers and often is isolated for medicinal purposes. Jalapeno, habanero, chili, and cayenne peppers all owe their spicy flavor to the capsaicin found in the placenta tissue surrounding their seeds. According to the Scoville Heat Index, a measure of capsaicin content, habaneros contain the highest concentration of capsaicin, with a variety in the Yucatan containing more than 300,000 Scoville units. Pure capsaicin reaches up to 16,000,000 Scoville units. The compound is an irritant to mucous membranes, and produces a painful burning sensation by binding to receptors in the cell membrane of sensory receptors. This action releases a chemical called "substance P," which sends the brain the same pain signal as an abrasion or burn might.

Despite its ability to invoke the sensation of pain, capsaicin is the critical ingredient in topical analgesics for chronic pain relief, used often for arthritis, peripheral neuropathy, fibromyalgia, and back pain. It causes an initial spike in the release of substance P which results in a brief burning sensation, but which also depletes neurons of this pain-signaling chemical so that the brain can no longer perceive messages of pain from affected neurons (De Silva., El-Metwally, Ernst, Lewith, & Macfarlane, 2011). Capsaicin creams also are recommended for some skin conditions that are accompanied by itchiness, such as psoriasis. Although these creams offer temporary relief from pain or itchiness, their effects are fairly mild and are not long lasting.

Research in laboratory animals suggests that capsaicin might contribute to heart health in several ways (American Chemical Society, 2012). It appears to help lower serum levels of LDL cholesterol, and even contribute to the regression of atherosclerotic plaques. Capsaicin also seems to block the activity of a gene that causes the small muscles around arteries to contract, which increases blood pressure because of increased resistance to blood flow. By blocking this action, capsaicin allows blood vessels to open and accommodate more blood flow at a lower pressure, thus lowering arterial blood pressure. Capsaicin also shows antioxidant activity.

Interesting research on capsaicin and cancer suggests that pure capsaicin inhibits activation of carcinogens and induces cancer cell apoptosis (cell death) in human cancers in vitro and in human cancers transplanted onto laboratory rodents (Bley, Boorman, Mohammad, McKenzie, & Babbar, 2012). These results counter epidemiological research that had suggested that capsaicin actually might act as a carcinogen in humans. The carcinogenic culprits appear not to be capsaicin per se, but rather the pesticides, insecticides, herbicides, fertilizers, molds, and other contaminants that can enter the body with hot peppers. In one analysis, 55% of hot peppers in the United States was found to be contaminated with a variety of 51 different pesticides (Environmental Working Group, 2010). In any case, research on capsaicin and cancer is too preliminary to recommend specific cancer prevention intakes of either capsaicin or hot peppers. Indeed, the U.S. FDA issued a warning against this action to a dietary supplement manufacturer in 2011 (US FDA, 2011). Consumers who enjoy spicy foods should use organic sources of hot peppers.

Capsaicin is available as a supplement that sometimes is referred to as cayenne pepper in its over-the-counter form. It stimulates digestion by increasing the production of gastric juices. Although evidence is not conclusive, capsaicin also might help increase the body's metabolic rate and therefore contribute to weight-loss efforts.

Patricia M. Cipicchio and Barbara A. Brehm

See Also: Cancer and nutrition; Dietary supplements.

Further Reading

American Chemical Society (2012). Hot pepper compound could help hearts. *ScienceDaily*. Retrieved from http://www.sciencedaily.com/releases/2012/03/120327215605.htm

Bley, K., Boorman, G., Mohammad, B., McKenzie, D., & Babbar, S. (2012). A comprehensive review of the carcinogenic and anticarcinogenic potential of capsaicin. *Toxicologic Pathology, 40* (6), 847–873. doi: 10.1177/0192623312444471

De Silva, V., El Metwally, A., Ernst, E., Lewith, G., & Macfarlane, G. J. (2011). Evidence for the efficacy of complementary and alternative medicines in the management of osteoarthritis: A systematic review. *Rheumatology, 50* (5), 911–920. doi: 10.1093/rheumatology/keq379

Environmental Working Group. (2010). *EWG's shopper's guide to pesticides compiled from USDA (Pesticide Data Program) and FDA (Pesticide Monitoring Database)*

data from 2000–2008. Retrieved from http://static.foodnews.org/pdf/2010-foodnews-data.pdf

U.S. Food and Drug Administration (US FDA). (2011). Inspections, compliance, enforcement, and criminal investigations: Millennium bioceutics 2/17/11. Retrieved from http://www.fda.gov/ICECI/EnforcementActions/WarningLetters/ucm244906.htm

Carbohydrate Loading

Carbohydrate loading refers to the practice of manipulating diet and physical activity to maximize the storage of glycogen in the liver and skeletal muscles. Glycogen is a type of starch consisting of many glucose units, and is the body's primary form of carbohydrate storage. The body manufactures glycogen from dietary carbohydrates. Carbohydrate loading is practiced primarily by endurance athletes before important contests, with the goal of beginning the contest with optimal glycogen stores. Carbohydrate loading sometimes is recommended to patients prior to surgery, so that they begin the recovery period with a good energy supply. Carbohydrate-loading practices can stimulate muscle and the liver to store greater than normal amounts of

Maintaining Optimal Energy Stores

Athletes vary in their response to carbohydrate-loading protocols. Many athletes are disappointed with carbohydrate-loading results, or think that the minimal results are not worth the time and effort required by the protocols. Success in endurance athletic events is more related to months of well-planned training and nutrition support rather than carbohydrate loading for a short period before a contest.

Suggestions for maintaining optimal glycogen stores throughout the training process include the following (ADA, 2009).

- Train regularly for the sport. Training increases the ability of muscles to store and use glycogen, thus the muscles required for the sport become very good at storing and using energy. Muscles also get better at using fat for energy, which results in a "glycogen-sparing" effect; the glycogen stores last longer.
- Consume food or drink with plenty of carbohydrate and some protein within an hour following each practice or competition. The muscles' glycogen storage chemistry is in high gear following exercise, so give them the carbohydrate they need to pack in energy for the next workout or competition. It can take 24 to 48 hours to replenish glycogen stores, so start right away.
- Be sure to include carbohydrate foods in meals or snacks that follow vigorous exercise. Include carbohydrate foods in other meals as well.
- Alternate difficult and easy training days, and give the body at least one day of rest each week. Taper off before important contests. Rest allows glycogen stores to build to optimal levels, in addition to allowing the body adequate time for recovery.

glycogen. People vary in their responses to carbohydrate-loading regimens, but the bulk of the evidence suggests that the practice generally improves both glycogen stores and athletic performance (ADA, 2009).

Importance of Glycogen for Endurance Activity

The body's primary sources of energy for physical activity are glycogen and fat. Muscle glycogen provides fuel for muscle contraction, and liver glycogen provides a steady supply of glucose to maintain optimal blood glucose (blood sugar) levels. The brain relies primarily on glucose delivered by the blood for fuel, therefore when blood glucose levels fall hypoglycemia results, presenting symptoms such as nausea, disorientation, fatigue, and confusion. These symptoms interfere with performance.

The body relies heavily on glycogen for moderate- to high-intensity exercise. Low-intensity activities such as walking primarily rely on stored fat for energy, and low to moderately intense activities such as jogging use both fat and glycogen for fuel. About 50% to 60% of energy used during one to four hours of continuous, moderately vigorous activity comes from carbohydrates (ADA, 2009). The rest is supplied by fat and some protein.

On average, people can store roughly 2,000 kilocalories of energy as glycogen, although this varies considerably with a person's size, training status, and diet. Liver and muscle glycogen stores can run low after about 90 minutes of endurance activity. It is important to note that glycogen stored in non-exercising muscles is not readily available to the exercising muscles. This means that the body can't really access all of the stored muscle glycogen.

Endurance athletes are particularly concerned about maximizing glycogen stores for training and performance. Optimal glycogen stores depend on an adequate intake of dietary carbohydrates. Research suggests that many athletes could improve their performance by consuming greater amounts of carbohydrate (ADA, 2009). Glycogen stores need not be depleted to be suboptimal. Some athletes consistently might consume somewhat less than optimal carbohydrate intakes for the energy demands of their sport.

Carbohydrate Loading and Pre-Surgery Nutrition

For surgical patients, glycogen loading appears to reduce risk of surgical complications, speed recovery, and reduce the length of a hospital stay. Carbohydrate loading usually is employed as a component of optimal preoperative nutrition that also includes immune-enhancing foods and supplements. Researchers have found that entering surgery in a fed rather than a fasted state (patients usually are told to fast at least eight hours prior to surgery), by using special carbohydrate drinks, does not interfere with anesthesia procedures. It also helps keep the body in an anabolic state (building tissue up rather than breaking it down), which enhances healing and reduces the lean body mass loss associated with bed rest (Kratzing, 2011).

Carbohydrate Loading and Athletic Performance

Many endurance and ultra-endurance athletes engage in carbohydrate loading in hopes of boosting their glycogen stores to even greater levels than normal. Another word for carbohydrate loading is "glycogen supercompensation." The idea is to stimulate production of the enzymes responsible for storing glycogen by sending the message that energy demands are high and that current glycogen stores are inadequate. Early experiments in glycogen loading had athletes "strip" glycogen supplies by exercising to exhaustion a week before a major competition, and then follow with three days of a low-carbohydrate diet with moderate training, leaving the muscles and liver glycogen depleted. Three days of high-carbohydrate intake followed, with little exercise performed. This resulted in increased glycogen stores (Ahlborg, Bergström, Ekelund, et al., 1967).

Most people find this procedure difficult and fatiguing. Many athletes report feeling lethargic and depressed if they train when carbohydrate intake is low. Researchers also have expressed concern that such extreme dietary manipulation could lead to the loss of muscle tissue and to other negative health effects, including increased risk for upper-respiratory infections because of immune-system suppression.

Fortunately, the low-carbohydrate diet phase does not appear to be essential for stimulating extra glycogen storage. A gradual combination of tapering exercise volume and increasing carbohydrate intake seems to be just as effective for improving athletic performance. Most endurance athletes who use carbohydrate loading simply incrementally reduce exercise, and maintain a high intake of carbohydrates (approximately 10 g/kg body weight/day) for three or four days before competition.

Some researchers have experimented with other loading methods. One interesting study had seven male cyclists perform three minutes of very hard cycling, and then consume a very high carbohydrate diet (about 10 g carbohydrate per kg body weight) during the following 24 hours (Fairchild et al., 2002). The researchers found that glycogen stores doubled from the previous day's pre-exercise levels.

Individual responses to carbohydrate loading and, indeed, to any type of dietary manipulation vary tremendously. Several studies have questioned whether any kind of carbohydrate loading—aside from providing adequate carbohydrate in the diet—improves performance. Results regarding the effectiveness of carbohydrate loading for female athletes have been somewhat mixed, but experts suggest that women generally do improve performance when extra calories along with extra carbohydrates are added to the diet for several days before competition (ADA, 2009).

Carbohydrate loading can have several potentially negative effects. Athletes must practice any type of dietary change during training, not during competition. Athletes who add new foods or change the volume or timing of food intake can experience abdominal cramps or diarrhea. Successful carbohydrate loading adds two to four pounds (one to two kg) of body weight. This is mostly water weight, because each gram of carbohydrate is stored with three grams of water, but the extra weight bothers some athletes.

Barbara A. Brehm

Research Issues

Most carbohydrate-loading studies have used male subjects, partly because female subjects can vary somewhat in their glycogen-storing capacities depending upon the phase of their menstrual cycle, and researchers don't want this variable to interfere with the results (ADA, 2009). Data on female subjects also have been more variable, as some study subjects restrict calorie intake and thus could fail to achieve adequate carbohydrate intake.

See Also: Blood sugar regulation; Carbohydrates; Glycemic index and glycemic load; Hypoglycemia; Sports nutrition.

Further Reading

Ahlborg, B., Bergström, J., Ekelund, L. G., Hultman, E., & Maschio, G. (1967). Human muscle glycogen content and capacity for prolonged exercise after different diets. *Forvarsmedicin, 3,* 85–99

American Dietetic Association, Dietitians of Canada, and American College of Sports Medicine (ADA). (2009). Position stand: Nutrition and athletic performance. *Medicine & Science in Sports & Exercise, 41* (3), 709–731. Retrieved from http://journals .lww.com/acsm-msse/Fulltext/2009/03000/ Nutrition_and_Athletic_Performance.27. aspx#P149

Burke, L. M., Hawley, J. A., Wong, S. H. S., & Jeukendrup, A. E. (2011). Carbohydrates for training and competition. *Journal of Sports Sciences, 29* (Suppl. 1), S17–S27. doi: 10.1080/02640414.2011.585473

Colombani, P. C., Mannhart, C., & Mettler, S. (2013). Carbohydrates and exercise performance in non-fasted athletes: A systematic review of studies mimicking real-life. *Nutrition Journal, 12,* (16). doi:10.1186/1475-2891-12-16

Fairchild, T. J., Fletcher, S., Steele, P., Goodman, C., Dawson, B., & Fournier, P. A. (2002). Rapid carbohydrate loading after a short bout of near maximal-intensity exercise. *Medicine & Science in Sports & Exercise, 34* (6), 980–986.

Kratzing, C. (2011). Pre-operative nutrition and carbohydrate loading. *Proceedings of the Nutrition Society, 70* (3), 311–315. http://dx.doi.org/10.1017/S0029665111000450

Carbohydrates

Carbohydrates are a large group of organic molecules that include sugars, starches, and some types of dietary fiber. The word "carbohydrate" comes from the raw materials from which carbohydrates are made. Plants make carbohydrates from carbon dioxide (source of the term "carbo") and water (hydrate), using energy from the sun. All carbohydrates contain only carbon, hydrogen, and oxygen.

The simplest carbohydrate structures are called "monosaccharides." Monosaccharides provide the basic units for other carbohydrate molecules. Monosaccharides also serve as components in genetic material and important compounds, such as adenosine triphosphate (ATP) involved in the metabolic pathways responsible for the production of energy in animals. Typical dietary sugars are composed of two monosaccharides, and are called "disaccharides." Larger structures composed of many monosaccharide units are called "oligosaccharides" (3 to 10 units) and "polysaccharides" (more than 10 units). Plant carbohydrates provide energy and dietary fiber to the animals that eat them. Animals also produce carbohydrates from the food they eat, primarily for the purpose of storing energy. Informally, the term "carbohydrate" (or "carbs") is used to refer to foods that contain relatively high concentrations of carbohydrate molecules. Most cultures of the world rely on carbohydrate foods for a majority of daily calories.

Simple Carbohydrates

Sugars, also known as "simple carbohydrates," are relatively small molecules of carbohydrate found naturally in fruits and vegetables, as well as milk. They are especially concentrated in sweeteners such as table sugar (usually made from sugar beets or sugar cane), honey, molasses, and maple syrup. Corn syrup is a sweetener made from the sugar in corn. Many food products contain added sweeteners.

The term sugars refer to monosaccharides and disaccharides. Monosaccharides are the simplest carbohydrate structures, containing three to seven carbon atoms. Monosaccharides generally contain carbon, hydrogen, and oxygen in a ratio of two hydrogen atoms and one oxygen atom to each carbon atom, for a molecular formula of $C_nH_{2n}O_n$. The most common monosaccharides in the human diet contain six carbons, and include glucose, fructose, and galactose.

Glucose is the most common monosaccharide found in nature. Glucose provides the types of chemical bonds from which people can capture energy. Glucose is carried in the bloodstream to all cells of the body to be used as an energy-production substrate. The term "blood sugar" refers to blood glucose level. Glucose rarely is found as a single unit in foods, but instead forms part of disaccharide structures. Fructose is the sweetest of the monosaccharides, and binds with glucose to form the disaccharide sucrose, found in many sweet foods. Galactose is the monosaccharide that is bound to glucose to form lactose, the disaccharide known as milk sugar.

The "pentoses" are five-carbon monosaccharide molecules. Best known of the pentoses are "ribose," a component of ribonucleic acid (RNA) and "deoxyribose," a component of deoxyribonucleic acid (DNA). The body synthesizes pentoses, therefore these monosaccharides need not be included in the diet.

The three most common disaccharides in the human diet are sucrose (composed of glucose plus fructose), galactose (glucose plus lactose), and maltose (two glucose units). Maltose is found in germinating grains and is a product of the breakdown of starch.

During digestion, simple sugars are broken down into monosaccharides that are transported into the bloodstream. The liver converts fructose and other monosaccharides into glucose or other molecules, including large chains of glucose called glycogen. Monosaccharides can also be converted into fats.

Complex Carbohydrates

Complex carbohydrates are larger molecules of carbohydrate and include starches and some types of dietary fibers. Oligosaccharides consist of 3 to 10 glucose units, and are found in a variety of foods. Common oligosaccharides include "raffinose" (3 glucose units) and "stachyose" (4 glucose units), found in legumes. Human digestive enzymes are unable to break the molecular bonds that hold the glucose units together, but intestinal bacteria can break these bonds, producing intestinal gas in the process. Human milk contains more than 100 different oligosaccharides that help babies in a number of ways, including binding with pathogens, serving as food sources for helpful bacteria, and promoting normal infant brain development. Oligosaccharides can serve as starches or dietary fibers, depending upon whether they can be broken down in the digestive tract.

Polysaccharides contain more than 10 glucose units and often are composed of hundreds of glucose units strung together in various formations. These formations determine the properties of the starch, including the speed at which it is digested and absorbed (a quality known as "glycemic index") and its behavior in recipes. The two primary starch formations in plants are "amylose" and "amylopectin." Amylose is composed of long straight chains of glucose units. Amylopectin contains long branching chains of glucose units. Starch polysaccharides are found in plant foods and products made from plants. Grains and grain products; root vegetables, such as potatoes, carrots, beets, and cassava; and vegetables that are the seeds of plants, such as corn, peas, and beans are high in starch. During digestion, starches are broken down into glucose units.

Glycogen is a form of starch manufactured by animals. Humans manufacture and store glycogen primarily in the liver and in skeletal muscles. Glycogen serves as a source of glucose when the body needs fuel. Liver glycogen is converted to glucose and released into the bloodstream when blood glucose levels fall too low. Skeletal muscles use glucose liberated from glycogen to fuel muscle contraction. Many athletes are careful to consume adequate amounts of carbohydrate to maximize glycogen stores so that they have adequate energy for training and performance. Athletes preparing for important endurance events even might consume significant amounts of carbohydrate for a few days prior to an event to maximize their glycogen stores.

Dietary fiber refers to structures that are not broken down by the digestive system. Dietary fiber comes primarily from plants. Some types of dietary fiber—such as cellulose—are composed of carbohydrates. Humans lack the necessary digestive enzymes to break down these structures, and fiber instead passes through the digestive system, adding bulk to the stools. Adequate intake of dietary fiber contributes to good health. Most dietary guidelines encourage people to consume adequate amounts of vegetables, fruits, legumes, and whole grains to promote a healthy intake of dietary fiber.

All types of fiber increase food volume without adding a significant number of calories. High-fiber meals generally provide feelings of satiety with fewer calories than low-fiber meals. A high-fiber diet could promote colon health by providing an environment inside the GI tract that favors the growth of beneficial bacteria—the probiotics.

Barbara A. Brehm

Research Issues

Many people regard carbohydrate foods as "bad." Yet carbohydrates are contained within a wide range of foods. Some of these foods, such as most vegetables, generally are regarded as very nutritious. Other foods high in carbohydrates, such as cakes, cookies, and soft drinks, obtain a majority of their calories from processed grains and sugars, and typically are higher in empty calories (calories that deliver little nutritive value). The dietary reference intake for carbohydrates is at least 130 g per day for children and adults. Most North Americans consume at least 50% of their calories as carbohydrates, which amounts to more than 250 g per day. What do public health experts say about making good choices for foods that provide carbohydrates? What are the characteristics of "good carbs"? What are the characteristics of "bad carbs"?

See Also: Blood sugar regulation; Fiber; Fructose; Glucose; Glycemic index and glycemic load; High-fructose corn syrup.

Further Reading

Centers for Disease Control and Prevention. (2012). *Carbohydrates*. Retrieved from http://www.cdc.gov/nutrition/everyone/basics/carbs.html

Harvard School of Public Health. (2013). *Carbohydrates: Good carbs guide the way*. Retrieved from http://www.hsph.harvard.edu/nutritionsource/carbohydrates-full-story/

Mayo Clinic Staff. (2011). *Carbohydrates: How carbs fit into a healthy diet*. Mayoclinic.com. Retrieved from http://www.mayoclinic.com/health/carbohydrates/MY01458/METHOD=print

Cardiometabolic Syndrome

Cardiometabolic syndrome (CMS) is an umbrella term for a combination of medical disorders. In the United States, it affects approximately 25% of adults age 20 and older, and up to 45% of adults age 50 and older (Kumar, Vishal, & Nema, 2013). Cardiometabolic syndrome is widely referred to as "metabolic syndrome X," "syndrome X," "metabolic syndrome," and "Reaven's syndrome." According to the scientific statement of the American Heart Association and the National Heart, Lung, and Blood Institute, CMS is diagnosed in men and women who possess three or more of the following risk factors: central adiposity, elevated fasting glucose levels, elevated resting blood pressure, high triglyceride levels, and low HDL cholesterol levels. The more risk factors individuals possess, the greater their risk for the development of serious medical conditions such as Type 2 diabetes, heart disease, and stroke.

History

Although cardiometabolic syndrome is a relatively new concept, researchers have noted the clustering of cardiovascular risk factors associated with the syndrome since the 1920s. In 1988, Dr. Gerald Reaven noted several risk factors that commonly cluster together and increase the risk for cardiovascular disease, which he called "syndrome X" (Grundy et al., 2005). Reaven noted that insulin resistance is the underlying factor of CMS.

Central Adiposity

Central adiposity, or central obesity, is the accumulation of excess body fat in the torso, especially around the internal organs. This is identified as having an "apple" shape. Central adiposity is a key causal factor in the development of insulin resistance, the main feature in the development of cardiometabolic syndrome. For diagnostic purposes, waist circumferences of 40 inches (102 cm) or more in men, and of 35 inches (89 cm) or more for a woman are considered risky. The body mass index (BMI) system of measurement, which uses weight and height, is the typical diagnostic tool for obesity. Although the presence of central adiposity is more highly correlated with cardiometabolic risk factors than with elevated BMI numbers, the prevalence of CMS has been shown to increase across BMI categories with approximately a much higher prevalence for severe obesity compared with non-obese.

Blood Sugar Levels

High blood sugar levels are a major component of cardiometabolic syndrome. Fasting blood glucose tests measure the blood glucose level after eight hours of fasting. High blood sugar levels are defined by a fasting blood glucose test result of greater than or equal to 100 milligrams per deciliter (mg/dL). Fasting blood glucose levels of 100 to 125 mg/dL are considered "prediabetes," or a condition likely to lead to type 2 diabetes. A fasting glucose of 126 mg/dL or greater suggests the person has diabetes mellitus.

Glucose is the energy source for cells. It is derived from food broken down during digestion. Blood glucose levels increase when the digestive system absorbs glucose, activating the hormone insulin to help control blood glucose levels. Impaired fasting glucose levels indicate that the cells are responding to insulin inadequately, a condition known as insulin resistance. This condition often develops into type 2 diabetes, which is the most common form of diabetes. In later stages of type 2 diabetes, insulin resistance is coupled with inadequate insulin production by the pancreas.

High blood glucose levels can contribute to the formation of atherosclerotic plaques, the hallmark of artery disease. Atherosclerotic plaques build up in the arteries, restricting oxygenated blood flow to major organs. Obesity and high blood sugar levels are associated with inflammation in the arteries. Inflammation can cause plaques to rupture, and plaque material to break off and interrupt blood flow. Artery disease is the leading cause of heart attack and stroke.

Hypertension

Hypertension, commonly referred to as "high blood pressure," affects approximately one-third of the total U.S. population (AHA, 2013). High blood pressure is strongly associated with obesity and commonly occurs in insulin-resistant persons, linking it to CMS. It contributes significantly to cardiovascular disease and is the leading global risk factor for premature mortality. Hypertension is diagnosed when resting blood pressure is ≥130/85 mmHg. (One or both of these numbers can be high for a diagnosis of hypertension.)

Atherogenic Dyslipidemia

Atherogenic dyslipidemia refers to blood lipid levels that are associated with an increased risk of artery disease. Atherogenic dyslipidemia frequently is characterized by the combination of three lipid abnormalities: elevated triglycerides, low levels of high-density lipoprotein (HDL) cholesterol, and high levels of low-density lipoprotein (LDL) cholesterol.

Triglycerides are the most common form of fat found in the diet and in the blood. The body manufactures triglycerides from excess calories, and stores the excess triglycerides to be used for energy. A serum triglyceride level of 150 mg/dL or greater contributes to a diagnosis of CMS. High-density lipoprotein cholesterol is inversely related to artery disease risk; that is, higher levels of HDL cholesterol are associated with lower risk. Low levels of HDL cholesterol contribute to a diagnosis of CMS—less than 40 mg/dL for men and less than 50 mg/dL for women. Although not a component of a CMS diagnosis, higher LDL levels put an individual at risk for CMS. Low-density lipoprotein is the major cholesterol carrier in human blood. High LDL cholesterol in the blood is a strong CVD risk factor because oxidized LDL compounds can enter the arterial wall and contribute to the formation of atherosclerotic plaque. LDL cholesterol levels of 130 to 159 mg/dL are considered borderline high, and levels of more than 160 mg/dL are considered high by the National Cholesterol Education Program (DHHS, 2005).

Causes and Risk Factors

Experts are unsure exactly why cardiometabolic syndrome develops. It is understood, however, that various risk factors contribute to the different causes. CMS is closely linked to the body's metabolism and insulin resistance. Insulin resistance is present in the majority of people diagnosed with cardiometabolic syndrome, and believed by researchers to be the underlying cause. Insulin resistance generally increases with the severity of obesity, although this resistance can exist at any given level of body fat. Given that obesity commonly is associated with insulin resistance, the two risk factors both influence the development of other cardiometabolic risk factors.

Additional factors contribute to the development of CMS, such as advancing age. Advancing age commonly affects all levels of pathogenesis, thus increasing the likelihood for the development of CMS as a person ages and among an older cohort. A pro-inflammatory state, reflected in an elevation of C-reactive protein, also is associated with insulin resistance and atherogenesis. Excess adipose tissue releases inflammatory cytokines that increase one's pro-inflammatory state. Sedentary lifestyle and family history—especially having a sibling or parent with diabetes—increase risk of CMS. A personal history of diabetes, including gestational diabetes, also increases risk.

Polycystic ovarian syndrome (PCOS) is an endocrine disorder characterized by hormone imbalance and affecting a woman's fertility. A woman is diagnosed with PCOS if she reports at least two of the following symptoms: an excess of androgen production, menstrual abnormalities, and polycystic ovaries. Obesity is associated with an increase in hyperandrogenism and menstrual irregularity in women, both of which are symptoms of PCOS. ("Hyperandrogenism" refers to greater than normal levels of male sex hormones, often accompanied by symptoms such as acne and excess facial hair). There is a discrepancy between whether PCOS or obesity comes first, but women with either risk factor are more likely to develop cardiometabolic syndrome. A study on cardiometabolic risk confirmed that the prevalence of CMS is approximately four times higher in women with PCOS compared to the general population (Cussons, 2008).

Women of African-American and Mexican-American ethnicity are more likely to develop CMS than are men from those groups. This could be because women generally have a greater number of risk factors, including central adiposity, PCOS, and obesity, and thus are more susceptible to the development of cardiometabolic syndrome. In combination with genetic and behavioral factors, hormonal changes at menopause contribute to the prevalence of CMS in women (Yu et al., 2013).

Treatment

There is no single treatment to cure cardiometabolic syndrome, however risk factors can be reduced though pharmacological therapies and therapeutic lifestyle changes. To best treat the totality of CMS, it is important to focus on the suggested treatments for each risk factor. The primary treatment of CMS is lifestyle therapy, including increased physical activity and an anti-atherogenic diet. Lifestyle intervention can reduce the risk of heart disease, diabetes, and stroke (Kumar, Vishal, & Nema, 2013). Pharmacological therapies frequently are used to improve lipid profile, blood pressure, and blood glucose regulation. Gastrointestinal surgeries for weight loss also are recommended in some cases.

Diet

Obesity is a central feature of the syndrome that is linked to the majority of risk factors attributing to CMS, therefore weight loss can greatly assist in the management of the syndrome. Diet intervention can drastically alter one's fasting glucose levels and, in turn, can decrease a person's risk for or severity of type 2 diabetes. When combined, diet and exercise are among the most effective treatments for obesity.

The Mediterranean Diet, based on the typical diet of Mediterranean cultures, is rich in omega-3 fatty acids, vegetables, whole grains, and nuts. Research suggests that the antioxidant rich and highly anti-inflammatory diet provides specific benefit for individuals affected by cardiometabolic syndrome (Blaha & Tota-Maharaj, 2012).

The "DASH-style" diet plan, or "Dietary Approaches to Stop Hypertension," was developed to reduce blood pressure without medication for patients with hypertension (Salehi-Abargouei et al., 2013). The diet is rich in fruits, vegetables, and low-fat dairy. It includes grains, especially whole grains; lean meats, fish, and poultry; nuts and beans. It is high fiber and low to moderate in fat. The DASH diet lowers blood pressure through a rich source of nutrients associated with reduced blood pressure levels, such as potassium, calcium, and magnesium (Salehi-Abargouei et al., 2013).

Allison M. Felix

Research Issues

As obesity rates in childhood and adolescence increase worldwide, so does the prevalence of cardiometabolic syndrome (CMS). How should CMS be diagnosed and treated in children and adolescents? The International Diabetes Federation has good information on this emerging topic.

International Diabetes Federation. (2014). *IDF definition of metabolic syndrome in children and adolescents.* Retrieved from http://www.idf.org/metabolic-syndrome/children

Zimmet, P., Alberti, G., Kaufman, et al. (2007). The metabolic syndrome in children and adolescents. *Lancet, 369,* 2059–2061.

See Also: Bariatric surgery; Blood sugar regulation; Cardiovascular disease and nutrition; Cholesterol; Diabetes, type 2; Hypertension and nutrition; Inflammation; Insulin; Lipoproteins; Obesity, definition and health effects; Triglycerides.

Further Reading

American Heart Association (AHA). (2013). *High blood pressure.* Retrieved from http://www.heart.org/idc/groups/heart-public/@wcm/@sop/@smd/documents/downloadable/ucm_319587.pdf

Blaha, M. J., & Tota-Maharaj, R. (2012). *Metabolic syndrome: From risk factors to management.* Torino: SEEd.

Cussons, A. J., Watts, G. F., Burke, V., Shaw, J. E., Zimmet, P. Z., & Stuckey, B. G. (2008). Cardiometabolic risk in polycystic ovary syndrome: A comparison of different approaches to defining the metabolic syndrome. *Human Reproduction, 23* (10), 2352–2358. doi: 10.1093/humrep/den263

Grundy, S., Cleeman, J. I., Daniels, S. R., et al. (2005). *Diagnosis and management of the metabolic syndrome.* An American Heart Association/National Heart, Lung, and Blood Institute Scientific Statement. Executive summary. *Cardiology in Review, 13* (6), 322–327.

Kumar, J., Vishal, B., & Nema, R. K. (2013). A review on metabolic syndrome: Plethora of disease. *Advances in Pharmacology & Toxicology, 14* (2), 29–42.

National Heart, Lung, and Blood Institute. (2011, November 3). *What is metabolic syndrome?* Retrieved from http://www.nhlbi.nih.gov/health/health-topics/topics/ms/

Salehi-Abargouei, A., Azadbakht, L., Shirani, F., & Maghsoudi, Z. (2013). Effects of Dietary Approaches to Stop Hypertension (DASH)-style diet on fatal or nonfatal cardiovascular diseases—Incidence: A systematic review and meta-analysis on observational prospective studies. *Nutrition, 29* (4), 611–618.

U.S. Department of Health and Human Services (DHHS). (2005). *High blood cholesterol: What you need to know.* Retrieved from http://www.nhlbi.nih.gov/health/public/heart/chol/wyntk.htm

Yu, R., Yau, F., Ho, S. C., & Woo, J. (2013). Associations of cardiorespiratory fitness, physical activity, and obesity with metabolic syndrome in Hong Kong Chinese midlife women. *BMC Public Health, 13* (1), 1–10. doi:10.1186/1471-2458-13-614

Cardiovascular Disease and Nutrition

Cardiovascular disease (CVD) refers to diseases of the heart and the blood vessels. It includes all types of heart disease, stroke, and artery disease. In the United States, cardiovascular disease is the leading cause of death among both women and men, causing one in three deaths per year (Go et al., 2013). The most common form of heart disease is coronary artery disease (CAD), also called "coronary heart disease," in which the arteries supplying the heart muscle with blood become thickened with plaque deposits. Coronary artery disease is the cause of death for about 380,000 people per year in the United States (CDC, 2014).

Another form of CVD is a stroke, which occurs when there is an interruption of blood flow to the brain, because of either a blockage or a break in an artery supplying the brain. In the United States, stroke causes about 1 in 19 deaths per year, with approximately 795,000 strokes occurring each year (Go et al., 2013). Artery disease is the most common cause of stroke. Of all types of cardiovascular disease, artery disease is most influenced by nutrition as well as by other lifestyle factors. People can slow and even reverse the progression of artery disease and reduce their risk of heart attack and stroke by consuming a healthful diet and making other lifestyle changes. A healthy diet also can help control several risk factors for CVD, including diabetes, hypertension, blood lipid profile, and obesity.

The Process of Atherosclerosis

Artery disease, or atherosclerosis, is a condition that develops when fatty deposits build up gradually within the inner walls of arteries. These fatty deposits are called plaques and are composed of cholesterol, cellular waste, calcium, immune cells, blood platelets, and other substances. Plaque buildup narrows the arteries, inhibiting blood flow; it also damages the arterial lining, so the arteries are unable to respond appropriately to signaling molecules that help to regulate blood flow and blood pressure. Over time plaques can become inflamed and unstable. If plaques rupture, then blood clots can form as the body attempts to repair artery damage. When blood clots block blood vessels they can cause a heart attack or stroke.

To understand the relationship between diet and artery disease, it is helpful to understand the process of atherosclerosis. Atherosclerosis begins with the oxidation of the compounds that carry fat and cholesterol in the blood stream, the lipoproteins. In particular, oxidation of low-density lipoproteins (LDLs) causes the LDLs to bind to the artery lining. The cells lining the arteries respond to this binding as an injury, signaling immune cells to come in and repair the damage. As immune cells called "macrophages" (a type of white blood cell) try to ingest the LDLs, the process of inflammation accelerates. The cells lining the artery proliferate in an attempt to heal the damaged area. Over a period of years, this process of plaque deposition leads to artery disease. The processes of oxidation and inflammation contribute to the development of atherosclerosis. Factors—including dietary nutrients and phytochemicals—that reduce LDL levels in the bloodstream, reduce the oxidation of LDLs, and limit the body's inflammatory response can help to slow the process of atherosclerosis.

Risk Factors

Artery disease does not appear to have one simple cause. Instead, the process is influenced by a number of variables, known as "risk factors." Dozens of risk factors have been identified. Some risk factors are outside of a person's control, including age (risk increases with age); genetics (having close relatives who experienced a heart attack before the age of 55 for males; 65 for females); and gender (women develop artery disease later in life than men).

Some risk factors are somewhat modifiable, including metabolic disorders that accelerate the progression of artery disease. Such disorders include diabetes (high blood sugar levels increase arterial inflammation and injure the artery lining); hypertension (high blood pressure injures the artery lining); and harmful blood lipid levels (higher levels of LDLs and lower levels of high-density lipoproteins [HDLs] are associated with artery disease). Obesity, especially excess fat in the abdominal region, increases risk of the cardiometabolic syndrome and the previously listed disorders. Obesity also is associated with increased levels of inflammation. These disorders are somewhat modifiable in the sense that they can be at least partially controlled by medications and lifestyle change, including dietary change.

Other modifiable risk factors include tobacco use (smoking increases oxidation of LDLs, increases blood pressure, and damages the artery lining); sedentary lifestyle (regular physical activity helps to normalize blood sugar regulation and blood pressure, raise HDL levels, and improve emotional health); chronic stress; and poor emotional health (chronic stress, anger, anxiety, and depression increase artery disease risk through a variety of mechanisms).

Diet and Cardiovascular Disease

Researchers have been interested in a possible relationship between lifestyle (including diet) and cardiovascular disease since the 1950s, when cardiovascular disease began to emerge as a leading cause of death in many countries. Early epidemiological studies suggested that countries with a Western diet suffered from higher rates of CVD than other countries. A Western diet is characterized by a higher intake of animal products and processed foods, with a lower intake of plant foods. This observation led to decades of research and speculation regarding which specific elements of the Western diet might be responsible for the development of artery disease. Researchers, the food industry, and consumers have hoped that by eliminating the causal elements from the Western diet, eating could go on with relatively minor changes in food choices. For example, in the 1980s, cholesterol and fat consumption were believed to be the primary drivers of the development of atherosclerosis, so people were urged to choose low-fat and low-cholesterol versions of familiar foods, for example, low-fat dairy rather than high-fat dairy products, low-fat meats, and even low-fat cookies. Ongoing epidemiological research using advanced statistical analyses revealed associations between trans fatty acids and glycemic load with increased risk of CVD (Jakobsen et al., 2009). Recent research continues to debate whether specific dietary components—such as carbohydrates or saturated fats—contribute to the development of artery disease (Chowdhury et al., 2014; Jakobsen et al., 2009). Such research is the basis for the dietary recommendations created by the U.S. Department of Agriculture (the U.S. Dietary Guidelines) and the American Heart Association (see sidebar).

Many experts have argued that it might be unrealistic to blame one or two dietary components for the progression of artery disease, and that it is likely that dietary pattern is more important. In epidemiological studies, for example, diets high in saturated fat have been associated with higher rates of artery disease. A statistical association, however, does not prove causation. This association might also be explained by other factors associated with a diet high in saturated fat, such as a high intake of animal protein or a low intake of plant foods, along with a low intake of dietary fiber, phytochemicals, and certain vitamins and minerals. Some researchers have argued that examining overall dietary pattern would be more applicable in terms of generating dietary recommendations.

A Healthy Diet to Help Prevent Heart Disease

A good, healthy diet can help to prevent heart (cardiovascular) disease. As the National Library of Medicine's Medline *Heart Disease and Diet* (2013) website suggests, making these types of changes in what adults eat can make a real difference.

- Add Fruits and Vegetables. They provide fiber, vitamins, and minerals. Eat five or more servings a day.
- Choose Good Grains. Low-fat breads, cereals, crackers, rice, pasta, and starchy vegetables (e.g., peas, potatoes, corn, winter squash, lima beans) are high in B vitamins, iron, and fiber and low in fat and cholesterol. Whole-grain foods should include at least half of daily grain intake. Grain products provide fiber, vitamins, minerals, and complex carbohydrates. Avoid refined grains, such as that found in white bread, pasta, and baked goods.
- Eat Healthy Protein. Meat, poultry, seafood, dried peas, lentils, nuts, and eggs are good sources of protein, B vitamins, iron, and other vitamins and minerals.
- Avoid High-Fat Meats. These include prime cuts of steak, duck, goose, kidneys, and liver, and processed meats such as sausage, hot dogs, and high-fat lunch meats.
    - Eat no more than 5 to 6 cooked ounces of lean meat, poultry, and fish daily.
    - Eat two servings of fish per week.
    - Consume lower-fat versions of milk and other dairy products; they have protein, calcium, the B vitamins niacin and riboflavin, and vitamins A and D.
- Beware of Trans Fatty Acids. These are found in fried foods, commercial baked foods (donuts, cookies, and crackers), processed foods, and hard margarines.
- Consume Sugar and Alcohol Sparingly. Women should have no more than one alcoholic drink daily; men should not have more than two alcoholic drinks daily.

National Institutes of Health. (2013). *Heart disease and diet*. Medline. National Library of Medicine. http://www.nlm.nih.gov/medlineplus/ency/article/002436.htm

Relatively few well-controlled experimental studies have been conducted to examine the effect of diet and lifestyle change on the progression of artery disease. The best of these studies have been led by cardiologist Dean Ornish. Dr. Ornish was the first to demonstrate that a program of lifestyle change—as compared with standard treatment—actually could lead to regression of atherosclerotic plaques in the coronary arteries in subjects with CAD, something thought to be impossible until the results of these studies were published (Ornish et al.,1990). Subsequent studies by Ornish and his colleagues have continued to support these initial observations (Silberman et al., 2010). Ornish's dietary guidelines for reversing atherosclerosis emphasize a whole food, plant-based diet. The diet is low in fat, cholesterol, animal products, sugar, caffeine, sodium, and alcohol, and is high in fiber, phytochemicals, vitamins, and minerals. Specific guidelines for reversal of heart disease include the following.

- Low fat—Less than 10% of calories in this diet come from fats. This goal is achieved by severely restricting all added fats in the diet, even "healthful" fats such as oils, nuts, and avocadoes.

- Cholesterol—The 10-mg limit is achieved by eliminating all meats and egg yolks.
- Animal products—Only 0 to 2 servings per day of nonfat dairy and egg whites are included.
- Sugar—Permitted in moderation; two or fewer servings per day of non-fat sweets.
- Caffeine—The only caffeine source included in this diet is green tea, because its antioxidant benefits outweigh its risk for most people, although Ornish cautions that people with cardiac arrhythmias and elevated stress levels should avoid all caffeine.
- Sodium—Moderate levels permitted unless other medical reasons, such as hypertension, suggest that the level should be very low.
- Alcohol—One drink per day is allowed but is "not encouraged."
- Soy—One serving of soy per day is encouraged.
- Supplements—A low-dose multivitamin and mineral supplement and a marine omega-3 fatty acid supplement are recommended. Depending on one's health risks, calcium also could be recommended.

Ornish advises that following the low-fat diet is only one part of the heart-disease reversal treatment protocol used in his studies. Participants also increase physical activity and stress-reduction practices, and engage in group counseling to improve emotional health and social support. Because of the strength of the evidence Ornish and his colleagues have collected to support the efficacy of the program, the Ornish program now is reimbursed by some insurance companies for people with demonstrated CAD who want to avoid surgical procedures, if possible.

Some experts argue that because a very low-fat diet is difficult to follow, a Mediterranean-type diet also could help to reduce risk of CVD (Estruch et al., 2013). Epidemiological and some experimental evidence suggests that people who consume a Mediterranean diet could have lower rates of heart disease than people who consume a Western diet, but experiments have not yet demonstrated reversal of heart disease with regression of plaque when following such a diet. It should also be noted that the Ornish diet offers less-stringent recommendations for apparently healthy people who simply want to prevent heart disease (as opposed to people who have documented artery blockage or who already have had a cardiovascular event, such as a heart attack or stroke) (Ornish Spectrum, 2014).

Dietary recommendations for the prevention of stroke echo those for artery disease, because artery disease causes about 2 in 3 strokes. Hypertension increases risk for the other type of stroke that is caused by an aneurism, a tear or break in the artery. Dietary recommendations for reducing hypertension are similar to those for the prevention of artery disease. Additionally, a very low sodium (salt) intake is recommended (1,500 mg or less), along with a high intake of potassium, magnesium, and calcium through consumption of vegetables, fruits, and low-fat dairy products. The Dietary Approaches to Stop Hypertension (DASH) diet has been shown to help control hypertension (National Heart, Lung, and Blood Institute, 2014).

Barbara A. Brehm, Karishma L. Parikh, and Jessica M. Backus

Research Issues

Recent research on the association of a compound called tri-methylamine-N-oxide (TMAO) with increased risk of heart disease suggests that a high intake of animal products might accelerate the progression of atherosclerosis. Tri-methylamine-N-oxide is synthesized by the liver from trimethylamine (TMA). Trimethylamine is made by bacteria residing in the colon from the precursors choline and carnitine. Choline is a nutrient plentiful in egg yolks. Carnitine is an amino acid plentiful in meat, especially red meat. It is not known whether TMAO contributes to cardiovascular disease, but the higher levels of TMAO observed in meat eaters compared with vegetarians has been suggested as a possible explanation for the link between a Western diet and cardiovascular disease (Koeth et al., 2013). Some researchers suggest that a high intake of animal protein, more than the saturated fat and cholesterol found in animal products, could be one of major causes of atherosclerosis (Campbell, 2014).

See Also: Antioxidants; Cardiometabolic syndrome; Carnitine; Cholesterol; Choline; Diabetes, type 2; *Dietary Guidelines for Americans*; The French paradox; Glycemic index and glycemic load; Hypertension and nutrition; Lipoproteins; Mediterranean diet; Obesity, definition and health effects; Phytochemicals; Trans fatty acids; Vegetarian and vegan diets.

Further Reading

American Heart Association. (2014, February). *The American Heart Association's diet and lifestyle recommendations*. Retrieved from http://www.heart.org/HEARTORG /GettingHealthy/NutritionCenter/HealthyEating/The-American-Heart-Associations -Diet-and-Lifestyle-Recommendations_UCM_305855_Article.jsp

Campbell, T. C. (2014, April 18). *A fallacious, faulty, and foolish discussion about saturated fat*. Center for Nutrition Studies. Retrieved from http://nutritionstudies.org /fallacious-faulty-foolish-discussion-about-saturated-fat/

Centers for Disease Control and Prevention (CDC). (2014, February 19). *Heart disease facts*. Retrieved from http://www.cdc.gov/heartdisease/index.htm

Chowdhury, R., Warnakula, S., Kunutsor, S., et al. (2014). Association of dietary, circulating, and supplement fatty acids with coronary risk. *Annals of Internal Medicine, 160* (6), 398–406.

Estruch, R., Ros, E., Salas-Salvadó, J., et al. (2013). Primary prevention of cardiovascular disease with a Mediterranean diet. *New England Journal of Medicine, 368*, 1279–1290. doi: 10.1056/NEJMoa1200303

Go, A. S., Mozaffarian, D., Roger, V. L., et al. (2013). AHA statistical update: Heart disease and stroke statistics—2013 update. *Circulation, 127*, e6-e245. doi: 10.1161 /CIR.0b013e31828124ad

Jakobsen, M. U., O'Reilly, E. J., Heitmann, B. L., et al. (2009). Major types of dietary fat and risk of coronary heart disease: A pooled analysis of 11 cohort studies. *American Journal of Clinical Nutrition, 89*, 1425–32.

Koeth, R. A., Wang, Z., Levison, B. S., et al. (2013). Intestinal microbiota metabolism of L-carnitine, a nutrient in red meat, promotes atherosclerosis. *Nature Medicine, 19*, 576–585. doi:10.1038/nm.3145

National Heart, Lung, and Blood Institute. (2014). *What is the DASH eating plan?* Retrieved from http://www.nhlbi.nih.gov/health/health-topics/topics/dash/

Ornish, D., Brown, S. E., Billings, J. H., et al. (1990, July 21). Can lifestyle changes reverse coronary heart disease? *The Lancet, 336*, 129–133.

Ornish Spectrum (The). (2014). *Nutrition: Spectrum of choices.* Retrieved from http://www.ornishspectrum.com/proven-program/nutrition/

Silberman, A., Banthia, R., Estay, I. S., Kemp, C., Studley, J., Hareras, D., & Ornish, D. (2010). The effectiveness and efficacy of an intensive cardiac rehabilitation program in 24 sites. *American Journal of Health Promotion, 24* (4), 260–266.

Carnitine

Carnitine is a compound that can be found in most cells in the human body. It is synthesized—mainly in the liver, but also in the kidneys—from the amino acids lysine and methionine. Carnitine is a generic term that includes L-carnitine, propionyl-L-carnitine, and acetyl-L-carnitine. Carnitine is significant for the body's energy production because it helps transport long-chain fatty acids into the mitochondria where they can be metabolized for energy. Carnitine also carries toxic metabolic byproducts out of the mitochondria, and thus helps keep this important organelle functioning at an optimal level. Carnitine is most concentrated in tissues of the body where fatty acids are the major source of energy, such as skeletal and cardiac muscle.

Generally, the human body synthesizes sufficient carnitine to satisfy its daily need; however some people do not make sufficient carnitine, and others are unable to transport carnitine into the tissues that need it. Dietary sources highest in carnitine include red meats such as steak and ground beef. Much lower amounts are found in dairy products, fish, and poultry. Dietary carnitine is absorbed by the small intestine then enters the bloodstream. The kidneys can conserve carnitine efficiently, as they are estimated to reabsorb 95% of serum carnitine (Hidgon & Drake, 2012). As a result, the excretion of carnitine generally is minimal.

Several conditions can cause a deficiency of carnitine in the body. One such condition is primary systemic carnitine deficiency, which is a rare autosomal recessive disorder that results from genetic mutations. The genetic mutations cause a carnitine-transporter protein to lose its ability to transport carnitine through the plasma membrane. People who have this disorder have a high urinary loss of carnitine and low intestinal absorption of dietary carnitine. Primary systemic carnitine deficiency causes serious symptoms, such as skeletal myopathy, hypoglycemia, and progressive cardiomyopathy. Primary systemic carnitine deficiency is fatal if it is not treated; treatment for this disorder requires a high supplemental intake of carnitine. Unlike primary systemic carnitine deficiency, secondary carnitine deficiency can be caused by either acquired or genetic conditions. Dietary management is the main treatment for secondary carnitine deficiency. People who have secondary carnitine deficiency are advised to follow a high-carbohydrate and low-fat diet, which decreases the need for the oxidation of fat, thereby decreasing the need for carnitine.

Potential Benefits

Carnitine has been studied extensively by scientists and researchers, as it has shown potential for the prevention and treatment of various diseases and conditions. Evidence is strongest for carnitine's role in helping to treat cardiovascular disease. A meta-analysis of 13 studies examining the effect of L-carnitine treatment versus placebo or control treatments on the outcome of 3,629 participants who had experienced a heart attack found that those receiving carnitine showed a 27% reduction in all-cause mortality, a 40% reduction in chest pain symptoms, and a 65% lower rate of heart rate arrhythmias (DiNicolantonio, Lavie, Fares, Menezes, & O'Keefe, 2013). Some studies have found that carnitine treatments can be helpful for reducing symptoms of heart failure and peripheral vascular disease (Ehrlich, 2011). Studies examining the effect of acetyl-L-carnitine in treating diabetic neuropathy suggest that acetyl-L-carnitine might be effective in improving neurophysiological parameters and in reducing pain over a one-year period (Ehrlich, 2011).

Carnitine is a popular supplement among athletes because it is thought to be able to improve performance by making fat more available for energy production. Research, however, generally has not found a performance benefit associated with carnitine supplementation.

Evidence suggests that the concentration of carnitine in body tissues decreases as people age (NIH, 2013). Researchers have suggested that the decline in the concentration of carnitine might lower the integrity of the mitochondrial membrane; mitochondrial decay is believed to be a factor in the aging process. Experiments with aged rats have shown that the supplementation of carnitine reduces mitochondrial decay and improves performance on memory-demanding work (NIH, 2013). Further studies in humans are needed to determine whether the same effect would be observed in people.

Risks

Recent research on the association of a compound called tri-methylamine-N-oxide (TMAO) with increased risk of heart disease suggests that further research is needed to clarify possible risks associated with carnitine supplementation. TMAO is synthesized by the liver from trimethylamine (TMA). Trimethylamine is made by bacteria residing in the colon from the precursors choline and carnitine. It is not known whether TMAO contributes to cardiovascular disease, but the higher levels of TMAO observed in meat eaters compared to vegetarians has been suggested as a possible explanation for the link between higher intakes of red meat and cardiovascular disease (Koeth, Wang, Levison et al., 2013).

Fei Peng

See Also: Choline.

Further Reading

DiNicolantonio, J. J., Lavie, C. J., Fares, H., Menezes, A. R., & O'Keefe, J. H. (2013). L-carnitine in the secondary prevention of cardiovascular disease: Systematic review and meta-analysis. *Mayo Clinic Proceedings, 88* (6), 544–551. doi: 10.1016/j.mayocp.2013.02.007

Ehrlich, S. D. (2011, March 31). *Carnitine.* University of Maryland Medical Center. Retrieved from http://www.umm.edu/altmed/articles/carnitine-l-000291.htm

Higdon, J., & Drake, V. J. (2012). *L-carnitine.* Linus Pauling Institute, Oregon State University. Retrieved from http://lpi.oregonstate.edu/infocenter/othernuts/carnitine/

Koeth, R. A., Wang, Z., Levison, B. S., et al. (2013). Intestinal microbiota metabolism of L-carnitine, a nutrient in red meat, promotes atherosclerosis. *Nature Medicine, 19,* 576–585. doi:10.1038/nm.3145

National Institutes of Health (NIH). (2013, May 10). *Carnitine.* Office of Dietary Supplements. Retrieved from http://ods.od.nih.gov/factsheets/Carnitine-HealthProfessional/

Carotenoids

Carotenoids are a class of phytochemicals that includes more than 600 natural pigments. These compounds give fruits and vegetables their vibrant yellow, orange, and red colors, such as those seen in sweet potatoes, melons, tomatoes, papayas, and pumpkins. In the human diet, carotenoids are associated with a number of health benefits. All of the carotenoids have antioxidant activity. Less than 10% of the carotenoids can be converted by the body into vitamin A. Many studies have found associations between the increased consumption of foods high in carotenoids and a reduced risk of heart disease and some types of cancer. Because carotenoids are fat soluble, consumption along with dietary fats such as olive oil is recommended.

Carotenoids are categorized into two major groups, carotenes and xanthophylls. Carotenes are hydrocarbons. The most common carotenes in the human diet are alpha-carotene, beta-carotene, and lycopene. Alpha-carotene and beta-carotene can be transformed into vitamin A, and the human body produces the most vitamin A from beta-carotene. Many studies have found strong associations between a high beta-carotene intake from food and several health benefits. Studies using beta-carotene supplements, however, generally have failed to find health benefits. Several well-designed experiments have even found an increased risk of lung cancer in smokers who consume beta-carotene supplements. Lycopene is a red-orange pigment plentiful in tomatoes and watermelon. Lycopene appears to be more bioavailable in cooked rather than raw foods. Diets high in foods containing lycopene have been associated with a reduced risk of prostate cancer in men; it is unknown whether supplements containing lycopene have the same association.

Xanthophylls are composed of oxygen, carbon, and hydrogen. They have anti-oxidant properties that limit photo-oxidative damage in plants and protect humans from free radical damage. The most common xanthophylls in the human diet are beta-cryptoxanthin, lutein, and zeaxanthin. Beta-cryptoxanthin can be converted to vitamin A. Lutein and zeaxanthin are stored in the retina and lens of the eye. Consumption of foods with high concentrations of these xanthophylls appears to exert protective effects on the eye, slowing the progression of macular degeneration and the formation of cataracts. Food high in lutein and zeaxanthin include dark leafy greens such as spinach and kale.

In various studies, foods high in carotenoids—including many fruits and vegetables—have been associated with a reduced risk of cancer and heart disease. The antioxidant activity of the carotenoids might protect the lining of arteries and fat in blood from free radicals and oxidative stress. In vitro studies have shown that carotenoids appear to influence intercellular signaling. Carotenoids also might improve immune function, although this could be an effect of vitamin A activity. Because carotenoids play a substantial role in the production of vitamin A, ingestion of foods with these pigments is necessary to maintain proper levels of vitamin A.

Deborah B. Ok and Jennifer Najera

See Also: Antioxidants; Beta-carotene; Eye health, and nutrition; Lutein; Lycopene; Phytochemicals; Vitamin A; Zeaxanthin.

Further Reading

Higdon, J., & Drake, V. J. (2009). *Carotenoids*. Linus Pauling Institute, Oregon State University. Retrieved from http://lpi.oregonstate.edu/infocenter/phytochemicals/carotenoids/index.html∞tro

International Carotenoid Society. (2013). *Carotenoids*. Retrieved from http://www.carotenoidsociety.org/carotenoids

Simon, H., & Rieve, D. (2013). Carotenoids. *The New York Times Health Guide*. Retrieved from http://health.nytimes.com/health/guides/nutrition/vitamins/carotenoids.html

Carrageenan

Carrageenan is a substance extracted from the red seaweed commonly found off the coast of North America, Great Britain, and Continental Europe. Although carrageen has no nutritional value, it is added to food products to thicken, emulsify, stabilize, and improve the overall texture of the food. It often is used in dairy products and dairy substitutes, such as ice cream, yogurt, cottage cheese, soy milk, rice milk, and almond milk. It also is found in other foods and products, such as tooth-paste, cosmetics, and processed meats. Carrageenan currently is labeled by the FDA as being "Generally Recognized as Safe." Even though it is permitted in many products, however, some scientific studies have led researchers to question the overall safety of this additive and its effect on the digestive system. In response to these studies, some physicians advise individuals with gastrointestinal symptoms and conditions to eliminate carrageenan from their diets.

Since the 1930s, carrageenan has been used in many food products. In France, acid is added to carrageenan at high temperatures to create a product that is sold as a treatment for peptic ulcers and as a bulk laxative (Therapeutic Research Faculty, 2009). Products containing carrageenan have been used in North American to treat cough, bronchitis, peptic ulcers, and constipation, although the evidence to support such uses is fairly weak. Carrageenan does appear to pull water into the intestine, contributing to its laxative effect (Therapeutic Research Faculty, 2009).

Although presently there are few studies to support the claims of carrageenan's health benefits, multiple studies—primarily led by Joanne Tobacman, MD, a physician-scientist at the University of Illinois College of Medicine—suggest that carageenan could have harmful physiological effects. Studies from Dr. Tobacman's lab have found that carrageenan and its breakdown in the body can lead to intestinal inflammation that can contribute to many chronic illnesses, such as irritable bowel syndrome, ulcerative colitis and other inflammatory bowel disorders, and colon cancer (Bhattacharyya et al., 2012). Tobacman and colleagues argue that it is the foreign chemical structure in carrageenan that stimulates an innate immune response that can lead to these symptoms, as well as to chronic inflammation. There are two forms of this additive, undegraded and degraded. Undegraded carrageenan is used in food products (Weil, 2012). Degraded, low molecular weight carrageenan is recognized as a "possible human carcinogen" by the International Agency for Research on Cancer, and has been used in the medical research community for decades to induce acute inflammation in lab animals to test anti-inflammatory drugs. Although undegraded carrageenan is listed as safe, studies have shown that carrageenan in food has contained trace amounts of degraded carrageenan, and that the acidic environment of the stomach could convert undegraded carrageenan to the degraded form. Research groups such as the Cornucopia Institute, a non-profit food- and farm-policy research organization, have advised consumers—especially those with gastrointestinal conditions—to completely avoid products containing carrageenan.

Elizabeth Kleisner

See Also: Food additives.

Further Reading

Bhattacharyya, S., Borthakur, A., Dudeja, P. K. & Tobacman, J. K. (2008). Carageenan induces cell cycle arrest in human intestinal epithelial cells in vitro. *Journal of Nutrition, 138* (3), 469–475.

Bhattacharyya, S., Liu, H., Zhang, A., et al. (2010). Carrageenan-induced innate immune response is modified by enzymes that hydrolyze distinct galactosidic bonds. *Journal of Nutritional Biochemistry, 21* (10), 906–913.

Cornucopia Institute. (2013). *Carageenan: how a "natural" food additive is making us sick.* Retrieved from http://www.cornucopia.org/wp-content/uploads/2013/02/Carrageenan -Report1.pdf

Therapeutic Research Faculty (2009). *Carageenan.* WebMD. Natural Medicines Comprehensive Database. Retrieved from http://www.webmd.com/vitamins-supplements /ingredientmono-710-CARRAGEENAN.aspx?activeIngredientId=710&activeIngredient Name=CARRAGEENAN

Weil, A. (2012, October 1). *Is carrageenan safe?* DrWeil.com. Retrieved from http://www .drweil.com/drw/u/QAA401181/Is-Carrageenan-Safe.html

Catechins

Catechins are a type of polyphenols, organic compounds composed of phenol groups, known for their distinct aroma. Sometimes referred to as tannins, catechins are well-known components of green and white teas and also are found in many fruits, potatoes, garlic, and some nuts. These polyphenols are secondary metabolites, or flavonoids, which are molecules that do not contribute directly to the body's life-sustaining processes, but the absence of which could cause a variety of long-term impairments. Catechins are found in their highest natural concentrations in green tea leaves with epigallocatechin gallate (EGCG) being the most abundant, making up 65% of the total catechin concentration (Holloway & Oshimi, 2006).

The potential health benefits of catechins are numerous. Research shows strong evidence for their support in the immune system where they prevent the adherence of bacteria and viruses to cell membranes (Murase et al., 2002). In vitro experiments suggest that some catechins could stimulate apoptosis of human cancer cells, and a number of trials of catechin treatment for cancer patients are under way (National Cancer Institute, 2014). Catechins are especially active in the vascular system where they help reduce blood pressure and cholesterol levels, as well as prevent the growth of new blood vessels that help feed tumorous growth (Zaveri, 2005). As powerful antioxidants, catechins scavenge reactive oxygen species, helping to reduce inflammation and oxidative damage that interferes with proper cell functioning. In laboratory rats, catechins have been shown to reduce the liver damage associated with alcohol intake (Bharrhan et al., 2011).

Tea catechin supplements have been shown to reduce the weight gain that occurs in rats with high fat diets (Lu, Zhu, Shen, & Gao, 2012). Although it is too soon to recommend catechin supplements, drinking several cups of green tea a day appears to be safe for most people, although people sensitive to caffeine might need to modulate their intake. A number of human cancer trials are under way, using EGCG and other catechins. Descriptions of these trials can be accessed at the National Cancer Institute's website (http://www.cancer.gov/drugdictionary?cd rid=506041).

Patricia M. Cipicchio

See Also: Antioxidants; Cancer and nutrition; Tea.

Further Reading

Bharrhan, S., Koul, A., Chopra, K., and Rishi, P. (2011). Catechin suppresses an array of signaling molecules and modulates induced endotoxin mediated liver injury in a rat model. *PLoS One, 6* (6), e20635. doi: 10.1371/journal.pone.0020635

Holloway, M & Oshimi, T. (2006). Health Benefits of Green Tea. *Health Hokkaido.* Retrieved from http://www.healthhokkaido.com/files/Articles_Oshimi/greentea.cfm

Lu, C., Zhu, W., Shen, C. L., & Gao, W. (2012). Green tea polyphenols reduce body weight in rats by modulating obesity-related genes. *PLoS One, 7* (6), e38332. doi: 10.1371/journal.pone.0038332.

Murase, T., Nagasawa, A., Suzuki, J., Hase, T., & Tokimitsu, I. (2002). Beneficial effects of tea catechins on diet-induced obesity: Stimulation of lipid catabolism in the liver. *Nature, 26* (11), 1459–1464.

National Cancer Institute. (2014, November 29). *NCI drug dictionary.* Retrieved from http://www.cancer.gov/drugdictionary?cdrid=506041

Zaveri, N. T. (2005). Green tea and its polyphenolic catechins: Medicinal uses in cancer and noncancer applications. *Life Sciences, 78,* 2073–2080.

Celiac Disease

Celiac disease is an autoimmune condition that can affect both children and adults. It is also referred to as "celiac sprue" and "gluten sensitive enteropathy" (GSE). If a person with this disorder consumes gluten—a mix of proteins that are stored in the seeds of wheat, barley, and rye—then the individual's immune system reacts by attacking the lining of the small intestine and, consequently, the body is unable to obtain the nutrients that it needs. It is a lifelong condition that affects approximately 1 in 133 people in the United States. Research continues in an effort to better understand the condition and to find possible treatments for the disease. This is extremely important because the condition can be both physically and emotionally taxing. Celiac disease is a condition that greatly affects the individual's daily life but can be managed with some increased effort.

History

Celiac disease is thought to have first developed when people changed their diets from those of simple hunter/gatherer cultures to those of agrarian societies

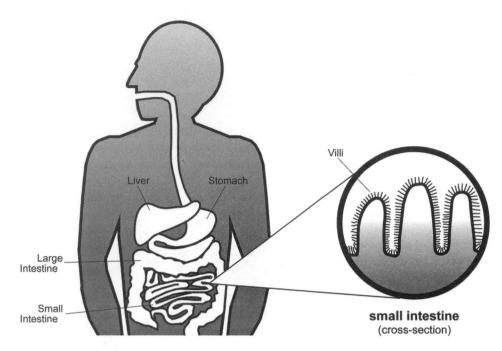

Villi are part of the lining on the intestine wall that aids in digestion. (ABC-CLIO)

when new crops were added to the food supply, including grains. Most people were able to adapt to the new food antigens, but food intolerances appeared in those who could not. Celiac disease was not identified or named, however, until about 8,000 years after people began eating wheat. In the first century CE, Aretaeus of Cappadocia, a Greek physician, wrote about "The Coeliac Affection." He named it after the Greek word, "koelia," meaning "abdomen" (Guandalini, 2007). In the early 19th century, Dr. Mathew Baillie wrote about a chronic diarrheal disorder causing malnutrition. It was not until about 75 years later that an English physician, Samuel Gee, described the "celiac affection" and presented the modern definition of the disease. After much research and many years, celiac disease was accepted as an autoimmune condition with a known trigger and autoantigen around the year 1990 (Guandalini, 2007).

Autoimmune diseases in general affect 3.5% of the U.S. population. In the United States, the prevalence of celiac disease is 1 in 133, or almost 1%. The prevalence for African Americans, Asian Americans, and Hispanic Americans is estimated to be 1 in 236. Researchers think that celiac disease affects at least 3 million Americans, but about 95% of these people are undiagnosed (University of Chicago Celiac Disease Center, 2012). It often takes several years for people with celiac disease to be diagnosed.

Physiology

The cause of celiac disease is still unknown. Researchers have discovered that it is partly hereditary. The prevalence of celiac disease in people with first-degree relatives who also have the disease is 1 in 22. Certain genes also seem to play a role in this disease. Two specific genes, HLA-DQ2 and HLA-DQ8, correlate with a person's risk of having the condition; and HLA-DQ2 is found in about 95% of individuals with celiac disease (Schoenstadt, 2013). About 30% of people without the disease have one of the two genes. This means that other factors must be involved. For example, situations such as surgery, pregnancy, childbirth, viral infection, or severe emotional stress might trigger the disease. Researchers believe that the cause of celiac disease most likely is a combination of genetic and environmental factors.

Although the symptoms of celiac disease vary among individuals, they often occur in the digestive system as well as in many other parts of the body. Young children and infants commonly suffer from digestive symptoms caused by the disease. Symptoms include abdominal bloating and pain; chronic diarrhea; vomiting; constipation; pale, foul-smelling, or fatty stool; and weight loss. Along with these, children also could suffer from irritability, delayed growth, delayed puberty, or dental enamel defects due to malabsorption of nutrients.

Adults often have symptoms unrelated to the digestive system. These symptoms include unexplained iron-deficiency anemia, fatigue, bone or joint pain, arthritis, bone loss or osteoporosis, depression or anxiety, tingling numbness in hands and feet, seizures, missed menstrual periods, infertility or recurrent miscarriage, canker sores inside the mouth, and a skin rash. Symptoms can vary in severity. Some people might show no symptoms but could develop complications over time, including malnutrition, liver diseases, and cancers of the intestine.

Researchers are studying the reasons for such variation of symptoms and severity. Symptom severity could be related to the age that the individual started eating foods containing gluten and the amount of these foods eaten. Studies show that symptoms appear later in individuals who were breast-fed longer. Symptoms also depend on a person's age and the amount of damage done to the small intestine. Individuals have a greater chance of developing long-term complications if they go for a long period without diagnosis.

Celiac disease is difficult to diagnose because it is characterized by symptoms that are similar to those of other diseases. It is sometimes confused with irritable bowel syndrome, iron-deficiency anemia, inflammatory bowel disease, diverticulitis, intestinal infections, or chronic fatigue syndrome. Because of this, celiac disease often is underdiagnosed and misdiagnosed. Doctors now are more aware of the symptoms, however, and there now are more reliable tests—this causes diagnosis rates to increase. The first tests performed to diagnose the disease often are blood tests. These measure the levels of two antibodies whose levels increase with celiac disease: anti-tissue transglutaminase antibodies and anti-endomysium antibodies. Additional blood tests are performed if the results come back negative and the disease still is suspected. For these tests to be accurate, it is important that the person being tested continues to eat a diet containing gluten. Otherwise, they might test negative for celiac disease even if it is present. To confirm the diagnosis an intestinal biopsy is performed. The doctor uses an endoscope to remove small pieces of tissue from the small intestine to check for damage to the villi. Screening for celiac disease is sometimes recommended to family members of a person with the disease as a precautionary measure.

Treatment

Although there is no known cure for the disease, treatment options do exist. Currently the only treatment is a gluten-free diet. Many individuals work with a dietician to create a gluten-free diet plan. People with the disease must learn to read the ingredients on the labels of all foods and identify those that contain gluten. Most people see improvement just days after starting the diet. In almost all cases, the symptoms disappear, intestinal damage heals, and further damage is prevented. In children, the small intestine takes about three to six months to heal, but it could take a couple years for adults. To stay healthy, individuals with celiac disease must stick to a gluten-free diet for the rest of their lives. In rare cases intestinal injury continues even when on a strict gluten-free diet; this is called refractory celiac disease, and it occurs when the intestines have been severely damage. In such cases, the patient might need to receive nutrients intravenously.

A gluten-free diet means eliminating foods that contain wheat, rye, and barley. "Plain" meat, fish, rice, fruits, and vegetables do not contain gluten. To maintain a healthy gluten-free diet, a person must use non-gluten containing ingredients when cooking and baking. Potato, rice, soy, buckwheat, or bean flour, for example, can be used instead of wheat flour. Gluten-free products also are available from many organic and mainstream food stores. It is important, though, that individuals with the disease verify that their foods were not contaminated with gluten during processing or preparation. For example, a person with celiac disease should not use a toaster that has been used to toast regular wheat bread. Individuals should be extremely cautious when eating out, and should ask a waiter or chef when uncertain about the ingredients used in a meal. Gluten also is used in some medications and other products, such as lipstick and play dough. Reading product labels therefore is crucial. This diet might seem difficult at first, but people are able to adjust and get used to the new lifestyle.

Emotional Adjustments

Many people with celiac disease suffer emotionally because diagnosis often is prolonged. When first diagnosed, the individual might experience anxiety, insecurity, isolation, fear of the unknown, and lack of information. There are celiac support groups that help people adjust to this way of life and to address such problems. As individuals struggle to become accustomed to a new way of eating, they experience emotions such as relief at finally finding out what was wrong, grief over the loss of their former lifestyle, and difficulty in finding appropriate food. These feelings don't last forever, but one must continually explain the disease to those around them. Staying healthy takes personal determination, family support, and a doctor who knows how to treat celiac disease.

Rebecca E. Ryder

Research Issues

Currently, a diagnosis of celiac disease is only considered confirmed following a biopsy of the small intestine. These biopsies usually are accomplished with an endoscopy procedure, in which a tube is snaked down the esophagus, through the stomach, and into the small intestine, where a tissue sample is taken. Although it is not extremely painful, most patients find the procedure uncomfortable. New diagnostic techniques are being studied including capsule endoscopy, in which the patient swallows a capsule containing a small video camera that records the small intestine. Additionally, researchers are experimenting with the idea of breeding new grains that lack key gluten proteins. New celiac disease treatments on the horizon include devising ways to retrain the immune system to no longer respond to gluten. A number of new drug treatments also are being evaluated.

See Also: Food allergies and intolerances; Small intestine.

Further Reading

Celiac Disease Foundation. (2014, November 29). Retrieved from http://www.celiac.org/

Guandalini, S. (2007). *A brief history of celiac disease.* The University of Chicago Celiac Disease Center. Retrieved from http://www.cureceliacdisease.org/wp-content/uploads/2011/09/SU07CeliacCtr.News_.pdf

National Foundation for Celiac Awareness. (2011). *Celiac disease.* Retrieved from http://www.celiaccentral.org/Celiac-Disease/21/

National Foundation for Celiac Awareness. (2014, November 29). *What is celiac disease?* Retrieved from http://www.celiaccentral.org/SiteData/docs/NFCAWhatis/97976cf09194b986/NFCA%20-%20What%20is%20Celiac%20Disease%202-2011.pdf

National Institute of Diabetes and Digestive and Kidney Diseases (NIDDK). (2012, January 27). *Celiac disease.* Retrieved from http://digestive.niddk.nih.gov/ddiseases/pubs/celiac/

Schoenstadt, A. (2013, October 31). *Causes of celiac disease.* Celiac Disease Channel. eMedTV. Retrieved from http://celiac-disease.emedtv.com/celiac-disease/causes-of-celiac-disease-p2.html

University of Chicago Celiac Disease Center. (2012). *Celiac disease facts and figures.* Retrieved from http://www.uchospitals.edu/pdf/uch_007937.pdf

Chamomile

Chamomile is an herb. The term "chamomile" refers to two species of plant that have daisy-like flowers, German Chamomile (*Matricaria recutita*) and Roman Chamomile (*Chamaemelum nobile*). Both species of plants originate from the Mediterranean region and were widely used in antiquity in Egypt, Greece, and Rome. Today chamomile also is grown in North America and is recognized as a popular ingredient in herbal tea. Chamomile is believed to work as a mild sedative as well as a digestive aid.

The origins of chamomile date back to 1550 BCE where it can be found on the Eber's medical papyrus. It was celebrated by the ancient Egyptians as a gift from the sun god, Ra, and was an ingredient in embalming oil. It was the Greeks who gave this herb the name "chamomile" and it was used medicinally to treat headaches, female disorders, and digestion problems. By the 17th century, the English herbalist Nicholas Culpeper put forth the idea that it could be used to remedy digestive problems. Chamomile is believed to have arrived in North America in the 16th century with European immigrants. Since that time it has gained popularity for its medicinal, therapeutic, and cosmetic benefits (Gahagan, 2013).

The German Chamomile plant can be found in areas that provide full sun and well-drained soil. It is the variety that is most widely used in North American. The flowering tops of chamomile plants are used in various forms, including tea bags, tinctures (alcoholic extract), and aromatic oils. The use of the tea is believed to help with minor cases of digestion problems such as nausea, abdominal pain, bloating, and irritable bowel syndrome (National Center for Complementary and Alternative Medicine, 2013). Chamomile also is used to help with sleeping problems, muscle tension, and anxiety. Laboratory studies suggest that chamomile extracts provide a helpful effect in both mild to moderate anxiety and mild to moderate depressive disorders (Amsterdam et al., 2012). For cosmetic use, chamomile is used to soothe the skin from burns, acne, puffiness, mouth sores, and eczema. It is found in lotions, sprays, and facial cleansers.

Chamomile appears to be safe for most people. Because chamomile has anticoagulant properties, however, people taking an anticoagulant drug are advised not to drink or use chamomile. People who have experienced prior allergic reactions to plants in the daisy family—which includes ragweed—also could experience allergic reactions to chamomile.

Angelica O. Patlan

See Also: Herbs and herbal medicine.

Further Reading

Amsterdam, J. D., Shults, J., Soeller, I., Mao, J. J., Rockwell, K., & Newberg, A. B. (2012). Chamomile (Matricaria recutita) may provide antidepressant activity in anxious, depressed humans: An exploratory study. *Alternative Therapies in Health and Medicine, 18* (5), 44–49.

Gahagan, M. (2013). *The history of chamomile.* The English Chamomile Company. Retrieved from http://www.chamomile.co.uk/history.htm

National Center for Complementary and Alternative Medicine. (2012). *Chamomile.* Retrieved from http://nccam.nih.gov/health/chamomile/ataglance.htm

Srivastava, J. K., Pandey, M., & Gupta, S. (2009) Chamomile, a novel and selective COX-s inhibitor with anti-inflammatory activity. *Life Sciences 85* (19–20), 663–669.

Therapeutic Research Faculty. (2014, 27 October). *Roman chamomile.* Natural Medicines Comprehensive Database. MedlinePlus. Retrieved from http://www.nlm.nih.gov /medlineplus/druginfo/natural/752.html

Childhood Nutrition

A healthy, balanced diet is essential during childhood for proper growth and development, including organ formation and function, cognitive and neurological development, and a strong immune system. Ensuring that a child receives adequate nutrition, however, is not always easy. Children can be picky eaters and caregivers are not always sure how much food children need as compared to adults. Both undernutrition and obesity continue to be critical issues affecting children worldwide. Conflicting information regarding food allergies, as well as the effects of additives in food also cause concern and confusion.

Nutritional Requirements

Infants have unique nutritional needs, but by the time babies are a year old, a wide variety of foods can be incorporated into their diets, as long as the foods do not pose a choking risk. The average one-year-old child requires between 850 and 1,000 kilocalories per day. This amount increases gradually until it doubles by age 10. The USDA recommends 6 ounces of grains, 2½ cups of veggies, 1½ cups of fruit, 2 to 3 cups of milk, and 5 ounces of protein foods per day for kids aged 6 to 11 years. Children have small stomachs, therefore 6 small meals a day often is a more appropriate meal plan than 3 big meals.

A balanced diet generally meets all of a child's nutritional requirements, and both the American Medical Association and the Academy of Nutrition and Dietetics recommend that children get nutrition from healthy foods rather than from vitamin supplements. Deficiencies in calcium, iron, and certain vitamins, however, are a concern for children who do not eat a balanced diet. Multivitamin supplements might be recommended for children who are failing to thrive, have severe food allergies or a chronic disease, or follow a restrictive diet, such as a vegan diet. The most common nutrient deficiency around the world is iron. Iron deficiency can affect a child's mood, energy level, attention span, and ability to learn. A healthy diet is the best way to prevent and treat iron deficiency. Good sources of iron include leafy green vegetables, oatmeal, meats, eggs, legumes, peanut butter, liver, baby formula with iron, breast milk, and iron-fortified cereal.

Picky Eaters

Children can be picky eaters and often dislike certain textures, colors, or flavors, such as particularly rich or spicy foods. Young children's taste buds are more sensitive than adults', which is one reason that mild flavors appeal to young children. Sometimes "picky eating" is simply less appetite resulting from a slowing growth rate. This is particularly common for children at around ages 3 and 4 years; other times it is an expression of independence for children who want to exert some control over their environment. Nutritionists recommend that caregivers be patient with picky eaters, set a healthy example, and continue to expose them to a wide variety of nutrient-rich foods. It could take eight to ten food exposures before the child accepts the new food. When given some autonomy in choosing foods and amounts, however, children usually outgrow these eating habits. Caregivers who are concerned about a picky eater becoming malnourished should talk to the child's health care provider.

Malnutrition

Malnutrition is caused by inadequate food intake or a diet lacking one or more nutrients; it can also be caused by problems with absorption and digestion that are linked to certain medical conditions. Hunger and malnutrition are responsible for 60% of child deaths worldwide (Insel, Ross, McMahon, & Bernstein, 2013). The signs and symptoms of malnutrition can vary, but they can include low energy, poor immune function, poor growth, muscle weakness, learning difficulties, and osteoporosis. Poverty, political crises, natural disasters, and epidemics all are common causes of malnutrition.

Vegetarian and Vegan Children

With careful planning, alternative diets such as vegetarianism or veganism can be healthy and safe for children. Vegetarian and vegan diets often are low in vitamins D and B12, calcium, zinc, and iron, but these nutrients can be absorbed through fortified products. Animal proteins can be replaced with wheat and rice products, as well as legumes and nuts. Vegan children also should consume dairy-free beverages that are fortified with calcium and B12.

Obesity

The number of obese children in the United States has more than doubled in the past 30 years, and was up to 18% in 2010 (CDC, 2013). Obese children are more likely to become obese adults, and have a higher risk of developing health problems later in life, such as heart disease, metabolic syndrome, and hormone-related cancers.

Diets that are high in sugar and fats, reliance on fast food, excessive snacking, limited physical activity, and environmental factors (such as no safe place to play) all have an impact on whether children become overweight or obese. Treatment should begin with assessing the child's physical activity and diet. The American Academy of Pediatrics recommends that children watch no more than 1 or 2 hours of entertainment media per day, and no television or other entertainment media is recommended for children younger than 2 years of age (American Academy of Pediatrics, 2014).

Many children spend significant time at childcare centers, therefore care providers have just as great an influence on children's diets as home care providers do. For this reason, childcare providers should go through nutrition and physical activity trainings to help prevent unhealthy eating habits that could lead to diet-related illnesses and obesity. Children should be taught how to make healthy choices regarding food and physical activity.

Allergies

From 1997 to 2011, the number of food allergies increased in children younger than age 18; they are now thought to occur in 6% to 8% of children (Branum & Lukacs, 2008). Six foods (milk, egg, peanuts, tree nuts, fish, and shellfish) cause 90% of all allergic reactions to foods. Considerable research is examining the increase. A common hypothesis, referred to as the "hygiene hypothesis," is that living in more-sterile environments interrupts the immune system function and development, leading to an increase in allergic reactions and autoimmune diseases.

Another hypothesis is that delaying giving children foods that commonly cause allergic reactions might increase the risk of developing an allergy. The American Academy of Pediatrics formerly recommended that pregnant women and young children avoid eating common-allergy foods. The Academy, however, changed this recommendation because of lack of evidence (Greer, Sicherer, & Burks, 2008). Studies of countries where pregnant women and young children eat common-allergy foods have much lower rates of food allergies than countries where these foods are delayed (like the United States and the United Kingdom). Many scientists now believe repeated exposure to a common-allergy food at a young age teaches the body to tolerate the allergens, thus decreasing the likelihood of an allergic reaction. The LEAP Study (Learning Early about Peanut Allergy) is an international clinical research study based in London that is currently investigating the best way to prevent peanut allergy in young children. Researchers are testing both the avoidance of peanut in infancy and the measured, repeated consumption of peanut-containing foods in infancy (Immune Tolerance Network, 2013).

Hyperactivity

According to a comprehensive review of research connecting diet to attention-deficit disorder (ADD) and attention-deficit hyperactivity disorder (ADHD) in children, researchers Millichap and Yee (2012) conclude that diet can decrease

ADHD symptoms, particularly when complemented with medication. There is no single dietary trigger, however—diet is but one factor of many affecting children's behavior and cognitive function. Dietary changes supported by research include lessening consumption of refined sugar, sodium, and total fat; increasing long-chain polyunsaturated fatty acid consumption (omega-3 and omega-6 fatty acids); and limiting artificial colors.

Lisa P. Ritchie and Ava B. Castro

Research Issues

In both the United States and Canada, steroid-based growth hormones can be given to meat cattle to increase their size. In the United States—but not Canada or the European Union—protein-based hormones can be given to cattle to increase milk production. These practices have sparked considerable debate regarding their consequences to human health and for children in particular. The considerable research findings have been inconclusive, however, and the FDA continues to promote the safety of these practices. One concern is that the increasing number of girls reaching puberty before age 12 could be connected to meat and dairy consumption. How can this be determined? Is earlier puberty linked to an increase in meat and dairy consumption, or is earlier puberty linked to an increase in the consumption of meat and dairy that have been treated with growth hormones? The use of hormones is not the only change in the meat and dairy industry over the past 50 years. Cows are milked far more frequently than in the past, for example, including during late stages of pregnancy, when the levels of naturally occurring hormones are 33% higher than normal. Is this affecting not only early puberty, but other increased cancer rates as well? Is earlier puberty not a result of meat and dairy consumption, but of increasing rates of obesity and inactivity?

See Also: Breast-feeding; Food allergies and intolerances; Infant formula; Iron-deficiency anemia; Obesity, causes; Obesity, definition and health effects; Phenylketonuria (PKU).

Further Reading

Adams, L. (2011). Do growth hormones in food affect children? *LiveStrong*. Retrieved from http://www.livestrong.com/article/546411-do-growth-hormones-in-food-affect-children/

American Academy of Pediatrics. (2014, November 29). *Media and children*. Retrieved from http://www.aap.org/en-us/advocacy-and-policy/aap-health-initiatives/Pages/Media-and-Children.aspx

Branum, A. M., & Lukacs, S. L. (2008). *Food allergy among US children: Trends in prevalence and hospitalizations*. NCHS Data Brief, No. 10. Retrieved from http://www.cdc.gov/nchs/data/databriefs/db10.pdf

Centers for Disease Control and Prevention (CDC). (2013). *Childhood obesity facts*. Centers for Disease Control and Prevention. Retrieved from http://www.cdc.gov/healthyyouth/obesity/facts.htm

Gandhi, R., & Snedeker, S. M. (2003). *Consumer concerns about hormones in food*. Program on Breast Cancer and Environmental Risk Factors in New York State. Sprecher

Institute for Comparative Cancer Research, Cornell University. Retrieved from http:// envirocancer.cornell.edu/Factsheet/Diet/fs37.hormones.cfm

Greer, F. R., Sicherer, S. H., Burks, A. W., & Committee on Nutrition and Section on Allergy and Immunology. (2008). Effects of early nutritional interventions on the development of atopic disease in infants and children: The role of maternal dietary restriction, breastfeeding, timing of introduction of complementary foods, and hydro-lyzed formulas. *Pediatrics, 121* (1). http://www.aap.org/en-us/advocacy-and-policy /aap-health-initiatives/Pages/Media-and-Children.aspx?nfstatus=401&nftoken=0000 0000-0000-0000-0000-000000000000&nfstatusdescription=ERROR%3a+No+local+t oken. doi: 10.1542/peds.2007-3022

Immune Tolerance Network. (2013). *About the LEAP study*. Retrieved from http://www .leapstudy.co.uk/study_about.html

Insel, P., Ross, D., McMahon, K., & Bernstein, M. (2013). *Discovering nutrition* (4th ed.). Burlington, MA: Jones & Bartlett Learning.

Ireland, C. (2006). Hormones in milk can be dangerous. *Harvard University Gazette*. Retrieved from http://news.harvard.edu/gazette/2006/12.07/11-dairy.html

Millichap, J. G., & Yee, M. M. (2012). The diet factor in attention-deficit/hyperactivity dis-order. *Pediatrics, 129* (2). Retrieved from http://pediatrics.aappublications.org/content /early/2012/01/04/peds.2011-2199

Chlorella

Chlorella is a unicellular, freshwater green alga that has been hailed as a superfood with numerous benefits to the immune system. The species most commonly con-sumed by humans is *Chlorella pyrenoidosa*, which also is called "sun chlorella." Chlorella grows best on the surfaces of shallow ponds in warm air. When swal-lowed whole, chlorella is indigestible due to its tough cell wall. Most chlorella tablets contain chlorella growth factor (CGF), which comprises about 5% of a single chlorella specimen. Chlorella growth factor is water soluble and full of vita-mins and amino acids. It is extracted from the microbe and then can be taken orally or through an injection. Chlorella is very popular in Japan, where it is sold as a medicinal supplement and often is recommended by doctors.

In the decade following World War II, a hunger crisis seemed imminent as the world's population boomed and farmers struggled to keep up with the demand for crops. While looking for a cheap and easily produced alternative to traditional foods, scientists turned to potential non-agricultural sources of nutrition, such as chlorella. A single chlorella microbe contains an impressive amount of fats and calories, as well as fiber, vitamins, minerals, and all of the essential amino acids. In fact, more than half of the dried product is composed of protein.

The world population did indeed double between 1950 and 1990, but the pre-dictions that agriculture would be overwhelmed by the population were proven wrong. The farming of chlorella also turned out to be much more involved and inefficient than previously thought. In 1950, pharmaceutical company Pfizer esti-mated that a pound of chlorella would cost one dollar to produce, as opposed to the six cents required to produce a pound of soy (Belasco, 1997). The idea of chlorella as a mass-produced food source was abandoned. In the 1970s and 1980s, however, health food enthusiasts in Japan claimed that chlorella was a miracle supplement. Chlorella sold for up to $50 per pound in health food stores, and it was shipped to the Western world and marketed as an oriental herb (Belasco, 1997). The claims for chlorella's powers ranged from controlling weight and boosting the immune system to curing or preventing cancer.

The alleged health benefits of chlorella have been praised widely, but little scientific evidence exists to support the claims. A handful of small, preliminary studies suggest that additional research might find support for potential health benefits. In a 1990 study, for example, cancer patients with brain tumors were given chlorella tablets as supplements to their regular medications for two years. The chlorella did not have a significant effect on the patients' survival, but it did have a notable impact on their immune systems. Patients' lymphocyte and neutrophil counts were almost completely normal, which is unusual considering they were undergoing chemotherapy and taking immunosuppressant drugs (Merchant & Andre, 2001). Merchant and Andre conducted another study in 2001 in which they focused on chronic diseases. They found that a supplement of 10 g of chlorella tablets and 100 mL of chlorella extract daily for two months helped to ease the symptoms of fibromyalgia in some of the study participants (Merchant & Andre, 2001). In a separate clinical trial, participants showed a decrease in serum cholesterol level when taking chlorella supplements (Merchant & Andre, 2001). More evidence is needed, however, before chlorella supplements can be recommended for these effects.

Some people report that, for the first week after beginning to take chlorella tablets, they experience some gastrointestinal cramping and general discomfort, as well as diarrhea and mild nausea. Because chlorella could help stimulate the immune system, it should be avoided by people who have autoimmune diseases.

Siobhan M. Prout

See Also: Spirulina.

Further Reading

Belasco, W. (1997). Algae burgers for a hungry world? The rise and fall of chlorella cuisine. *Technology and Culture 38* (3), 608–634.

EBSCO CAM Review Board. (2014, September 18). *Spirulina*. Retrieved from http://saltlakegynecology.com/your-health/ condition_detail.dot?id=21606&lang=English&db=hlt&ebscoType=healthlibrary&widgetTitle=FOR+ALL+HOSTS+(DUPLICATE)+****+EBSCO+-+Condition+Detail+v2#ref20

Merchant, R. E., & Andre, C. A. (2001). A review of recent clinical trials of the nutritional supplement Chlorella pyrenoidosa in the treatment of fibromyalgia, hypertension, and ulcerative colitis. *Alternative Therapies in Health and Medicine, 7* (3), 79–90.

Therapeutic Research Faculty (2009). *Chlorella*. WebMD. Natural Medicines Comprehensive Database. Retrieved from http://www.webmd.com/vitamins -supplements/ingredientmono-907-CHLORELLA.aspx?activeIngredientId=907&activ eIngredientName=CHLORELLA

Chloride

Chloride is an essential mineral that helps maintain the balance of fluids within the body, and is an important ingredient in gastric juices secreted by glands in the stomach—especially hydrochloric acid. Chloride comprises 70% of the body's negatively charged particles, thus chloride plays a pivotal role in the conduction of electrical impulses that enable the nervous system to function. As a negative ion it often binds with cations such as sodium, which forms table salt (NaCl) and is the primary source of chloride for humans. Chloride also is found in many foods, especially seaweed, tomatoes, lettuce, celery, and olives.

Chloride deficiency is rarely observed. It is most likely to occur in conditions marked by frequent vomiting, which causes the loss of hydrochloric acid from the stomach contents. Frequent vomiting can occur with the eating disorder bulimia. When frequent self-induced vomiting occurs over a long period (several weeks or months), low blood chloride levels can occur, a condition known as "hypochloremia." Hypochloremia also can occur with other situations that involve extreme loss of bodily fluids through sweating, vomiting, or diarrhea. When the body is chloride deficient the pH of the blood increases. This condition is known as "alkalosis." Alkalosis is a life-threatening state that is accompanied by lethargy, irritability, muscle weakness, and dehydration. Occasionally, ingesting too much water also can result in hypochloremia, causing similar symptoms. Because healthy individuals with adequate water intake are able to excrete excess chloride in urine and sweat, the toxic effects of sodium and potassium typically are felt before those of chloride. High blood chloride levels are uncommon, except with severe dehydration or as a side effect of some medications.

The adequate intake of chloride for adults is 2.3 g per day, and ensures normal ion concentration. The adult upper limit for chloride intake is set at 3.6 g per day. The average daily intake of chloride from salt for people in North American, however, is about 4.5 g per day. Limiting the daily intake of salt—both as table salt and from prepared foods—can help people achieve a more desirable chloride intake.

Patricia M. Cipicchio

See Also: Electrolytes; Stomach.

Further Reading

Bodyventures. (2010). *Chloride*. Diet & Fitness Today. Retrieved from http://www .dietandfitnesstoday.com/chloride.php

Evert, A. (2011). *Chloride in diet*. Medlineplus. National Institutes of Health. Retrieved from http://www.nlm.nih.gov/medlineplus/ency/article/002417.htm

Insel, P., Ross, D., McMahon, K., & Bernstein, M. (2013). *Nutrition*. Burlington, MA: Jones & Bartlett.

Chocolate

Chocolate is a food or flavoring produced from the seeds of the cacao tree. Chocolate often is made into powdered, paste, or solid forms, usually with sweeteners and other ingredients added. Chocolate is especially popular in candy form, but is also added to other foods, such as milk. Chocolate's roots reach back to ancient Mesoamerica (a region that includes what is today parts of Mexico and Central America), where it was first used as a medicinal treatment. The cocoa produced then would be unrecognizable to modern-day connoisseurs. The cacao seed now undergoes a complex process of roasting, grinding, pressing, and mixing into a refined cocoa product.

The merits of chocolate long have been the subject of debate. For many years, chocolate was considered a junk food having no nutritive value. Cocoa, the main ingredient of chocolate derived from cacao seeds, however, has been shown to

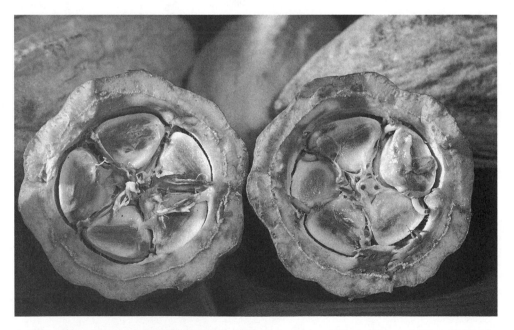

Cocoa or cacao beans in a cacao pod. The pod has a thick, rough rind. The white seeds inside turn brown as they dry. (U.S. Department of Agriculture)

contain compounds that could be beneficial to health. Chocolate contains flavonoids and other phytochemicals, which have recently sparked research interest. Some studies suggest chocolate may improve insulin resistance and cardiovascular health. However, the health effects of chocolate depend upon how it is prepared. A majority of commercial chocolate products, including most chocolate candy, has a low content of flavonoids and antioxidants in addition to high concentrations of sugar.

History of Chocolate

Mesoamerican civilizations are believed to have used cacao seeds and have produced cocoa as early as 600 BCE (Lippi, 2013). A cocoa beverage was used by these civilizations for medicinal purposes. Hernán Cortés was the first conquistador to document the existence of chocolate in 1528 and brought cocoa to Spain for sampling by King Charles. Much later, in 1753, Carl Linnaeus dubbed the *Theobroma* cocoa plant, from which cocoa is developed, the "Chocolate Tree."

Chocolate's euphoric, romantic effects were immediately observed upon its introduction to Europe (Lippi, 2013). The Catholic Church disapproved of chocolate due to these effects (Lippi, 2013). European doctors were quick to incorporate chocolate into medical treatments, citing observations of cocoa uses from Mesoamerica. The *Badianus Manuscript*, written in 1552 by M. De La Cruz, a Mexican teacher, describes the therapeutic uses of cocoa to treat a variety of indigenous disorders and diseases, especially angina, various digestive symptoms, and dental issues. These medical uses in the Americas inspired the European use of chocolate as a treatment for such things as weight loss, weight gain, and digestive issues. Additionally, cocoa was thought to be a nervous-system stimulant (Lippi, 2013).

Chocolate Production

Chocolate is typically divided into three varieties: dark, milk, and white. These chocolates are distinguished by their different ratios of cocoa liquor and cocoa butter. Chocolate production begins with the harvesting of cacao seeds (also referred to as "cocoa beans") from cacao trees. To produce cocoa liquor, the seeds are fermented, dried, cleaned, and roasted. The seeds then are cracked open to harvest the cocoa nibs, which are ground to produce the cocoa mass. Cocoa liquor is the paste made from the nibs of cocoa beans, and contains most of the nutritional components of interest. Cocoa butter is the fatty portion of chocolate refined from the cocoa liquor. The non-fatty portion of cocoa liquor, resulting from the ground and roasted nibs, often is called "nonfat cocoa solids." The nonfat cocoa solids have relatively high concentrations of polyphenols, vitamins, and fiber. Dark chocolate is distinguished by a greater percentage of cocoa liquor. Milk chocolate contains added dairy product (usually powdered milk or sweetened condensed milk) and a lesser percentage of cocoa liquor. White chocolate has no cocoa liquor; it simply is produced from cocoa butter and other additives.

The amount of cocoa liquor in the chocolate determines the percent cocoa, and ultimately what type of chocolate is produced. A minimum of 35% cocoa liquor is needed for the production of dark chocolate. In the United States, generally 10% to 12% cocoa liquor by weight is used for the production of milk chocolate (Katz, Doughty, & Ali, 2011).

Nutrition Content of Chocolate

The fatty acids of the cocoa butter are a combination of saturated and unsaturated fatty acids. There is an unusually high concentration of stearic acid, which has a neutral effect on the cholesterol profile, appearing to neither increase nor decrease serum cholesterol levels.

The nonfat cocoa solids (which make up the majority of chocolate liquor) include the bran of the cocoa seed, which contains fiber. Most fiber is lost in the processing of the cocoa seed; however about 1.7 to 0.6 grams of fiber are found in a 100 kcal portion of dark or milk chocolate (Katz, Doughty, & Ali, 2011). Cocoa contains mostly insoluble fibers. There are very low amounts of other vitamins and minerals in the nonfat cocoa solids. These micronutrients include copper, magnesium, potassium, and iron. A number of phytochemicals are found in the nonfat cocoa solids and are of particular interest in recent research.

Chocolate and Health

Modern studies of the possible health benefits of chocolate were inspired by studies of the Kuna Island natives. Kuna Island is located off the coast of Panama. Kuna Indians have an unusually low risk for heart disease and lower blood pressure than other groups having comparable salt intake and weight (NIH, 2011). It was noted that the Kuna consume more than ten times the amount of cocoa as compared to the average American. Additionally the Kuna people consume a much less processed form of cocoa, thought to be higher in flavonoids. Upon moving away from the island, Kuna natives experience an increased risk in heart disease, an increase in blood pressure, and a decrease in cocoa intake. It is unclear how much of the explanation for these observations can be attributed to chocolate. Nevertheless, the research generated by these studies has led to some interesting findings.

Antioxidants and Chocolate

Cocoa is a very flavonoid-rich food. Flavonoids are credited for the main antioxidant properties of chocolate, and flavonoid antioxidants are associated with the plasma's ability to better protect itself from oxidative damage. Plasma is the fluid component of human blood, and contains many molecular elements that are essential to nutrition, immune function, and clotting. Flavonoids also are being investigated for antibacterial, antiviral, anti-inflammatory, and anticancer roles, although these functions have not yet been linked specifically to chocolate's flavonoids.

Most flavonoids are found in the cocoa liquor and derive from the nonfat chocolate solids. Higher concentrations of cocoa liquor are correlated with higher amounts of flavonoids and more antioxidant properties. Flavonoid concentrations often vary greatly between different chocolates; this probably is due to variance in cocoa-seed processing.

Health Benefits of Chocolate

A recent meta-analysis supports the idea that cocoa flavonoids help reduce insulin resistance and improve blood glucose regulation (Hooper et al. 2012). These observations in part could be due to chocolate's effects on endothelial function. Endothelial function refers to the normal dilation and constriction of the arteries due to adequate responses to signaling molecules such as nitrous oxide. Improvements in endothelial function also could explain the association of chocolate consumption with reductions in resting diastolic blood pressure and with heart health. Researchers have proposed that the improved blood flow seen in chocolate studies might explain preliminary results observing better cognitive function with chocolate consumption. Consumption of chocolate has been shown to improve mood in many people, and chocolate appears to have an effect on the central nervous system, possibly through the release of neurotransmitters associated with positive affect in the reward system of the brain.

Recommendations for Chocolate Intake

People who enjoy chocolate and hope for health benefits from its consumption are advised to consume up to 3 oz (85 g) of dark chocolate daily. Chocolate should be labeled as containing at least 65% cocoa. This amount of chocolate can contain hundreds of calories, so people adding chocolate to their diets must subtract calories in other areas to avoid weight gain.

Robin E. Currens and Cheri M. Eschete

See Also: Antioxidants; Phytochemicals.

Further Reading

Beckett, S. T. (2009). Traditional chocolate making. In S. T. Beckett (Ed.), *Industrial chocolate manufacture and use* (4th ed.), pp. 1–9. Oxford, United Kingdom: Wiley-Blackwell.

Hooper, L., Kay, C., Abdelhamid, A., Kroon, P. A., Cohn, J. S., Rimm, E. B., & Cassidy, A. (2012). Effects of chocolate, cocoa, and flavan-3-ols on cardiovascular health: A systematic review and meta-analysis of randomized trials. *American Journal of Clinical Nutrition, 95,* 740–751. doi: 10.3945/ajcn.111.023457

Katz, D. L., Doughty, K., & Ali, A. (2011). Cocoa and chocolate in human health and disease. *Antioxidants and Redox Signaling, 15* (10), 2779–2811. doi: 10.1089/ars.2010.3697

Lippi, D. (2013). Chocolate in history: Food, medicine, and medi-food. *Nutrients, 5,* 1573–1584. doi: 10.3390/nu5051573

National Institutes of Health (NIH). (2011, August). Claims about cocoa: Can chocolate really be good for you? *NIH News in Health,* 1–2. Retrieved from http://newsinhealth. nih.gov/issue/aug2011/feature1

Zeratsky, K. (2012, February 4). *Can chocolate be good for my health?* Mayo Clinic: Nutrition and Healthy Eating. Retrieved from http://www.mayoclinic.com/health /healthy-chocolate/AN02060

Cholesterol

Cholesterol belongs to a group of chemical compounds called sterols and is found both in foods and in the human body. Cholesterol is made from four linked hydrocarbon rings with a hydrocarbon group at one end and a hydroxyl group at the other end. It is an important lipid involved in membrane permeability and fluidity, and is found in varying degrees in practically all animal membranes. Cholesterol is the precursor of steroid hormones such as progesterone, testosterone, estrogens, and cortisol. It also is the precursor of vitamin D. Cholesterol can be obtained from both animal products in a diet and be synthesized de novo by the body from its precursor acetyl CoA, an activated carrier molecule of great importance in cellular metabolism. The liver manufactures bile from cholesterol. Bile is important for the digestion and absorption of fats and fat-soluble vitamins. The liver is the major site of cholesterol synthesis in mammals. The small intestine also produces significant amounts of cholesterol. The rate of synthesis of cholesterol by the body can vary greatly, based on how much cholesterol is consumed in the diet. Blood levels of cholesterol and cholesterol-transport compounds are somewhat predictive of a person's risk for the development of artery disease and its complications, including heart attack and stroke. Overall diet patterns, as well as several dietary components, appear to influence blood cholesterol levels.

Cholesterol in both the diet and as a component of artery disease came under scrutiny in the 1950s as researchers began to investigate artery disease etiology. Observing that arterial plaque contains high concentrations of cholesterol and other lipids, researchers began to explore the association between dietary cholesterol and fats, serum cholesterol levels, artery disease development and progression, and end points such as heart attack and stroke. Researchers now believe that intake of dietary fat and cholesterol does influence artery disease development, but in complex ways, primarily through the behavior of cholesterol-carrying compounds known as lipoproteins.

Cholesterol is transported from its sites of synthesis or absorption to the sites of use, and finally to the liver for excretion by transport molecules called lipoproteins. Lipoproteins are composed of cholesterol, triglycerides, phospholipids, and proteins. They have nonpolar, hydrophobic regions in the center, with polar regions on the exterior, allowing the compounds to travel in the aqueous environment of the body. Lipoproteins exist in several forms; they are classified based on their increasing density in plasma. Higher levels of low-density lipoprotein (LDL) cholesterol are associated with increased risk of artery disease. Low-density lipoproteins appear to promote arterial damage when they become oxidized and bind with the artery lining. Higher levels of high-density lipoprotein (HDL) cholesterol, however, are associated with lower risk of artery disease; thus LDLs are known as the "bad" cholesterol, and HDLs are known as the "good cholesterol." The HDLs transport cholesterol from plasma and deliver it to the liver where cholesterol is converted to bile and excreted. Additionally, HDLs shuttle cholesterol throughout the body to the tissues where cholesterol is used to synthesize the steroid hormones.

Cholesterol and Artery Disease

High serum cholesterol levels increase artery disease risk. This risk was first observed in people with abnormally high serum cholesterol levels because of an inherited condition known as familial hypercholesterolemia. This condition is characterized by deposition of cholesterol in various tissues. Familial hypercholesterolemia is not due to diet failure, but rather to the inability the LDL receptors located throughout the body to take up triglycerides because of a defect in the LDL receptors.

As research continued to accumulate evidence that blood levels of total cholesterol, LDL cholesterol, and HDL cholesterol are related to artery disease risk, in 1985 the U.S. National Heart, Lung, and Blood Institute (NHLBI) launched the National Cholesterol Education Program (NCEP). The program has promoted public education regarding the importance of diagnosing and treating high cholesterol levels. High LDL cholesterol levels can be reduced by both lifestyle measures and medications. Lifestyle measures that promote healthful blood cholesterol levels include regular physical activity, weight control to achieve healthful body fat levels, and a heart-healthy diet.

Diet and Cholesterol

Studies on serum cholesterol, foods, and diet pattern have found that dietary change and cholesterol-lowering functional foods and dietary supplements are possible alternative therapies for lowering plasma total cholesterol and LDL cholesterol, especially for people whose blood cholesterol level is slightly high but not high enough to necessitate the prescription of cholesterol-lowering medication. Dietary patterns associated with improved blood cholesterol levels include almost any weight-loss diet, including low-carbohydrate diets (such as the Atkins diet), low-fat diets, and Mediterranean-type diets. Weight-loss diets are effective for short-term cholesterol reduction. For long-term weight-loss maintenance and blood cholesterol control, both low-fat and Mediterranean-type diets have strong support. Nutrition professionals recommend diets high in plant foods, including fruits, vegetables, and legumes. Consumption of foods high in saturated fats, such as high-fat

What Do Your Cholesterol Numbers Mean?

Lipoprotein cholesterol levels are predictive of heart disease risk, therefore adults are urged to monitor these levels. The National Heart, Lung, and Blood Institute (NHLBI) launched the National Cholesterol Education Program (NCEP) in November 1985. The following advice comes from NCEP's Web site. More-detailed information is available there.

Everyone age 20 years and older should have their cholesterol measured at least once every 5 years. It is best to have a blood test called a "lipoprotein profile" to determine cholesterol numbers. Cholesterol levels are measured in milligrams (mg) of cholesterol per deciliter (dL) of blood. This blood test is done after a 9- to 12-hour fast and gives information about the following.

- Total cholesterol
- LDL (bad) cholesterol—The main source of cholesterol buildup and blockage in the arteries
- HDL (good) cholesterol—Helps keep cholesterol from building up in the arteries
- Triglycerides—another form of fat in the blood

If it is not possible to get a lipoprotein profile done, knowing the total cholesterol and HDL cholesterol can provide a general idea about cholesterol levels. If total cholesterol is 200 mg/dL or more, or if HDL is less than 40 mg/dL, then a lipoprotein profile should be performed. For comparison, cholesterol numbers are provided in the tables below.

Table 1. Cholesterol Level Categories

Total Cholesterol Level	Category
Less than 200 mg/dL	Desirable
200–239 mg/dL	Borderline High
240 mg/dL and greater	High

* Cholesterol levels are measured in milligrams (mg) of cholesterol per deciliter (dL) of blood.

Source: U.S. Department of Health and Human Services. (2005). *High blood cholesterol: what you need to know*. Retrieved from http://www.nhlbi.nih.gov/health/public/heart/chol/wyntk.htm

Table 2. LDL Cholesterol Level Categories

LDL Cholesterol Level	LDL-Cholesterol Category
Less than 100 mg/dL	Optimal
100–129 mg/dL	Near optimal/above optimal
130–159 mg/dL	Borderline high
160–189 mg/dL	High
190 mg/dL and greater	Very high

Source: U.S. Department of Health and Human Services. (2005). *High blood cholesterol: what you need to know*. Retrieved from http://www.nhlbi.nih.gov/health/public/heart/chol/wyntk.htm

HDL (good) cholesterol protects against heart disease, thus, for HDL, higher numbers are better. A level less than 40 mg/dL is low and is considered a major risk factor because it increases the risk for developing heart disease. HDL levels of 60 mg/dL or more help to reduce the risk of heart disease.

Triglycerides also can increase heart disease risk. Levels that are borderline high (150–199 mg/dL) or high (200 mg/dL or more) could require treatment for some people.

U.S. Department of Health and Human Services. (2005). *High blood cholesterol: what you need to know.* Retrieved from http://www.nhlbi.nih.gov/health/public/heart/chol/wyntk.htm

meats and processed meats, should be reduced. Although intake of dietary cholesterol does not appear to have a strong effect on serum cholesterol levels in healthy people, some public health organizations continue to recommend keeping daily cholesterol intake below 300 mg. People with type 2 diabetes, obesity, or heart disease appear to be most sensitive to cholesterol intake and should try to limit foods such as eggs that are high in cholesterol.

Several specific foods and food components exert modest cholesterol-lowering effects. They appear to work through a variety of mechanisms; for example, many act as bile acid sequestrants. Excessive cholesterol can be eliminated from the body via formation of bile acids, and secretion of bile into the small intestine. Bile acid sequestrants bind bile acids in the intestine, and inhibit their reabsorption by producing an insoluble complex. Inhibition of bile acid reabsorption decreases hepatic cholesterol concentration, increases synthesis of bile acids from cholesterol, and causes an entry of plasma cholesterol into the liver, because the lowered level of hepatic cholesterol increases the expression of LDL receptors. Phytochemicals in a variety of foods also appear to interact at other steps in cholesterol pathways. Foods and food components that might influence serum cholesterol levels include the following.

- Foods with water-soluble dietary fibers—Non-digestible polysaccharides and fermentation-produced short chain fatty acids are the active ingredients in water-soluble fibers. They work by inhibiting bile acid reabsorption and cholesterol absorption. Oatmeal, oat bran, and other high-fiber foods contain water-soluble fiber.
- Fish and omega-3 fatty acids—These foods alter blood lipid profile. Walnuts, almonds, and other nuts also have beneficial fatty acids and fiber.
- Plant sterols and stanols—These phytochemicals often are added to margarines and other foods designed to help control blood cholesterol levels. They block the reabsorption of cholesterol.
- Olive oil—Using olive oil for cooking and for salad dressing is associated with reductions in blood cholesterol.
- Other phytochemicals: Garlic, soy foods, and green tea contain an abundance of phytochemicals that have shown cholesterol-lowering effects in some studies.

Many dietary supplements and herbal remedies claim to help reduce high blood cholesterol levels. One of the most effective is red yeast rice, a therapeutic agent from traditional Chinese medicine. Red yeast rice is prepared by fermenting a type of yeast over rice. This herbal medicine contains statins similar in nature to those in cholesterol-lowering medication. High-dose niacin supplements can also be helpful for reducing LDL cholesterol and raising HDL cholesterol. Some studies, however, have found increased stroke risk in patients already taking statins who were given high-dose niacin supplements. Because both red yeast rice and high-dose niacin supplements behave as drugs, use should be carefully monitored.

Djene Keita and Paulina M. Solis

See Also: Cardiovascular disease and nutrition; Gallbladder and gallbladder disease; Lipids; Lipoproteins; The liver; Niacin.

Further Reading

Chen, Z., Ma, K. Y., Liang, Y., Peng, C., & Zuo, Y. (2011). Role and classification of cholesterol-lowering functional foods. *Journal of Functional Foods, 3* (2), 61–69.

Cohen, J. S., Kamili A., Wat, E., Chung, R. W. S., & Tandy, S. (2010). Reduction in intestinal cholesterol absorption by various food components: Mechanisms and implications. *Atherosclerosis Supplements, 11* (1), 45–48.

Schekman, R. (2013). Discovery of the cellular and molecular basis of cholesterol control. *Proceedings of the National Academy of Sciences, 110* (37), 14833–14836. http://www.pnas.org/content/110/37/14833.full

U.S.D.A. Center for Nutrition Policy and Promotion. (2010). *Report of the DGAC on the Dietary Guidelines for Americans (2010). Part D. Section 3: Fatty Acids and Cholesterol.* Retrieved from http://www.cnpp.usda.gov/DietaryGuidelines

Choline

Choline is a substance that is similar in structure and function to vitamins, so it is commonly referred to as a "vitamin-like compound." It plays several significant roles in the human body. In healthy people the liver is able to synthesize most of the choline required for good health from the amino acid precursors methionine and serine. Because deficiency symptoms develop in some people (especially men) on a choline-free diet over time, however, choline is classified as an essential nutrient, meaning it must be obtained from the diet. A relative latecomer to the Dietary Reference Intakes table, choline was first recognized as an essential nutrient by the Institute of Medicine in 1998. The adequate intake for choline is 550 mg per day for adult men and 425 mg per day for adult women. Choline is plentiful in a mixed diet, as it is found in many foods, including meats, liver, eggs, nuts, beans, cauliflower, and spinach.

Functions

Choline forms part of the important neurotransmitter acetylcholine. It is also a component of bile, which aids in the digestion of lipids. Choline is a component of—and is required for—the synthesis of several phospholipids which serve as structural components of cell membranes, including a form of lecithin called phosphatidylcholine. Some of these phospholipids also are precursors for the intracellular messenger molecules diacylglycerol and ceramide. These messengers are important for healthy cellular function. Choline also serves as a donor of methyl groups (CH_3), a step in many important metabolic pathways. Researchers have explored possible health benefits related to choline intake.

Cognitive Function

Choline's role in the formation of the neurotransmitter acetylcholine has prompted research into the relationship between choline intake and cognitive function. Preliminary research with small groups of Alzheimer's disease patients found that those receiving supplemental choline showed a slight improvement in symptoms as compared to a control group (EBSCO, 2009). Similarly, research with a small group of stroke patients found slightly better chance of full recovery in the patients receiving choline as compared to those in the control group (EBSCO, 2009).

Liver Disease

When choline deficient, some people develop a condition called "fatty liver" and show signs of liver damage. Choline is required to form part of very low-density lipoprotein (VLDL) molecules which transport fat from the liver to tissues. Without choline, VLDL particles cannot be synthesized and fat accumulates in the liver, eventually leading to liver damage (Ziesel, 2009). In rats, a deficiency in choline also is associated with increased liver cancer and increased sensitivity to carcinogenic chemicals, although the implication of these observations for humans presently is unknown.

Neural Tube Defects

A few preliminary studies suggest that higher than recommended choline intakes might be beneficial for preventing birth defects known as "neural tube defects." Such neural tube defects include spina bifida, in which the developing spinal column fails to close properly, and anencephaly, in which the brain fails to develop properly. In a recent case-controlled study of pregnant women, higher dietary choline levels were associated with fewer neural tube defects in the children (Zeisel, 2009). The B vitamin folate is well known as a methyl donor, important for the high levels of cellular division that occur during fetal development. It is possible that future research will show that adequate choline levels also are important in this context.

Cardiovascular Disease

As a methyl group donor, choline might assist in the conversion of homocysteine to methionine. Higher serum homocysteine levels are associated with greater levels of systemic inflammation and an increased risk of artery disease. Researchers do not know whether elevated levels of homocysteine actually cause heart disease, and research linking serum choline levels to cardiovascular disease is weak.

Toxicity

High doses of choline result in a fishy body odor, vomiting, low blood pressure, and increased sweating. The fishy odor is due to excessive production and excretion of thimethylamine (TMA), a product of choline. The tolerable upper intake level of choline was set by the Food and Nutrition Board in 1998 at 3.5 g per day for adults.

Recent research on the association of a compound called tri-methylamine-N-oxide (TMAO) with increased risk of heart disease suggests that choline supplementation should be avoided unless medically necessary. TMAO is synthesized by the liver from TMA. Thimethylamine is made by bacteria residing in the colon from the precursors choline and carnitine. (Carnitine is an amino acid that is plentiful in meat.) It is not known whether TMAO contributes to cardiovascular disease, but the higher levels of TMAO observed in meat eaters as compared to vegetarians has been suggested as a possible explanation for the link between higher intakes of red meat and cardiovascular disease (Koeth, Wang, Levison et al., 2013).

Barbara A. Brehm and Emily Ohrtman

See Also: Carnitine; Lecithin; Lipids; Phospholipids.

Further Reading

Berkeley Wellness. (2010, November 11). *Should you boost your choline?* Retrieved from http://www.berkeleywellness.com/supplements/vitamins/article/should-you-boost-your -choline

EBSCO CAM Review Board. (2012). Choline. *Natural and Alternative Treatments.* Retrieved from http://healthlibrary.epnet.com/GetContent.aspx?token=e0498803-7f62 -4563-8d47-5fe33da65dd4&chunkiid=21658

Koeth, R. A., Wang, Z., Levison, B. S., et al. (2013). Intestinal microbiota metabolism of L-carnitine, a nutrient in red meat, promotes atherosclerosis. *Nature Medicine, 19,* 576–585. doi: 10.1038/nm.3145

Ziesel, S. H. (2009, August 18). *Choline.* Micronutrient Information Center, Linus Pauling Institute. Retrieved from http://lpi.oregonstate.edu/infocenter/othernuts/choline

Chromium

Chromium is a trace mineral that is essential for various biological processes. It is relatively abundant in the earth's crust and is a transition element, which means it can exist in many ionic forms (Chromium I-VI). It primarily is found in two forms, however, trivalent chromium (Cr III) and hexavalent chromium (Cr VI). The dietary form is trivalent chromium and essential to the human body. The hexavalent form generally is a by-product of industrial pollution and can be very hazardous to human health. This entry focuses on trivalent chromium. Chromium has been found to play an important role in insulin metabolism, and also in metabolizing carbohydrates, fats, and proteins.

Chromium was first discovered by French chemist Louis Nicolas Vauquelin in 1797; however, its nutritional value was not discovered until 1957, by NIH scientists Walter Mertz and Klaus Schwarz (Pazirandeh, Bums, & Griffin, 2014). Mertz and Schwarz discovered that a compound extracted from the kidneys of pigs was able to reverse hyperglycemia in rats and was termed "glucose tolerance factor" (Pazirandeh, Bums, & Griffin, 2014). This later was found to be chromium. Interestingly, one hospital found that several of their patients on parenteral nutrition feeds (a method of delivering nutrition intravenously with special formulas) developed signs of diabetes, including weight loss, neuropathy, and impaired glucose tolerance. This was reversed when 150 to 250 mcg per day of chromium was added to the feeding solution. Thus, chromium now is a standard component of intravenous nutrition for critically ill patients.

Chromium is required in very small amounts. True chromium deficiency is rare in the nonhospitalized patient population, and there are no well-documented diseases associated with chromium deficiency in the general population. Chromium is absorbed via the small intestine and transported in the circulation bound to albumin and transferrin. Intestinal absorption has been estimated to be less than 0.4% to 2.5% of the amount ingested; the rest is excreted in the feces (Pazirandeh, Bums, & Griffin, 2014). There is enhanced absorption of chromium in the setting of iron and zinc deficiency, likely because chromium competes with iron and zinc for intestinal absorption. Certain medications can interfere with chromium absorption, including nonsteroidal anti-inflammatory medications and antacids (Kroner, 2011). Vitamin C coadministration enhances the absorption of chromium. Chromium can be lost from the body in the urine if the diet contains an excessive amount of simple sugars (more than 35%), or in times of physical stress, such as during rigorous exercise, pregnancy, or illness (Kroner, 2011).

Chromium's role in the body is not entirely clear, but it does appear to play a role in glucose tolerance and it enhances the action of insulin. Chromium is taken up by insulin-dependent cells and goes through a series of steps that leads to activation of tyrosine kinase, an enzyme that propagates insulin activity (Kroner, 2011). Insulin, in turn, allows for entry of glucose into most cells; glucose then can be used to fuel various processes within the body.

The relationship between chromium and diabetes has been studied, and several studies have shown improvement in glucose tolerance with chromium supplementation both in vitro and in vivo. Two double-blind, placebo-controlled studies examining the effects of chromium on factors such as weight loss, metabolic syndrome, and glucose tolerance did not find a significant benefit for those participants taking chromium versus those who took a placebo (NIH, 2013; Igbal, Cardillo, & Volger, 2009). Another large analysis, however, suggested that supplementation with chromium picolinate could have a beneficial effect for patients with diabetes (Kroner, 2011). Patients had improvement in glucose levels, decreased LDL cholesterol and triglycerides, with improvement in HDL levels (Kroner, 2011). Because not all studies have found beneficial results, however, the American Diabetes Association cautions that chromium supplements probably only are helpful for people with a chromium deficiency.

The Institute of Medicine currently recommends a dietary intake of 30 mcg to 35 mcg of chromium per day for adult men, and 20 mcg to 25 mcg daily for adult women, with slightly higher doses for lactating and pregnant women (up to 45 mcg per day) (NIH, 2013). Dietary sources of chromium include some meats, vegetables including green peppers and black pepper, broccoli, and whole-grain products (*see* Table 1) (NIH, 2013). Likewise, toxicity from chromium intake has not been well documented, and at this time the Food and Nutrition Board has not defined a recommended upper limit. Some possible side effects of excessive chromium

Table 1. Selected Food Sources of Chromium

Food	Chromium (mcg)
Broccoli, ½ cup	11
Grape juice, 1 cup	8
English muffin, whole wheat, 1	4
Potatoes, mashed, 1 cup	3
Garlic, dried, 1 teaspoon	3
Basil, dried, 1 tablespoon	2
Beef cubes, 3 ounces	2
Orange juice, 1 cup	2
Turkey breast, 3 ounces	2
Whole wheat bread, 2 slices	2
Red wine, 5 ounces	1–13
Apple, unpeeled, 1 medium	1
Banana, 1 medium	1
Green beans, ½ cup	1

Source: National Institutes of Health. Office of Dietary Supplements. (2013). *Chromium. Dietary Supplements Fact Sheet.* http://ods.od.nih.gov/factsheets/Chromium-HealthProfessional/

References: Anderson, R. A., Bryden, N. A., & Polansky, M. M. Dietary chromium intake: Freely chosen diets, institutional diets and individual foods. *Biol Trace Elem Res 1992*, 32, 117–121; Cabrera-Vique, C., Teissedre, P.-L., Cabanis, M.-T., & Cabinis, J.-C. Determination and levels of chromium in French wine and grapes by graphite furnace atomic absorption spectrometry. *J Agric Food Chem 1997*, 45, 1808–1811; and Dattilo, A. M., Miguel, S. G. Chromium in health and disease. *Nutrition Today 2003*, 38: 121–133.

intake include decreased iron absorption, and there have been some case reports of renal failure, stomach irritation, liver problems, and stomach ulcers associated with high intake of chromium supplements, but these cases are rare and are potentially due to other coexisting variables.

Libi Z. Galmer

See Also: Minerals.

Further Reading

Ehrlich, S. D. (2013, May 7). *Chromium*. University of Maryland Medical Center. Retrieved from https://umm.edu/health/medical/altmed/supplement/chromium

Igbal, N., Cardillo, S., & Volger, S. (2009). Chromium picolinate does not improve key features of metabolic syndrome in obese nondiabetic adults. *Metabolic Syndrome Related Disorders, 7* (2), 143–150.

Kroner, Z. (2011). "Chromium." In Z. Kroner (Ed.), *Vitamins and Minerals*. Santa Barbara, CA: ABC-CLIO.

National Institutes of Health (NIH), Office of Dietary Supplements. (2013, November 4). *Chromium*. Retrieved from http://ods.od.nih.gov/factsheets/Chromium -HealthProfessional/

Pazirandeh, S., Bums, D., & Griffin, J. (2014). *Overview of dietary trace minerals*. UpToDate. Retrieved from http://www.uptodate.com/contents/overview-of-dietary-trace -minerals?source=search_result&search=chromium&selectedTitle=1~51

Climate Change and Global Food Supply

The term "climate" refers to patterns of temperature, precipitation, humidity, wind, and seasons; the term "climate change" refers to changes in these patterns. The impacts of climate change can be seen not only on the weather system but in ecosystems as well. Both are linked to effects on the global food supply. Environmental changes have been on the forefront of political and scientific debate in how to handle policy and technology in preparation for the future. The world population has continued to increase, and because environmental changes suggest changes in food security, the relationship between climate change and food supply is especially relevant.

The earth has gone through—and continues to experience—climatic changes, and has been subject to many cycles of warm and cool periods. The earth currently is leaving a cool period and entering a warm period. The speed of the current warming trend is attributed to a variety of factors, including changes in solar activity and increased production of greenhouse gases that capture and accumulate heat from the sun. The present increase in average global temperature is predicted to continue, and will influence local climates, weather patterns, and ecosystems in many ways.

Climate Change and Agriculture

The interconnectedness between climate change and food supply is quite clear. Agricultural crops need a healthy and stable environment to provide for the human population. Because plants require specific water availability, temperatures, healthy soil, and insects for growth and reproduction, climate change has put many agricultural systems at risk. Natural ecosystems, as well as human economies and cultures, have emerged and have been sustained by stable climate patterns. Because so many systems are tied to climate, a change in climate therefore means a change in the ecosystems of people, plants, and animals.

To see the interconnection between climate change and ecosystems, imagine, for example, a change in the usual timing of rains or a change in seasonal temperatures. The blooming of plants and the production of fruits or the hatching of insects would be in disarray. This, in turn, would affect the synergy between pollination of crops, food for migrating birds, spawning of fish, water supplies for drinking and irrigation, forest health, and more. Climate change can increase diseases in crops and other plants, as well as in farm animals. Weeds and pests also are influenced by the weather and climate change.

Current climate-change patterns have been associated with an increase in extreme weather events, such as tornadoes, hurricanes, and other storms, usually accompanied by heavy precipitation, floods, and coastline storm surges. Heat waves and droughts also are becoming more common in various parts of the world. Weather extremes always have been a part of agriculture, but these extremes are predicted to become more common and thus more disruptive to food production. The effect of severe weather on agricultural production is familiar to most people. Increased temperatures can reduce crop yields. Droughts or heavy rains can destroy crops completely.

Climate Change and Freshwater Supplies

Climate change is likely to affect an already precarious freshwater supply in many world regions. Droughts influence not only agricultural crops, but also farm animals and people. Flooding can cause contamination of water supplies, as sewage and unsanitary groundwater infiltrate stores of drinking water. Increased temperatures have caused the melting of snow and ice in many regions, causing sea levels to rise. Rising sea levels threaten vulnerable coastline communities around the world. Coastline storm surges bring flooding and disruption of drinking-water supplies, along with damage to farms and other food production, storage, and transportation systems in a region.

Climate Change and Food Security

According to the World Health Organization, food security occurs "when all people at all times have access to sufficient, safe, and nutritious food to maintain a healthy and active life" (WHO, 2013). Food security relies not only on food production, but also on adequate storage and transportation systems—all of which can be disrupted by extreme weather, such as severe storms and flooding. Climate change not only affects food production directly through changes in ecological conditions, but also indirectly by affecting growth and distribution of incomes and thus demands for agricultural produce.

When food production or food availability declines, food prices increase. Individuals in richer countries enjoy a diverse food supply and are better able to handle an increase in food prices. People in poor countries, however, already have limited access to sufficient high-quality and nutritious foods. They might subsist on staple grains, consuming a single food such as rice or wheat as part of each meal and obtaining a majority of daily calories from that one food. A change in price or availability of that food staple is extremely disruptive to food security for such individuals. Families in some countries normally spend 75% of their income on food and cannot adapt to further increases in food prices (Carty, 2012). Increased food prices also often lead to civil unrest. In 2008, for example, food riots erupted in more than 20 countries, with unrest toppling the Haitian government (Gillis, 2012). Poorer countries are less able to cope with extreme weather or political events that disrupt the production, storage, and transportation of food to its citizens than are resource-rich countries. Therefore the increasing prices are not the only problem; sometimes food simply is not available in certain areas.

Future Directions

Scientists and environmental organizations are attempting to predict patterns of climate change using various models. Although no one can say exactly how climate change will proceed over the coming decades, change itself appears to be a certainty. Local, national, and world organizations must work together to diversify food production, storage, and transportation systems. Communities must invest in sustainable and resilient agriculture to increase local access to food and to increase food reserves that could become available to regions suffering from food insecurity. Communities at all levels must increase disaster preparedness so that they can respond as effectively as possible when severe weather strikes, and ensure that residents have access to clean water and food. Countries and nongovernmental funding agencies must support research on the effects of climate change and the managing of ecosystems under the influence of climate change and severe weather. Comprehensive study of specific regional and local effects of climate change must be performed to help understand and manage the state of the future food supply.

Erika S. Marin and Barbara A. Brehm

Research Issues

In the United States, Hurricane Katrina in 2005 and Hurricane Sandy in 2012 caused disruption of freshwater supplies and food availability. Use the Internet to access local news reports written during one of these disasters and find descriptions of how these storms influenced water and food availability for local residents. Examine the local and national response to these disasters. What actions appeared to be most effective? What should local and national governments do to reduce the negative impact of future storms?

See Also: Global hunger and malnutrition; Sustainable agriculture.

Further Reading

Carty, T. (2012, September). *Extreme weather, extreme prices*. Oxfam International. Retrieved from http://www.oxfamamerica.org/files/Extreme-Weather-Extreme-Prices.pdf

Gillis, J. (2012, September 6). Climate change and the food supply. *New York Times*. Retrieved from http://green.blogs.nytimes.com/2012/09/06/climate-change-and-the-food-supply/

Godfray, H. C. J., Crute, I. R., Haddad, L., et al. (2010). The future of the global food system. *Philosophical Transactions of the Royal Society: Biological Sciences, 365* (1554), 2769–2777. Retrieved from http://rstb.royalsocietypublishing.org/content/365/1554/2769.full.pdf+html

Schmidhuber, J., & Tubiello, F. N. (2007, December 11). Global food security under climate change. *Proceedings of the National Academy of Sciences of the United States of America, 104* (50), 19703–19708. Retrieved from http://www.pnas.org/content/104/50/19703.full

Washington State Department of Ecology. (2012). *Preparing for a changing climate.* Retrieved from http://www.ecy.wa.gov/climatechange/whatis.htm

World Health Organization (WHO). (2013). *Trade, foreign policy, diplomacy, and health; Food security.* Retrieved from http://www.who.int/trade/glossary/story028/en/

Coenzyme Q10

Coenzyme Q10 (CoQ10) is a naturally occurring compound found in the mitochondria of cells. It participates in pathways of cellular respiration and energy production, and is a member of the ubiquinone group of compounds. Forms of CoQ10 can function as both lipid-soluble antioxidants and as electron carriers in ATP production. As an antioxidant, CoQ10 reduces free radicals by giving up its outer shell electrons as well as accepting electrons from other atoms, thus preventing the production of lipid peroxyl radicals which can damage cellular components. In the electron transport chain, CoQ10 co-performs the role of an electron carrier with vitamin K2 in several enzyme complexes.

The term "ubiquinone" is derived from the words "ubiquitous"—chosen because early chemists observed these compounds in all animal cells—and "benzoquinone," which is a chemical group found in ubiquinone structures. Ubiquinones contain 1 to 12 5-carbon isoprene units. CoQ10 has 10 isoprene units, hence its name. CoQ10 was first isolated in 1957 by Frederick Crane (Crane, 2007). The name "ubiquinone" was coined in England by Professor R. A. Morton, who identified CoQ10 in rat liver. In 1958, scientist Karl Folkers discovered the exact chemical structure of CoQ10 and developed processes to synthesize it (Discovery, 2014). In 1978, Peter Mitchell received the Nobel Prize in Chemistry for his research on CoQ10 in mitochondrial energy transduction and his chemiosmotic hypothesis.

Mitchell's hypothesis suggested that most ATP synthesis in cells comes from the electron transport chain—the electrochemical gradient across the inner membranes of mitochondria—by using the energy from specialized electron carriers that are formed by breaking down energy-rich molecules (Press Release, 1978).

Because CoQ10 is produced by the body it is not considered an essential nutrient. The human body, however, also obtains CoQ10 from foods. The foods highest in CoQ10 include meat and fish, but CoQ10 also is found in oils, nuts, seeds, and some fruits and vegetables. Physiological CoQ10 levels decline with age and certain disease states. This has prompted researchers to investigate possible therapeutic benefits of supplementing with this compound. Research suggests that CoQ10 supplements could be effective for reducing high blood pressure and the symptoms of congestive heart failure (Mayo Clinic Staff, 2013). Preliminary evidence suggests that CoQ10 supplementation might be helpful for a number of other health problems, although more research is required to confirm these potential benefits. Researchers presently are exploring the use of CoQ10 supplements for many conditions, including the following (Mayo Clinic Staff, 2013).

- Age-related eye disease—CoQ10 might slow the development of age-related macular degeneration and cataracts, probably because of its antioxidant activity.
- Coronary artery disease—CoQ10 appears to reduce levels of inflammation in the arteries.
- Muscle weakness accompanying statin therapy—Statins reduce production of CoQ10, therefore supplementation might offset this effect.
- Parkinson's disease and other neurological disorders—CoQ10 appears to have neuroprotective effects.
- Male infertility—CoQ10 contributes to the production of healthy sperm.
- Asthma—CoQ10 might help counteract the inflammatory processes associated with an inappropriate immune response.
- Cancer—CoQ10 might reduce the risk of breast cancer. The role of CoQ10 in breast cancer carcinogenesis is unclear, but it might reduce the growth of cancer cells by reducing inflammation and oxidative stress. CoQ10 also has been used to reduce the side effects of chemotherapy, especially in children.
- Chronic fatigue syndrome—CoQ10 could enhance energy production for people with chronic fatigue syndrome.

Because of its important roles in energy production, CoQ10 supplements often are used by athletes, although research supporting this use is sparse. Supplements seem to be fairly safe up to doses of about 1,200 mg per day in healthy adults (Higdon, Drake, & Stocker, 2014). Typical doses are closer to 30 mg to 100 mg per day. Coenzyme Q10 has been known to negatively interfere with anticoagulant therapies. People taking CoQ10 for health problems should work with their health care providers to be sure the supplement is recommended for their situations.

Stephanie DeFrank and Barbara A. Brehm

See Also: Dietary supplements.

Further Reading

Crane, F. L. (2007). Discovery of ubiquinone (coenzyme Q) and an overview of function. *Mitochondrion, 7S*, S2–S7. Retrieved from https://www.grc.com/sr6dev/misc/coq10/The%20Discovery%20of%20Ubiquinone.pdf

Discovery of coenzyme Q10. (2014, January 9). *History of science.* Retrieved from http://historyofsciences.blogspot.com/2014/01/discovery-of-coenzyme-q10.html

Higdon, J., Drake, V. J., & Stocker, R. (2014, November 30). *Coenzyme Q_{10}.* Linus Pauling Institute, Oregon State University. Retrieved from http://lpi.oregonstate.edu/infocenter/othernuts/coq10/

Mayo Clinic Staff. (2013). *Coenzyme Q10.* Natural Standard Patient Monograph. Mayo Clinic. Retrieved from http://www.mayoclinic.org/drugs-supplements/coenzyme-q10/background/hrb-20059019

Press Release. *The 1978 Nobel Prize in Chemistry.* (1978). Nobelprize.org. Retrieved November 30, 2014, from http://www.nobelprize.org/nobel_prizes/chemistry/laureates/1978/press.html

Coffee

Coffee, as it is commercially sold and used, refers to the roasted seeds of the berries (also called "cherries") of the coffee tree. Coffee also refers to the beverages produced from the infusion of ground roasted coffee seeds with boiling water. The word "coffee" can also refer to the flavor of these beverages (as in "coffee ice cream"). Coffee is a popular beverage around the world and accounts for about 71% of adult caffeine intake in the United States (O'Keefe et al., 2013). Coffee often is imbibed for its beneficial effects on mental state, increasing alertness and productivity. Long-term coffee consumption is associated with a number of significant health benefits, and daily consumption of 2 to 3 cups appears to be safe for most adults. Coffee's negative short- and long-term effects, however, might outweigh its benefits for some groups.

Contrary to popular belief, coffee beans are not true beans. This common misconception comes from the seed's bean-like shape. Most coffee cherries contain two green seeds having flat sides that face each other. Within the Coffea genus, there are more than 6,000 species of shrubs and trees. Because of the wide range of characteristics expressed in coffee plants, botanists disagree on which plants can be accurately classified as coffee trees. There are 25 to 100 plants that are true coffee plants (NCA, 2014).

It is estimated that coffee was first brewed and drunk in the 13th century, but the first credible accounts come from the 15th century. Coffee was probably first brewed by Sufi monks in Yemen. The legend of Kaldi is widely recounted as the genesis of coffee. It is a story of a shepherd who noticed that when his goats ate a particular type of berry, they became exceptionally high-spirited. It is said that Kaldi then harvested the berries, roasted them, boiled them, and drank the resulting liquid (NCA, 2014).

Types of Coffee

Coffee beans sold for commercial use are one of two species, Coffea canephora, (more commonly called "robusta"), and Coffea arabica. Arabica beans account for approximately 70% of coffee beans sold globally. These plants are more disease-prone than the robusta species. The caffeine in arabica beans accounts for about 1% of the mass. Robusta beans produce coffee that has a distinctive taste and has 50% to 60% more caffeine than coffee made from arabica beans. Robusta coffee accounts for the other 30% of commercially grown and sold coffee.

Cultivation and Processing

Coffee plants require rich soil and they thrive in climates with frequent rain, mild temperatures, (between 59 and 75 degrees F), and shaded sun. The best regions for growing coffee are those that are subtropical. Arabica thrives at high altitudes between 1,800 and 3,600 feet, and robusta grows best at altitudes between sea level and 3,000 feet. Frequent rainfall causes the coffee plants to flower continuously, and allows for two harvesting seasons (NCA, 2014).

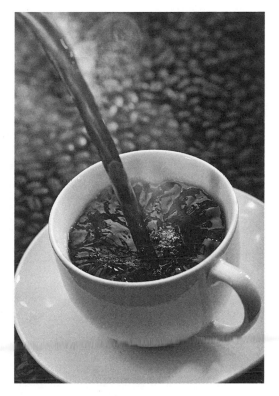

Cup of hot coffee. Black coffee has no calories. Some of the potential health benefits of coffee drinks may be blunted if large amounts of cream and/or sugary syrups are added. Some 16 oz. specialty coffee drinks have over 600 calories. (Johannes Gerhardus Swanepoel/Dreamstime. com)

Although some coffee trees can grow to be 20 to 30 feet tall, during cultivation they are commonly pruned to be short. It takes approximately 3 to 4 years for coffee trees to bear fruit. Once trees have started to bear fruit, the cherries are picked using one of two methods. In one method, the trees are strip-picked, and all cherries are harvested at one time. In an alternative, more labor-intensive method, cherries are selectively picked one at a time at peak ripeness. Selectively picked cherries are processed into beans that are usually more expensive than strip-picked varieties (ICO, n.d.).

Once picked, the coffee cherries are processed using one of two methods. The dry method of processing coffee, more frequently utilized in regions where water is scarcer, involves drying the cherries in the sun. While the cherries dry out, they are raked several times a day to prevent spoiling. When the cherries reach 11%

moisture content, usually after several weeks, they are gathered and stored (NCA, 2104).

An alternative to the dry method of processing coffee is the wet method. This process requires that the freshly harvested cherries be passed through a pulping machine, in which the skin and pulp are separated from the seed and washed away with water. The beans then are separated by weight using water; the heavy beans sink to the bottom of channels, and the lighter beans float to the top. Once separated by size, the beans are immersed in water-filled tanks to ferment for 12 to 48 hours. The fermentation process eliminates the slimy mucilage that remains attached to the beans after the skin and pulp are separated from the seed. After fermentation, the seeds are rinsed again and then sent to dry. The wet-processed beans can be machine dried in large tumblers, or be sun dried. Once dried the beans are ready for export (NCA, 2014).

Roasting

Roasting is the process by which green coffee seeds are turned into the brown coffee beans that are used in brewing and cooking. Before roasting the coffee seeds are green, grassy smelling, and spongy. Roasting brings out the oils and aromas that give coffee beans their unique qualities. There are very few industry-wide standards of roasting, therefore names and qualities of roasts often differ from roaster to roaster (NCA, 2014).

In general, coffee is categorized by the color of the beans as light, medium, medium-dark, or dark roasts. Light roasts are light brown in color. Because they are roasted for a shorter time and the oils inside of the beans do not break through to the surface, light-roast beans are not as shiny as are those which undergo other types of roasts. Medium roasts have a medium-brown color, a stronger taste, and are non-oily. In the United States, medium roasts are highly favored. Medium-dark roasts are characterized by a slightly oily outside, and a bittersweet aftertaste. Dark roast beans have a shiny oily surface and a pronounced bitter taste.

Decaffeination

There is significant demand for caffeine-free coffee by people who wish to enjoy the flavor, aroma, and health benefits, but do not wish to experience coffee's stimulant effects. Several techniques can be used to decaffeinate coffee. Some of these processes use chemicals to absorb or dissolve caffeine and others, such as Swiss water processing, use a series of water baths. Decaffeination processes remove about 97% of the caffeine naturally present in coffee.

Health Issues: Benefits and Risks

Coffee contains more than 1,000 components. Caffeine—the addictive component of coffee—is by far the most comprehensively researched of coffee's constituents and is associated with a myriad of symptoms, as well as both positive and negative health effects. Chlorogenic acid is one of coffee's polyphenolic compounds, and is associated with helpful antioxidant activity. Lignans in coffee are phytoestrogens, and could have beneficial health effects in this capacity. The most interesting studies of coffee's health effects, however, come not from examination of a single compound, but from large epidemiological studies. These studies have found several interesting associations.

- Cardiovascular disease—Epidemiological studies suggest that coffee intake is associated with slightly reduced risks of heart disease and stroke. These findings were somewhat surprising, as earlier studies suggested that coffee might increase harmful blood lipids and increase blood pressure. Subsequent research found that the diterpenes cafestrol and kahweol do increase serum low-density lipoprotein cholesterol levels, but are effectively removed by paper coffee filters. Research also has shown that caffeine does cause a transient increase in resting blood pressure, but that this increase is small in regular coffee drinkers. Coffee might improve arterial health because of its antioxidants or its positive effects on blood glucose regulation.
- Diabetes mellitus type 2 and cardiometabolic syndrome—Both decaffeinated and regular coffee consumption are associated with improved insulin sensitivity and glucose regulation. Coffee consumption is associated with lower risk of type 2 diabetes mellitus.
- Parkinson's disease—Consumption of both coffee and tea are associated with reduced risk of Parkinson's disease, at least in men, suggesting that caffeine might be the active agent. The effect in women is less robust. Some research suggests that coffee reduces risk for older women who are not taking estrogen medications, but not for older women taking estrogen medications.
- Alzheimer's disease—Epidemiological studies have shown that coffee intake over the course of decades can decrease risk of Alzheimer's. Researchers are unsure of the exact mechanisms through which coffee exerts this effect. Studies suggest that trigonelline, a constituent of coffee, has been shown to regenerate axons and dendrite of neurons in vitro (Butt & Sultan, 2011). Antioxidant activity of phytochemicals also could play a role in the prevention of Alzheimer's disease.
- Liver disease—Coffee drinkers have a lower risk of cirrhosis and liver cancer.

Although coffee consumption is associated with many health benefits, research also shows that coffee can increase risk for some conditions. Many individuals are sensitive to caffeine and experience a variety of negative effects, including anxiety, heart palpitations, irritability, nervousness, tremor, and insomnia. Other negative effects include the following.

- Elevated serum LDL cholesterol levels—elevation in atherogenic blood lipids primarily is observed in people who drink large amounts of unfiltered coffee.
- Heartburn—Overconsumption of coffee can cause heartburn from gastro-esophageal reflux in vulnerable individuals.

- Reduced iron absorption—People with iron-deficiency anemia should avoid consuming coffee with their supplements or with meals.
- Increased risk of miscarriage during pregnancy—High levels of coffee consumption (more than 1 to 2 cups per day) have been associated with a slightly increased risk of miscarriage.
- Osteoporosis—Coffee consumption is associated with a slightly increased risk of osteoporosis and hip fracture in older adults. Consuming adequate calcium and vitamin D could reduce this risk.

Gabriella J. Zutrau and Ga Hyun Moon

Research Issues

The worldwide coffee trade exerts an enormous impact on many countries, especially resource-poor countries. Because coffee growing and production is such a large industry, it also has large environmental impacts. Issues of environmental sustainability associated with coffee farming can be explored on the International Coffee Association's website, as well as by doing other research.

International Coffee Organization. (n.d.). *Developing a sustainable coffee economy*. Retrieved from http://www.ico.org/sustaindev_e.asp

See Also: Caffeine; Polyphenols.

Further Reading

Butt, M. S., & Sultan, M. T. (2011). Coffee consumption and its benefits. *Clinical Reviews in Food Science and Nutrition, 51,* (4), 363–373. doi: 10.1080/10408390903586412. Retrieved from http://www.tandfonline.com/doi/full/10.1080/10408390903586412#.UyO0rPSwLj4

Drake, V. J., (2007, December). *Is Coffee Harmful or Helpful?* Oregon State University, Linus Pauling Institute. Retrieved from http://lpi.oregonstate.edu/fw07/coffee.html

International Coffee Organization (ICO). (n.d.). *Harvesting*. Retrieved from http://www.ico.org/harvest_e.asp

National Coffee Association USA (NCA). (2014, November 30). *All about coffee*. Retrieved from http://www.ncausa.org/i4a/pages/index.cfm?pageid=30

O'Keefe, J. H., Bhatti, S. K., Patil, H. R., DiNicolantonio, J. J., Lucan, S. C., & Lavie, C. J. (2013). Effects of habitual coffee consumption on cardiometabolic disease, cardiovascular health, and all-cause mortality. *Journal of American College of Cardiology, 62* (12), 1043–1051. Retrieved from http://www.medscape.com/viewarticle/810989_2

Cognitive Restructuring

Cognitive restructuring is a step-by-step technique used to recognize, challenge, and eventually change distorted thoughts, assumptions, and predictions. It can be utilized to avoid automatic maladaptive thinking patterns that negatively affect a person's behavior. By avoiding distorted ways of thinking, individuals learn to approach situations in a less rigid and more productive way. Cognitive restructuring can be especially helpful in regard to nutrition. By changing maladaptive thought patterns, individuals can master the skills needed to practice healthy eating and exercise habits.

History

Albert Ellis and Aaron T. Beck are two major figures accredited with cognitive restructuring techniques. In 1957, Albert Ellis devised the beginnings of Rational Emotive Behavioral Therapy (REBT), an approach that targeted irrational beliefs to change negative psychological outcomes. Ellis relied on what he called the "ABC Model." The ABC model contains three elements: A (activating event), B (beliefs), and C (consequences). "A" represents an activating event; "B" represents the underlying beliefs regarding the activating event; and "C" represents the emotional and behavioral consequences of one's interpretations. Ellis demonstrated that psychological distress often results from negative interpretations of an event, rather than the event itself.

Ellis's work became a foundation for Aaron T. Beck's cognitive therapy (CT), which is at the core of what is known today as cognitive behavioral therapy (CBT). Beck was particularly interested in studying ways in which negative thinking contributed to depression. Beck observed that his patients possessed a negative bias toward reality, something he referred to as the "cognitive triad": distorted negative views of the self, life experience, and future. Testing the reliability of these "automatic thoughts" through cognitive restructuring, he thought, could help his patients overcome depression.

Procedure

There are several approaches to cognitive restructuring. Below is a simplified version that illustrates the procedure step by step.

1. Identify the situation.
2. Identify negative emotions associated with the event.
3. Identify thoughts, beliefs, or assumptions associated with these emotions.
4. Evaluate the evidence for and against those beliefs.
5. Challenge these automatic thoughts with rational responses.

The first step in cognitive restructuring is to pinpoint the triggering event for one's negative or uncomfortable emotions. Being as specific as possible when identifying these emotions can assist in recognizing distorted thinking. Evaluating the evidence encourages individuals to observe their thoughts from an objective standpoint. For example, "Would these rules apply to my friends and family?" "What is the worst thing that could happen?" Using constructive doubt about negative thinking can serve as a helpful reality check.

The goal of the last step—challenging the automatic thoughts with rational responses—is to determine a more realistic way of thinking that, while helpful, validates the emotions associated with the original maladaptive thought. Even if the individual understands the rationale of the new thought, it might not feel true right away. Negative thinking patterns often result from years of reinforcement, and therefore can take time to reverse. It is important to practice this new way of thinking to make these new thoughts feel more believable. This will allow for the development of new coping strategies and, it is hoped, a change in behavior. Table 1 gives an example of cognitive restructuring.

Cognitive Distortions

Cognitive distortions are distorted or irrational thinking patterns about the self, world, or future. They often stem from a fear of failure. Clinging to these beliefs allows for very little flexibility and can have a significant effect on one's motivation, self-esteem, and ultimately, behavior. Below are some examples of cognitive distortions.

- All-or-nothing thinking / black-and-white thinking. People or situations are perceived as either "good" or "bad," and anything falling short of perfect feels like failure. Example: If I don't follow my meal plan perfectly this week, I can officially say I'm a hopeless case.
- Overgeneralization: Perceiving an isolated negative event as a never-ending pattern of defeat. Example: I was too tired to run for more than 20 minutes today . . . I'll never be a good athlete!
- Mental filter: Dwelling on a single negative detail exclusively until the perception of the entire event is darkened. Example: My doctor complimented my efforts because my glucose levels have been better with my dietary changes, but said I should consume more leafy greens. I'm clearly not trying hard enough.
- Disqualifying the positive: Disregarding positive experiences by insisting that they "don't count." It doesn't matter that I made healthy food choices today, because yesterday's meals were a disaster.
- Jumping to conclusions: Negatively interpreting any event without substantial evidence to support it.
- Mind reading: Irrationally concluding that someone is reacting negatively without substantial evidence. Example: Everyone in this restaurant thinks I have no self-control over what I'm eating.
- Fortune-teller error: Predicting a negative event and insisting that it will come true. Example: I will never develop healthy eating patterns.
- Magnification (catastrophizing) or minimization: Exaggerating the significance a negative event or minimizing the significance of a positive one. Example of magnification: I miscalculated the amount of carbohydrates I consumed today! My day is ruined. Example of minimization: Why would I thank her for baking me a birthday cake? I have a gluten intolerance.

Table 1. Cognitive Restructuring

Situation	Emotions	Automatic Thought	Supporting and Refuting Evidence	Rational Response
I ate a donut at today's meeting even though I have been trying to eat less junk food.	Frustration Shame Disappointment Anger Hopelessness	I already strayed from my meal plan so I might as well forget about following it for the rest of the day.	Support: Given that I ate the donut, I will not have followed 100% of my meal plan by the end of the day. Refute: Eating more junk food won't bring me any closer to my goal, and it certainly won't undo my actions.	Today's eating will not be perfect, but just because things didn't go according to plan doesn't mean I have to throw myself completely off track. I can start over at any point and still make my day's efforts count.

- Emotional reasoning: Forming beliefs based on emotional, rather than logical, aspects or events. Example: I feel like I've gained five pounds, so it must be true.
- "Should" statements: Holding rigid beliefs that things ought, or ought not, be a certain way. Example: I should have gone to the gym today despite feeling ill.
- Labeling and mislabeling: Replacing an error or negative event with oneself or someone else by affixing a label to the individual. Example: I didn't achieve my weight goal. I'm such a failure.
- Personalization: Blaming oneself for the negative outcome of an event for which the individual is not responsible. Example: If I had encouraged healthier eating habits, my child wouldn't have developed an eating disorder.

When Can People Use It?

Cognitive restructuring can be used to live a healthier, more productive life. It often is used to treat mental illness, and also can help manage eating and exercise behaviors related to acute or chronic illnesses. Examples include the following.

- Diabetes
- Obesity
- Eating disorders
- Heart disease

- Digestive diseases such as celiac disease, irritable bowel syndrome, ulcers, and gastric reflux
- Allergies and sensitivities (e.g., soy, gluten, lactose)
- Stroke
- Cancer
- High blood pressure
- Autoimmune disorders
- Osteoporosis

Efficacy

Studies have shown cognitive restructuring to be a reliable and effective method for minimizing levels of distress. It has been proven to be highly effective for individuals of different age groups, backgrounds, and medical histories. Cognitive restructuring is used widely in CBT for treatment of depression, anxiety disorders, post-traumatic stress disorders, eating disorders, and autism. Recent studies also have shown benefits of cognitive restructuring in adults with ADHD. Frequent use of strategies for coping, homework compliance, and willingness resulted in reduced rates of symptoms. People with certain skills and personality traits, however, might be more apt to practice the technique successfully. It has been questioned whether cognitive restructuring is as effective in older adults, whose executive functioning skills often decline with age, as it is in the younger population. Executive functioning includes cognitive processes such as working memory, verbal reasoning, planning, problem solving, inhibitory control, and self-monitoring. Impairment or deficits in any one of these areas can drastically affect an individual's aptitude for cognitive restructuring.

Criticisms

- It's not enough. Although many individuals find cognitive restructuring helpful in their day-to-day lives, some find it difficult to do alone. In some cases, these maladaptive thought patterns can be indicative of a more serious condition for which it is imperative that one seek help from a health care provider.
- It's an escape tactic. Some critics argue that cognitive restructuring teaches individuals to suppress, rather than confront, their thoughts. This allows them to avoid pain and anguish associated with the uncomfortable event, and to distance themselves from their experiences.
- The chicken or the egg? The sequence of steps in cognitive restructuring has been questioned. Do emotions stem from beliefs or are beliefs a response to emotions?

Nicole D. Teitelbaum

See Also: Eating disorders; Obesity, treatment.

Further Reading

Burns, D. D. (1980). *Feeling good: The new mood therapy*. New York: William Morrow and Company, Inc.

Burns, D. D., & Nolen-Hoeksema, S. (1991). Coping styles, homework compliance, and the effectiveness of cognitive-behavioral therapy. *Journal of Consulting and Clinical Psychology, 59* (2), 305–311.

Castle, P., & Buckler, S. (2009). Is talking to yourself the first sign of "madness"? Self-talk and cognitive restructuring. In P. Castle, & S. Buckler, *How to Be a Successful Teacher: Strategies for Personal and Professional Development* (pp. 149–160). London, UK: SAGE Publications Ltd.

David, D. (n.d.). *Rational emotive behavior therapy in the context of modern psychological research*. The Albert Ellis Institute. Retrieved from http://albertellis.org/rebt-in-the -context-of-modern-psychological-research/

Johnco, C., Wuthrich, V., & Rapee, R. (2013). The role of cognitive flexibility in cognitive restructuring skill acquisition among older adults. *Journal of Anxiety Disorders, 27* (6), 576–584.

Mueser, K. T., Rosenberg, S. D., & Rosenberg, H. J. (2009). Cognitive restructuring II: The 5 steps of CR. In K. T. Mueser, S. D. Rosenberg, & H. J. Rosenberg (Eds.), *Treatment of posttraumatic stress disorder in special populations: A cognitive restructuring program*, 121–162. Washington, DC: American Psychological Association.

Colostrum

Colostrum, also known as "first milk," is a nutrient-rich mammary secretion, produced by female mammals in late pregnancy and the few days after giving birth. It is a great source of nutrients such as protein, fat, carbohydrates, vitamins, and minerals. Additionally, it is full of immune, growth, and tissue-repair factors, which are all beneficial to the development of the newborn. Colostrum has numerous antimicrobial agents, such as lactoferrin, lysozyme, and lactoperoxidase, which are responsible for helping the newborn's immune system to mature. Colostrum is particularly rich in antibodies that are able to provide a passive immunity for newborns. The health benefits of colostrum are one reason that health organizations around the world encourage mothers to breast-feed their infants. Two major growth factors—insulin-like growth factors 1 and 2, and transforming growth factors alpha and beta—are found in colostrum. These growth factors have regenerative effects on many structural body cells, and they stimulate wound healing and muscle and cartilage repair in vitro.

In 1912, L.W. Famulener showed that immunized goats were able to pass on their immunity to their offspring through colostrum (Wheeler, Hodgkinson, Prosser, & Davis, 2007). In 1922, colostrum was found to have a greater concentration of antibodies than found in mature milk. In the same year, Theobald Smith and Ralph B. Little performed an experiment on calves that demonstrated the importance of colostrum in providing protection against bacterial infections (Smith &

Little, 1922). In the experiment, 22 calves were separated into two groups. One group of 10 calves received colostrum after birth, and they all survived. Another group of 12 calves did not receive colostrum and 8 of the 12 died, mostly due to bacterial infections. It was discovered that calves that did not receive colostrum lacked specific agglutinins in the blood, which made them vulnerable to infectious bacteria. By 1930, it was confirmed that mammary glands accumulate and secrete agglutinating antibodies that are directed against pathogens, to give the newborns protection.

Because of the large amount of nutrients and antibodies in colostrum, it often is used by people both as medicine and supplement. Bovine colostrum has been used as a raw material for immunonoglubulin-rich commercial products and supplements. Some animal studies have shown that growth factors in bovine colostrum can promote cell growth in the intestine. These immunonoglubulin products therefore sometimes are used as treatments for patients who have gastrointestinal tract infections, and are used as supplements by those who want to prevent gastrointestinal infections.

Northfield Laboratories, for example, produces a product called "Gastrogard" that is designed to prevent diarrhea caused by rotavirus in young children. This product is a special type of colostrum known as hyperimmune bovine colostrum, in which cows are exposed to a particular microbe so that they will manufacture antibodies for the microbe, which then make their way into the colostrum. This type of colostrum can be effective for the treatment of several types of infectious diarrhea. Colostrum supplements have demonstrated some positive effects on athletic performance, especially for sprint-event athletes. Bovine colostrum products appear to be safe, although long-term comprehensive studies have not been conducted.

Fei Peng

See Also: Breast-feeding.

Further Reading

EBSCO CAM Review Board. (2014, September 18). *Colostrum.* Retrieved from http://healthlibrary.epnet.com/GetContent.aspx?token=e0498803-7f62-4563-8d47-5fe33da65dd4&chunkiid=21692

Smith, T., & Little, R. B. (1922). The significance of colostrum to the new-born calf. *Journal of Experimental Medicine, 36* (2), 181–198. Retrieved from http://www.ncbi.nlm.nih.gov/pubmed/19868663?dopt=Abstract

Therapeutic Research Faculty. (2009). *Colostrum.* WebMD. Natural Medicines Comprehensive Database. Retrieved from http://www.webmd.com/vitamins-supplements/ingredientmono-785-COLOSTRUM.aspx?activeIngredientId=785&activeIngredientName=COLOSTRUM

Wheeler, T. T., Hodgkinson, A. J., Prosser, C. G., & Davis, S. R. (2007). Immune components of colostrum and milk—a historical perspective. *Journal of Mammary Gland Biology and Neoplasia, 12* (4), 237–247.

Copper

Copper (Cu) is an essential trace mineral. It is an important component of the enzymes involved with iron metabolism. Copper helps with collagen formation (a component of many organs in the body, such as bone and muscle), myelination of nerve cells, immune function, and cardiovascular function. Copper converts ferrous iron to ferric iron to be transported into the blood by transferrin, thus helping to prevent anemia. Copper is a component of the antioxidant enzymes, the superoxide dismutases. The human body, however, does not require large amounts of copper, and most cases of deficiency result from too much supplementation with other minerals, such as zinc.

Researchers identified the essential need for copper with experimental animals in 1928. Evidence regarding copper deficiency, however, in humans did not emerge until the 1960s. Research on two genetic disorders involving copper metabolism, including Wilson's disease (a very rare condition which causes copper toxicity) and Menke's syndrome (causes copper deficiency) inspired interest in copper and led to new discoveries about its metabolism and physiological functions.

The small intestine absorbs approximately 50% of dietary copper, but this depends on the amount of copper found in the food and additional dietary factors. Albumin helps transport copper from the intestinal cells to the liver where approximately two-thirds is involved with ceruloplasmin, the enzyme that catalyzes the oxidation of iron. Research indicates healthy adult bodies have 100 mg of copper with distribution to the liver, brain, blood, and bone marrow. The body stores limited amounts of copper and excretes the excess amounts.

Food Sources and Dietary Recommendations

The recommended dietary allowance (RDA) for both adult men and women is 900 micrograms per day. Copper is found in a limited variety of foods; the richest sources include organ meats such as liver, shellfish, nuts, seeds, legumes, peanut butter, and chocolate. Soymilk, black beans, pistachios, spinach, blackberries, baked potatoes with skins, and lean slices of ham also are good sources. Dietary surveys in the United States suggest adults consume about 1.2 milligrams of copper each day.

Copper Deficiency and Menke's Syndrome

Humans rarely experience high levels of copper deficiency, but this commonly occurs among premature infants due to their limited copper stores at birth and their rapid growth rate. Excessive supplementation with additional minerals (zinc and iron) can cause a secondary copper deficiency, leading to iron-deficiency anemia. Young children with a copper deficiency can suffer from bone abnormalities, likely caused by poor synthesis of connective tissue. Additionally, copper-deficient individuals experience elevated blood cholesterol, impaired glucose tolerance, and heart-related issues. During pregnancy, fetal growth and development is negatively impacted if the woman is copper-deficient.

Menke's syndrome is rare (1 in 50,000 live births) (Insel, Ross, McMahon, & Bernstein, 2014), but can be fatal and irreversible if copper-histidine treatment (increases copper absorption) is not administered within the first days of life. This genetic disorder occurs when copper is not absorbed in the bloodstream, creating a lack of functional copper-containing proteins. Copper accumulates in the intestinal wall, causing buildup that could lead to neurological degeneration; brittle, depigmented, kinky hair; abnormal connective-tissue development; low bone density; osteoporosis; and poor growth.

Copper Toxicity and Wilson's Disease

Copper toxicity is uncommon. The Tolerable Upper Intake Level (UL) is 10,000 micrograms per day. Copper poisoning can develop if people consume beverages that have absorbed copper from containers. The U.S. Environmental Protection agency limits copper levels in drinking water to 1.3 mg per liter (Higdon, Delage, & Prohaska, 2014). Copper often is found in well water, which should be tested for mineral content. Individuals can consume copper unknowingly from using copper cookware (copper pots and pans lined with other metals such as stainless steel, however, are safe) or consuming water that has traveled through copper pipes, especially untreated hot water.

Wilson's disease is rare genetic disorder, occurring among 1 in 200,000 individuals (Insel, Ross, McMahon, & Bernstein, 2014). This disorder limits copper excretion in bile, causing toxic buildup in the liver, brain, kidneys, and eyes. Accumulation of copper in the red blood cells triggers the onset of anemia. The symptoms of Wilson's disease are often undetected until adolescence or early adulthood. Without treatment, individuals develop liver and neurological complications. Chelation therapy helps reduce copper toxicity by binding and eliminating copper and supplementing the diet with zinc, which decreases the absorption of copper.

Carolyn Gross

See Also: Minerals; Zinc.

Further Reading

Ehrlich, S. D. (2011, March 6). *Copper.* University of Maryland Medical Center. Retrieved from https://umm.edu/health/medical/altmed/supplement/copper

Higdon, J., Delage, B., & Prohaska, J. R. (2014, January). *Copper.* Linus Pauling Institute, Oregon State University. Retrieved from http://lpi.oregonstate.edu/infocenter/minerals /copper/

Insel, P., Ross, D., McMahon, K., & Bernstein, M. (2014). *Nutrition.* Burlington, MA: Jones & Bartlett Learning.

Cordyceps Sinensis

Cordyceps are a group of parasitic fungi that parasitize, kill, and then grow on a variety of insects. There are many species of cordyceps, and each grows on a single insect host species. The most common types of cordyceps for consumption is cordyceps sinensis, a type of cordyceps that has been part of traditional Chinese medicine for more than 700 years. Cordyceps sinensis officially was classified as a drug in the Chinese Pharmocopoeia in 1964. Cordyceps supplements also have become popular around the world, although scientific research documenting health benefits is preliminary. In this entry the word "cordyceps" refers to cordyceps sinensis, the type of cordyceps used in Chinese medicine and in dietary supplements.

Cordyceps sinensis is produced in nature when a host caterpillar ingests fungal spores which grow inside the caterpillar, eventually causing the host organism to die. After the host's death, the fungus continues to grow and eventually emerges from the corpse. Cordyceps are harvested mainly in the high-altitude regions of the Tibetan plateau. The time frame for harvesting is very short, as the cordyceps needs to be harvested right after the fungus emerges from the corpse of the host and before the fungus releases spores, which causes the cordyceps to shrivel up and become useless. Wild cordyceps are very expensive in the market. In international trade, (wild) cordyceps were priced at anywhere between US$20,000 and US$40,000 per kg in 2013, with typical consumption in the scale of grams. Cordyceps can also be grown in the laboratory on cultures in a controlled environment replicating the temperatures and high-altitude conditions of Tibet.

Although popular in traditional Chinese medicine for many years, the potential health effects of cordyceps only have recently garnered interest in the West, where it is viewed as a type of alternative medicine and herbal supplement. The interest was sparked when, in 1993, three female runners set world records in the 1,500-, 3,000-, and 10,000-meter races at the National Games in Beijing, China. The runners tested negative for typical performance-enhancing drugs, however cordyceps sinensis extracts were revealed to be part of the runners' diets. Traditional Chinese medicine typically prescribes cordyceps as a general strengthening tonic, especially for use after a serious illness, and to improve the health of the lungs and kidneys. It also has been used to treat ailments ranging from bronchitis to diabetes to eyesight problems. In North America, cordyceps supplements are marketed with properties such as antiaging, "pro-sexual," anti-cancer, and immune boosting. Preliminary studies suggest that cordyceps might deserve further investigation for possible effectiveness in controlling high blood pressure, high blood cholesterol levels, and high blood glucose levels, and for reducing cancer risk.

Studies on cordyceps are a relatively new endeavor, therefore the potential side effects of taking cordyceps are not well known. There have been rare cases of dry mouth, nausea, diarrhea, and systemic drug allergy. Clinical trials on rabbits for a period of 3 months used 10 g per kilogram of weight ingested daily and resulted in no significant side effects on the liver, kidney, and blood (Chen, Wang, Nie, & Marcone, 2013). That dosage (10g/kg) is much more than typically is consumed by humans. Anecdotal information on the use of cordyceps for cancer patients was based upon a dosage of 3 g to 5 g daily. Consuming too much cordyceps is not necessarily better, as studies have shown that the effectiveness of cordyceps in rats peaked at 8 mg per kilogram of weight per day and decreased at 10 mg per kilogram of weight per day (Chen, Wang, Nie, & Marcone, 2013). There is a concern regarding heavy-metal contamination, however, if wild cordyceps are not sourced from the right place. Due to the significant cost of cordyceps, unscrupulous sellers might insert heavy metal into the fungi to increase its weight and its selling price.

Yuxin Li

See Also: Dietary supplements.

Further Reading

Chen, P. X., Wang, S., Nie, S., & Marcone, M. (2013). Properties of Cordyceps sinensis: A review. *Journal of Functional Foods, 5,* 550–569.

Das, S. K., Masuda, M., Sakurai, A., & Sakakibara, M. (2010). Medicinal uses of the mushroom Cordyceps militaris: Current state and prospects. *Fitoterapia, 80,* 961–968

EBSCO CAM Review Board. (2013). *Cordyceps.* Retrieved from http://ent.med.nyu.edu/content?ChunkIID=104680

Lo, H., Hsieh, C., Lin, F., & Hsu, T. (2013). A systematic review of the mysterious caterpillar fungus Ophiocordyceps sinensis in DongChongXiaCao and related bioactive ingredients. *Journal of Traditional and Complementary Medicine, 3* (1), 16–32.

Russell, R., & Paterson, M. (2008). Cordyceps—A traditional Chinese medicine and another fungal therapeutic biofactory? *Phytochemistry, 69* (7), 1469–1495. doi: 10.1016/j.phytochem.2008.01.027

Creatine

Creatine is an amino acid made naturally by the body that helps to supply energy to all cells, especially muscle cells. It also is available as a dietary supplement and generally is used as an ergogenic aid. A nutritional ergogenic aid is any supplement, food product, chemical, or dietary manipulation that enhances a person's physical performance ability. The body uses creatine to produce the molecule phosphocreatine, which helps to replenish adenosine triphosphate (ATP), the body's primary energy molecule. Phosphocreatine is especially important for energy production during the first few seconds of exercise. Ninety-five percent of the body's creatine is stored in skeletal muscles. The body's remaining creatine reserves are found in the brain and other tissues with heavy energy demands.

In 1847, German scientist Justus von Liebig discovered more intramuscular creatine in wild foxes than in captive foxes, providing evidence for its role in energy production in skeletal muscles. Later, a nutritional supplement, called "Fleisch

Extrakt," was made from beef and created as a cheap substitute for people who were unable to get enough meat in their diet. The extract essentially became the first creatine supplement. Today, a variety of creatine supplements claim to promote the body's muscle-building processes and contribute to greater muscle strength, volume, and power.

A 150-pound male adult requires approximately 2 g of creatine daily for normal functioning. The greater a person's muscle mass, the greater the daily need. Because the body can make creatine from amino acid precursors, there is no recommended dietary allowance for creatine. Creatine can be obtained from meat, such as beef, pork, chicken, and fish; relatively small amounts of creatine also are available from milk and cranberries. Heat contributes to creatine degradation, therefore overcooked meat tends to have reduced creatine content. Creatine also is synthesized by the liver, pancreas, and kidneys from the amino acids L-arginine, glycine, and L-methionine and then is transported throughout the body in the blood. Omnivores generally obtain about 1 g of creatine from their diets and make another gram from other amino acid precursors. Strict vegetarians and vegans ingest almost no creatine, as the exclusion of meat in one's diet eliminates the primary source of creatine. Vegetarians and vegans do make creatine, given adequate protein intake, although the extent of creatine production depends on the person's diet.

In tissues, creatine serves as a critical energy storage component of the phosphagen—or creatine-phosphate—energy system, which is utilized for brief, high-intensity activity. In its active form, creatine combines with a phosphate group to form a molecule called "phosphocreatine." For instantaneous energy, such as a powerful muscle contraction, phosphocreatine readily gives up its phosphate group to adenosine-diphosphate (ADP) to form ATP, a process facilitated by the enzyme creatine kinase. A high-energy bond between two phosphate groups in this molecule provides a burst of energy when broken. The reserves of phosphocreatine in muscles typically last for up to 15 seconds of intense activity, and then take 5 minutes of rest to be fully restored. Fast twitch, type-II muscle fibers use creatine most, as they split ATP at a high rate. These muscle fibers are recruited for fast, high-intensity exercise. Slow twitch, type-I fibers use creatine sparingly, as they are utilized more frequently for endurance exercises.

Creatine supplementation for muscle-building purposes has increased in popularity in recent years. Numerous studies have shown that creatine supplementation combined with appropriate exercise training can improve anaerobic capacity and increase lean muscle mass. The method by which creatine promotes synthesis of new muscle, known as "myogenesis," is not fully understood. One theory is that creatine's volumizing properties might allow muscles to retain more fluid. In the first few weeks of a supplementation regimen, 2 lbs to 5 lbs of increased body mass are gained strictly due to fluid retention. This increased fluid could make more of the molecular building blocks of muscles, especially amino acids, accessible for immediate use (Francaux & Poortsmas, 2006). A second theory suggests that creatine simply might help generate the capacity for more exercise by making more phosphocreatine available to muscles and helping muscles recover more quickly from exertion. This would allow for more muscle growth due to an increased ability to train. A third theory suggests that creatine might contribute to hyperplasia, the creation of entirely new muscle cells from progenitor cells. Lastly, increased creatine levels could influence other anabolic hormone concentrations in the body that encourage muscle cell growth.

The effectiveness of creatine supplementation for females is not well established, as most recommendations and research focus on its use in adult males. Further, 20% to 30% of users do not significantly respond to creatine supplementation in any way. Individuals who respond best to creatine have low initial levels of creatine and phosphocreatine and a greater quantity and cross-sectional area of type II muscle fibers. Vegetarians and vegans usually benefit from creatine supplementation. The elderly population has shown marked improvement in strength and fat-free mass when using creatine along with resistance training.

The American Academy of Pediatrics (AAP) strongly discourages use of creatine supplements in children and adolescents (Metzl, Small, Levine, & Gershel, 2001). Although creatine supplements appear to be relatively safe for healthy, young adults, no long-term safety data are available. Additionally, the AAP is concerned that using ergogenic aids such as creatine often leads to the use of more dangerous supplements and drugs by children and teens (Eisenberg, Wall, & Neumark-Sztainer, 2012).

Too much creatine can have negative health effects and puts undue stress on the kidneys. Short-term effects of creatine can include diarrhea, muscle cramping, dehydration, and asthmatic symptoms. Some researchers have expressed concern about altered kidney and liver function. Consequently, creatine supplementation requires careful calculation and development of a well-planned regimen. Creatine interferes with several prescription drugs, therefore people using prescriptions drugs—and, indeed, anyone with medical issues—should consult their physicians before beginning a creatine-supplementation program.

Although evidence is not strong, creatine supplementation shows some promise for aiding in disorders characterized by cachexia ("wasting syndrome"), including muscle atrophy. Creatine use by people with muscular dystrophy has revealed increased lean body mass and improved voluntary muscle contraction. Results of creatine use have been disappointing for patients with human immunodeficiency syndrome. Limited success has been observed in some studies of patients with chronic obstructive pulmonary disease and congestive heart failure.

Additional applications for creatine in relation to its role in the brain also have been explored. High-dose creatine has been shown to have some neuroprotective effects in neurodegenerative disorders such as Huntington's Disease and Parkinson's Disease (Gualano, Artioli, Poortmans, & Lancha, 2010). Supplementation might help to stabilize creatine kinase levels, or decrease the need for it if the enzyme is not functioning properly. Creatine also has been shown to block the formation of aggregates within cells that are thought to trigger apoptosis, or cell death. More evidence is needed to confirm or refute the benefits of creatine supplementation in these disease states.

Patricia M. Cipicchio

Research Issues

Some of the problems reported with creatine supplementation could be related to other ingredients—such as caffeine and ephedra—found in supplement preparations. Researchers are exploring the interactions between creatine and other supplement ingredients. Research continues to explore creatine's therapeutic uses in disease states.

See Also: Dietary supplements; Energy balance.

Further Reading

Eisenberg, M. E., Wall, M., & Neumark-Sztainer, D. (2012). Muscle-enhancing behaviors among adolescent girls and boys. *Pediatrics, 130* (6), 1019–1026. doi: 10.1542/peds .2012-0095

Francaux, M., & Poortsmas, J. R. (2006). Side effects of creatine supplementation in athletes. *International Journal of Sports Physiological Performance, 1* (4), 311–23.

Gualano, B., Artioli, G. G., Poortmans, J. R., & Lancha, A. H., Jr. (2010). Exploring the therapeutic role of creatine supplementation. *Amino Acids, 38*, 31–44.

King, J. (2011). *The negative consequences of creatine.* Livestrong.com. Retrieved from http://www.livestrong.com/article/466417-the-negative-consequences-of-creatine/

Metzl, J., Small, E., Levine, S. R., & Gershel, J. C. (2001). Creatine use among young athletes. *Pediatrics, 108* (2), 421–425. doi: 10.1542/peds.108.2.421

Curcumin

Curcumin is the principal component of turmeric, giving turmeric its yellow color and contributing to its characteristic flavor. Turmeric is derived from the rhizomes of *Curcuma longa,* a member of the ginger family. A rhizome is a modified stem of a plant that spreads underground and is capable of allowing the growth of new shoots and roots. Turmeric is a common component of curry and mustard preparations. It is used widely in the cuisine of South Asian cultures and the yellow mustard commonly used in North America. The bright yellow color of turmeric comes from phytochemical pigments known as "curcuminoids," several of which are thought to be therapeutic; the most studied curcuminoid is curcumin. Curcumin comprises approximately 75% of turmeric's curcuminoid content (Higdon, Drake, & Yang, 2009).

Curcumin supplements commonly contain a substance called piperine, which comes from black pepper and enhances the absorption of curcumin from the small intestine. In the laboratory, in vitro, and in animal studies, curcumin exhibits antioxidant and anti-inflammatory effects. Curcumin also has been shown to inhibit several carcinogenic processes in vitro. Researchers therefore are studying its usefulness in treating a variety of chronic illnesses, including Alzheimer's disease, rheumatoid and osteoarthritis, and cancer.

The progression of Alzheimer's disease is associated with inflammation and oxidative damage. Alzheimer's disease is characterized by the formation of clumps of proteins in the brain that appear to inhibit normal nerve activity. These clumps, also called "plaques," are composed of proteins called amyloid beta. Studies show that curcumin inhibits amyloid beta formation in vitro. When injected into mice, curcumin crosses the blood-brain barrier (BBB) and significantly decreases biomarkers for inflammation and oxidative damage, amyloid plaque, and amyloid beta-induced memory deficits. Clinical trials currently are underway to determine whether curcumin crosses the human BBB and whether it is as efficacious in humans.

Curcumin treatment has shown some effectiveness for the treatment of joint pain associated with both rheumatoid and osteoarthritis. In one study, curcumin supplements were found to be about as effective as ibuprofen in the treatment of knee pain caused by osteoarthritis, reducing pain and increasing mobility (Kuptniratsaikul et al., 2009). Researchers hypothesize that these results come from curcumin's anti-inflammatory activity.

In vitro, curcumin appears to induce apoptosis (cell death) in a wide range of cancer cells. Human trials using curcumin for cancer treatment are under way. Thus far, curcumin has been most promising for cancers of the gastrointestinal tract, including colorectal cancers. Once curcumin is absorbed from the small intestinal, its bioavailability is quite low. Researchers are exploring ways to deliver curcumin intravenously as an anticancer drug.

Some researchers have suggested that it is premature for consumers to take curcumin supplements in hopes of preventing health problems (Burgos-Moron et al., 2010). Curcumin is metabolized by the liver and intestine and has low bioavailability. This means that high doses of curcumin are required if administered orally to achieve adequate tissue levels of the substance for a therapeutic effect. No research has evaluated the long-term safety of such high intakes, however. Like many phytochemicals, curcumin could behave as an antioxidant at low doses, but be a pro-oxidant at high doses and contribute to cellular activity that potentially could encourage—rather than discourage—processes that increase cancer risk.

Curcumin can act as a blood thinner and slows the formation of clots; it is should not be taken with anticoagulants or by those who have pre-existing bleeding disorders. Because it also can cause increased bleeding during surgery, curcumin supplementation must be discontinued two weeks prior to surgery. Curcumin eases the flow of bile from the liver to the gallbladder, thus preventing the formation of gallstones. If gallstones already exist, however, then curcumin can exacerbate the problem by flushing them into the bile duct, thereby causing additional blockage (Higdon, Drake, & Yang, 2009). The safety of curcumin supplements has not been established for pregnant women. South Asian cultures consume about 0.15 g of curcumin per day as part of a normal diet, year after year. This level is associated with beneficial health effects and appears to be safe for most people (Burgos-Moron et al., 2010).

Sonya Bhatia and Barbara A. Brehm

See Also: Alzheimer's disease and nutrition; Arthritis and nutrition; Cancer and nutrition; Inflammation; Phytochemicals.

Further Reading

Burgos-Moron, E., Calderon-Montano, J. M., Salvador, J., Robles, A., & López-Lázaro, M. (2010). The dark side of curcumin. *International Journal of Cancer, 126* (7), 1771–1775.

EBSCO CAM Review Board. (2012). *Turmeric.* Natural and Alternative Medicine. Retrieved from http://www.consumerlab.com/tnp.asp?chunkiid=21874#ref32

Goel, A., Kunnumakkara, A. B., & Aggarwal, B. B. (2008). Curcumin as "curecumin": From kitchen to clinic. *Biochemical Pharmacology, 75* (4), 787–809.

Higdon, J., Drake, V. J., & Yang, C. S. (2009). *Curcumin.* Linus Pauling Institute, Oregon State University. Retrieved from http://lpi.oregonstate.edu/infocenter/phytochemicals /curcumin/

Kuptniratsaikul, V., Thanakhumtorn, S., Chinswangwatanakul, P., Wattanamongkonsil, L., & Thamlikitkul, V. (2009). Efficacy and safety of Curcuma domestica extracts in patients with knee osteoarthritis. *Journal of Alternative and Complementary Medicine, 15* (8), 891–897. doi: 10.1089/acm.2008.0186

Weil, A. (2013). *3 reasons to eat turmeric.* Drweil.com. Retrieved from http://www.drweil .com/drw/u/ART03001/Three-Reasons-to-Eat-Turmeric.html

D

Daily Values

The following information is adapted from the U.S. Food and Drug Administration *Guidance for Industry: A Food Labeling Guide* (2013). "Daily values" are a set of dietary standards used on food labels to help consumers understand the nutrient content of food products. The daily values were established in 1993 and do not always match current "Daily Recommended Intake" (DRI) values. The Food and Nutrition Board of the National Academy of Sciences, along with Health Canada, establishes recommended intake level for a variety of nutrients for 22 different population groups, based on age, gender, and, for women, conditions of pregnancy and lactation. The daily values are a single set of values drawn from this information that is useful for food labeling. Food labeling in the United States is overseen by the Food and Drug Administration.

According to the FDA (2014), there are two sets of reference values for reporting nutrients in nutrition labeling: daily reference values (DRVs), and reference daily intakes (RDIs). These values assist consumers in interpreting information about the amount of a nutrient that is present in a food, and comparing nutritional values of food products. The DRVs are established for adults and children four years of age or older, as are RDIs, except for protein. The DRVs are provided for total fat, saturated fat, cholesterol, total carbohydrate, dietary fiber, sodium, potassium, and protein. The RDIs are provided for vitamins, minerals, and for protein for children younger than four years of age and for pregnant and lactating women.

To limit consumer confusion, however, labels include a single term (i.e., daily value [DV]) to designate both the DRVs and the RDIs. Specifically, the label includes the percent DV except for protein. Protein information is not required unless a protein claim is made for the product or if the product is to be used by infants or children younger than four years of age. The following table lists the DVs based on a caloric intake of 2,000 calories, for adults and children four years of age and older.

To calculate the percent DV, determine the ratio between the amount of the nutrient in a serving of food and the DV for the nutrient.

Barbara A. Brehm

See Also: Dietary Reference Intakes.

Table 1. Daily Values

Food Component	Daily Value
Total Fat	65 grams (g)
Saturated Fat	20 g
Cholesterol	300 milligrams (mg)
Sodium	2,400 mg
Potassium	3,500 mg
Total Carbohydrate	300 g
Dietary Fiber	25 g
Protein	50 g
Vitamin A	5,000 International Units (IU)
Vitamin C	60 mg
Calcium	1,000 mg
Iron	18 mg
Vitamin D	400 IU
Vitamin E	30 IU
Vitamin K	80 micrograms (µg)
Thiamin	1.5 mg
Riboflavin	1.7 mg
Niacin	20 mg
Vitamin B6	2 mg
Folate	400 µg
Vitamin B12	6 µg
Biotin	300 µg
Pantothenic acid	10 mg
Phosphorus	1,000 mg
Iodine	150 µg
Magnesium	400 mg
Zinc	15 mg
Selenium	70 µg
Copper	2 mg
Manganese	2 mg
Chromium	120 µg
Molybdenum	75 µg
Chloride	3,400 mg

Source: U.S. Food and Drug Administration. (2013). *Guidance for Industry: A Food Labeling Guide*. Retrieved from http://www.fda.gov/Food/GuidanceRegulation/GuidanceDocumentsRegulatoryInformation/LabelingNutrition/ucm064928.htm

Further Reading

U.S. Food and Drug Administration. (2013). *Guidance for Industry: A Food Labeling Guide*. Retrieved from http://www.fda.gov/Food/GuidanceRegulation/GuidanceDocumentsRegulatoryInformation/LabelingNutrition/ucm064928.htm

Dairy Foods

Dairy products refer to food items that contain milk. Female mammals produce milk for the nourishment of their offspring. Throughout their lives, some people continue to drink milk and consume products made from the milk of animals, including cows, sheep, goats, horses, camels, yaks, and buffalo. Numerous essential nutrients are found in milk, including vitamins, minerals, and protein. Dairy products include yogurt, kefir, and cheese, produced by the fermentation of milk; frozen dairy desserts, such as ice cream, ice milk, and frozen custard; and butter and whipped cream, produced from churning milk or cream. Some people experience bloating, cramping, and other forms of digestive discomfort when they consume dairy products because they have an enzyme deficiency that results in lactose intolerance—difficulty digesting the sugar contained in milk. Many questions regarding the health benefits of dairy products have arisen over the past several decades, as consumers strive to make sense of public health dietary advice.

Nutritional Components of Milk

Cow's milk is approximately 87% water by weight. About 4.9% of milk is carbohydrate, primarily in the form of lactose, a disaccharide (sugar). About 3.4%

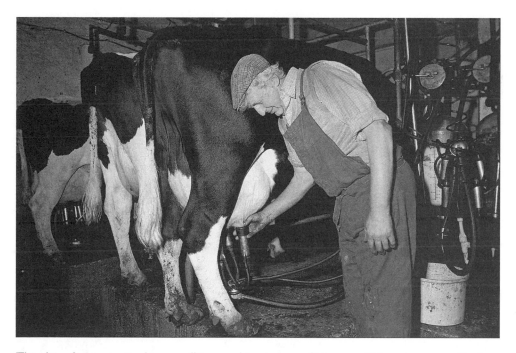

This dairy farmer is attaching a milking machine to one of his cows. Dairy cows are milked on a consistent schedule, usually twice daily, to maintain optimal milk production. (Corel)

of milk is composed of fats, and of this fat 65% is saturated, 29% is monounsaturated, and 6% is polyunsaturated fatty acids (Cornell, Nutritional components, 2014b). About 3.3% of milk is protein. Milk has all nine of the essential amino acids, as do other animal products (Cornell, Nutritional components, 2014b). Milk contains a number of vitamins, most notably vitamin A (an 8 oz serving of 2% milk provides about 15% of the DRI); riboflavin (35% of the DRI); and vitamin B12 (47% of the DRI) (Cornell, Nutritional components, 2014b). One cup of fortified milk contains about 20% of the DRI for vitamin D. For many people, milk is an important source of many minerals. One cup of 2% milk provides 30% of the DRI for calcium; 7% of the DRI for magnesium; 30% of the DRI for phosphorus; 8% of the DRI for potassium; 11% of the DRI for selenium; 7% of the DRI for sodium; and 10% of the DRI for zinc (Cornell, Nutritional components, 2014b).

Pasteurized versus Unpasteurized

When milk is pasteurized it goes through a heating process that kills microorganisms—many of which can cause serious and even potentially lethal foodborne illnesses. Unpasteurized milk is the same thing as "raw milk," and it has not gone through pasteurization. Although raw milk is preferred by some people for its flavor and potentially helpful microbes and other components, the U.S. Food and Drug Administration cautions that the benefits of consuming raw milk do not outweigh the risks of foodborne illness. It is highly recommended that women who are pregnant, children, and older adults avoid raw milk (FDA, 2013).

Lactose Intolerance and Dairy Allergies

Lactose is a monosaccharide carbohydrate found in milk. For the body to be able to digest lactose it uses lactase (an enzyme found in the small intestine) to break lactose down into simpler molecules that then are absorbed into the blood. People who produce little or no lactase are not able to digest lactose and are considered lactose intolerant. A majority of people from many ethnic groups, including people of African American, Asian American, and Native American descent are lactose intolerant. Although some lactose-intolerant individuals can ingest small portions of dairy products or consume dairy if they take lactase medication, high rates of lactose intolerance around the world have led many public health experts to question the validity of recommending daily dairy intake in dietary guidelines, such as the U.S. Dietary Guidelines.

People with dairy allergies develop allergic symptoms when they consume dairy products or the exacerbating proteins, such as whey and casein, from dairy products. Allergic symptoms include hives, difficulty breathing, nausea, and vomiting. People with milk allergies even can experience anaphylactic shock, a medical emergency marked by swelling of the airways and difficulty breathing.

Other symptoms of dairy allergies include diarrhea, abdominal cramps, and runny nose.

Dairy and Health

The health impacts of dairy consumption vary with the type of dairy product consumed. Products high in fat and added sugar (e.g., ice cream) can contribute many calories with little nutritive value; intake of these products should be limited. Research has explored the association and impact of milk and dairy-product consumption on a number of health issues, including those listed below.

Cardiovascular Disease

When scientists found an association between saturated fat intake and risky blood lipid levels (which are associated with artery disease, the most common form of cardiovascular disease), public-policy groups advised consumers to switch from whole milk, which is almost 3.5% fat (by weight) to milk with less fat (2%, 1%, or skim milk). Over time, researchers discovered that not all saturated fatty acids have the same effects in the body. For example, fatty acids with shorter chain lengths (10 or fewer carbons) are absorbed from the digestive tract and transported in the bloodstream differently from longer chain saturated fatty acids, and do not seem to cause harmful changes in blood lipid levels. Stearic acid, a saturated fatty acid with 18 carbons, also does not appear to negatively influence blood lipid levels. Therefore, although milk fat is composed of about 65% saturated fats, 10% of these are the shorter chain-length variety and 14% is stearic acid (Cornell, Human health, 2014a). Therefore, the impact of whole-milk consumption on artery disease might not be as harmful as was once believed (German et al., 2009). Nevertheless, public-health groups, including the U.S. Department of Agriculture (USDA), still urge consumers to choose lower fat milk varieties to limit saturated fats and calories. Dairy producers are experimenting with the types of food dairy cows consume, to determine whether the fatty acid profiles can become more healthful if cows consume organic or grass-based diets (Benbrook, Butler, Latif, Leifert, & Davis, 2013).

Hypertension

Increased intakes of low-fat dairy products are associated with small but significant decreases in blood pressure, especially in people with borderline hypertension and in African-Americans. The most effective version of the well-studied Dietary Approaches to Stop Hypertension (DASH) diet recommends 2 to 4 servings of low-fat or nonfat dairy products per day. Researchers believe that it could be the calcium found in dairy products that helps to normalize blood pressure, but the magnesium and potassium also are thought to be helpful. Bioactive proteins found in milk also could influence the activity of arteries, and thus contribute to a better blood pressure response (German et al., 2009).

Osteoporosis

Osteoporosis is characterized by low bone-mineral density and fragile bones prone to fracture. Early studies suggested that, because milk contains large amounts of calcium, dairy products should be helpful for the prevention of osteoporosis; research has generally found this to be the case (Cornell, Human health, 2014a). Especially important is calcium intake during childhood and adolescence, because peak bone mass is attained in young adulthood.

Theoretical concerns regarding the impact of a high protein intake on net endogenous acid production led to the questioning of whether milk's high protein content might mean that the risks of milk consumption outweigh its benefits. "Net endogenous acid production" refers to the metabolic effect of foods on physiological acid levels, normally well regulated by the kidneys in young people, but less well controlled in older adults—those most prone to osteoporosis. When the pH of the blood becomes too acidic, it is believed that calcium is drawn from the bones to neutralize pH. Well-controlled studies, however, support the positive effect of dairy consumption on bone density. Although calcium excretion does increase with a high protein intake, the calcium in milk contributes to a net calcium gain (Cornell, Human health, 2014a; Schardt, 2011). The protein in milk also can be helpful to frail older adults—the group most prone to debilitating fractures. Protein intake in this group is often too low. Bones are about 50% protein, and without adequate protein intake bone structure can be compromised (Cornell, Human health, 2014a). Vitamin D is another nutrient critical to bone health, and dairy products fortified with vitamin D can help people achieve better dietary intakes of this nutrient.

Cancer

Good evidence suggests that milk protects against colorectal cancer (Schardt, 2011). One meta-analysis found that people who drank at least one cup of milk a day had a 15% lower risk of being diagnosed with colorectal cancer than those who drank fewer than two glasses per week (Schardt, 2011). Both calcium and vitamin D are thought to contribute to the effect of dairy on colorectal cancer risk. Dairy consumption also might help reduce risk for bladder cancer. Conversely, high calcium intakes—especially intakes of more than 1,200 mg per day—have been associated with increased risk for prostate cancer. Greater dairy consumption is associated with increased levels of certain growth factors that have been linked to better bone density, but also are linked to an increased risk of certain cancers, including prostate cancer. Dairy consumption does not appear to be associated with breast cancer risk, however.

Weight Loss

Although early studies suggested that dairy products might be helpful for weight loss, other studies have been less supportive. Dairy products can be part of a healthful, low-calorie diet, but the key to losing weight is the reduction of calorie intake and the development of lifelong healthful eating behaviors.

Dairy Politics

Whether dairy foods should be part of a healthful diet often inspires passionate debate. Why? Many political and environmental issues are linked to dairy consumption. Some nutrition researchers bristle at the inclusion of daily dairy consumption in national dietary guidelines, because many people are lactose intolerant. Some people charge the USDA—which regulates the dairy industry—with catering to the dairy lobby rather than putting the public's health first. Groups concerned with sustainable agriculture and animal cruelty object to the treatment of dairy animals, especially the use of growth hormones to increase milk production, antibiotics to increase growth and prevent disease, and confinement feeding procedures. Even grass-fed dairy operations draw criticism from environmentalists, as the methane naturally excreted by cows and other dairy animals contributes to greenhouse gases thought to influence climate change. Water pollution and land conversion (from forest to pasture) also can exert negative environmental impacts.

Barbara A. Brehm and Brittney M. Blokker

Research Issues

Critics have charged that the U.S. Department of Agriculture, whose mission includes the promotion of agricultural products, could be influenced by special interests as it designs dietary guidelines. Some critics have suggested moving the design of dietary guidelines to a science-based department, such as the Centers for Disease Control and Prevention or the Institute of Medicine (Willett & Ludwig, 2011).

Willett, W. C., & Ludwig, D. S. (2011). The 2010 Dietary Guidelines—the best recipe for health? *New England Journal of Medicine, 365,* 1563–1565. doi: 10.1056/NEJMp1107075

See Also: Climate change and global food supply; Food allergies and intolerances; Hypertension and nutrition; Lactose intolerance; Microbiota and microbiome; Organic food and farming; Osteoporosis; Raw milk; Sustainable agriculture; Whey protein.

Further Reading

Benbrook, C. M., Butler, G., Latif, M. A., Leifert, C., & Davis, D. R. (2013). Organic production enhances milk nutritional quality by shifting fatty acid composition: A United States-wide, 18-month study. *PLoS One.* Retrieved from http://www.plosone.org/article/info%3Adoi%2F10.1371%2Fjournal.pone.0082429#pone.0082429-Ludwig1. doi: 10.1371/journal.pone.0082429

Cornell University. Milk Quality Improvement Program. (2014a, December 1). *Milk and human health*. Retrieved from http://www.milkfacts.info/Nutrition%20Facts/ Milk%20 and%20Human%20Health.htm

Cornell University. Milk Quality Improvement Program. (2014b, December 1). *Nutritional components in milk*. Retrieved from http://www.milkfacts.info/Nutrition%20Facts /Nutritional%20Components.htm

German, J. B., Gibson, R. A., Krauss, R. M., Nestel, P., Lamarche, B., et al. (2009). A reappraisal of the impact of dairy foods and milk fat on cardiovascular risk. *European Journal of Nutrition, 10*. Retrieved from http://link.springer.com/article/10.1007% 2Fs00394-009-0002-5/fulltext.html#Sec3

Louie, J. C. Y., Flood, V. M., Burlutsky, G., Rangan, A. M., Gill, T. P., & Mitchell, P. (2013). Dairy consumption and the risk of 15-year cardiovascular disease mortality in a cohort of older Australians. *Nutrients, 5* (2), 441–454. Retrieved from http://www.ncbi .nlm.nih.gov/pmc/articles/PMC3635204/. doi: 10.3390/nu5020441

Schardt, D. (2011, July). Dairy: Hero or villain? *Nutrition Action Healthletter.* Retrieved from http://www.thefreelibrary.com/Dairy%3A+hero+or+villain%3F-a0263156515

U.S. Food & Drug Administration (FDA). (2013, June). *Questions and answers: Raw milk*. Retrieved from http://www.fda.gov/food/foodborneillnesscontaminants /buystoreservesafefood/ucm122062.htm

Dental Caries (Cavities)

Dental caries commonly are known as cavities and are a symptom of tooth decay. Tooth decay occurs when acid produced by bacteria living in the mouth erode a tooth's protective enamel. Proper dental care and good oral hygiene are both important to one's oral health. Additionally, good oral health is also an important part of one's overall health. Routine dental care can prevent cavities from forming and enables dentists to treat cavities in their early stages. According to the American Dental Association ([ADA], 2013b) as many as 100 million Americans forego their routine dental care each year.

Cavities

Both helpful and harmful bacteria reside in the mouth. These bacteria live on teeth, gums, tongues, and other areas in the mouth. Most foods and drinks, such as cookies, soda, juice, and even milk, contain both natural and added sugars. The sugars provide a food source for these bacteria. The bacteria and sugars are part of a biofilm that forms around the teeth, better known as plaque. Acid is produced when the bacteria metabolize sugars. It is this acid that causes cavities.

A cavity destroys a tooth's enamel, which is the outer layer of the teeth. The destruction of the tooth's enamel causes it to lose minerals. A white spot forms on areas where minerals have been lost (NIH, 2014). If this process continues and the enamel is weakened and destroyed then a cavity forms; cavities can continue to grow and must be repaired with a filling by a dentist. This process,

The stages of tooth decay

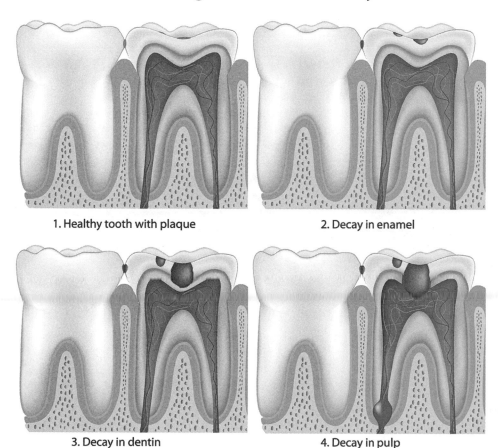

1. Healthy tooth with plaque

2. Decay in enamel

3. Decay in dentin

4. Decay in pulp

Tooth decay begins when bacteria living in the plaque on the teeth metabolize sugars, producing acid as a byproduct. Fluoride applications can reverse very early stages of tooth decay, but if left untreated, decay can spread to the interior of the tooth and cause pain and inflammation. (Shutterstock.com)

however, can be stopped or even reversed in its early stages by repairing the enamel with minerals from salvia, toothpaste with fluoride, and other fluoride treatments (NIH, 2014).

Dental Health Basics

To avoid cavities, it is important to follow the tips listed below as recommended by the ADA (2013d).

Dental Care Costs

It is important to take advantage of good dental care. Regular teeth cleaning performed by a dental professional can reduce the plaque and tartar (hardened plaque) that houses harmful bacteria. The expense of dental care, however, deters people from visiting a dentist regularly. The Affordable Care Act (ACA) (also commonly referred to as "Obamacare") offers dental coverage for adults via most of the state marketplaces (ADA, 2013a). The ACA Web site (www.healthcare.gov) can help people locate a plan that fits their budget.

Aside from the state marketplaces, dental-school clinics provide lower-cost dental care; some collect only partial payment to cover the cost of materials and equipment. Dentists and hygienists also might donate their services at no cost to those who cannot afford to pay. Overall, good oral care can prevent greater expense in the future. Dental caries can progress to a point where required treatments are much more costly. Regular dental care also is an important investment in overall health, as, in addition to dental caries, gum disease can result from poor oral hygiene.

- Brush for two minutes with a fluoride toothpaste at least twice a day
- Floss between teeth daily
- Consume a healthful diet
- Limit snacking, especially avoiding sticky, sugary foods.

In addition to a good home dental care routine, regular dental visits for professional cleaning and oral examination can prevent and catch small cavities when they are easier to treat.

Susana Leong

See Also: Fluoride; The mouth.

Further Reading

American Dental Association. (2013a). *Choosing a dental plan under ACA*. Retrieved from www.healthcare.gov

American Dental Association. (2013b). *Dental care concerns*. Retrieved from www .mouthhealthy.org/en/dental-care-concerns

American Dental Association. (2013). *Helpful resources: Paying for dental care*. Retrieved from http://www.mouthhealthy.org/en/dental-care-concerns/paying-for -dental-care/helpful-resources

American Dental Association. (2013). *Mouth healthy*. Retrieved from www.mouthhealthy .org

American Dental Association. (2013c). *Questions about going to the dentist*. Retrieved from www.mouthhealthy.org/en/dental-care-concerns/questions-about-going-to-the-dentist

American Dental Association. (2013d). *Teeth cavities*. Retrieved from www.mouthhealthy. org/en/az-topics/c/cavities

National Institute of Health (NIH). (2014, January). *The tooth decay process: How to reverse it and avoid a cavity*. National Institute of Dental and Craniofacial

Research. Retrieved from www.nidcr.nih.gov/OralHealth/OralHealthInformation /ChildrensOralHealth/ToothDecayProcess.htm

Depression and Nutrition

Depression is a broad term used to describe persistent feelings of sadness, hopelessness, and emptiness. The *Diagnostic and Statistical Manual of Mental Disorders* (DSM-5) is the handbook used to classify or diagnose mental disorders. It provides diagnostic criteria for the seven clinical depressive disorders, including major depressive disorder (MDD), dysthymia, premenstrual dysphoric disorder, substance/medication-induced depressive disorder, depressive disorder due to another medical condition, other specified depressive disorder, and unspecified depressive disorder. Depression affects about 7% of the U.S. population (American Psychiatric Association, 2013). Women are diagnosed with depression about twice as often as men. There is some evidence that nutrition plays a part in depression.

Major depressive disorder is the most representative of these types of depression. Its diagnostic criteria include constant depressed mood or loss of interest in the same two-week period; significant distress or impairment; mood is not due to effects of a substance or other medical or psychiatric condition; manic and hypomanic episodes have never occurred. Other symptoms include the following.

- Anhedonia (loss of ability to find pleasure in activities)
- Poor concentration and difficulty making decisions
- Insomnia
- Weakness or fatigue
- Aches and pains
- Significant weight loss (not attributable to dieting) or weight gain
- Irritability
- Anxiety
- Suicidal ideation or attempt
- Feelings of worthlessness

It is important to not underestimate the potential seriousness of depression. In extreme cases, people experiencing depression might commit suicide to end their suffering. Suicide is the third leading cause of death for individuals between 10 and 24 years old.

Depression often is treated with various forms of psychotherapy, medication, and electroconvulsive therapy (ECT). Hospitalization could be warranted, especially if people are at risk of harming themselves or others. Mild to moderate depression might respond to lifestyle measures, such as regular exercise, adequate sleep, and a healthful diet.

Depression and Overall Diet Quality

Some studies suggest that overall diet quality could be related to depression risk. One group of researchers conducted a five-year longitudinal study consisting of more than 3,000 middle-aged male and female participants (Akbaraly, Brunner, Ferrie, Marmot, Kivimaki, & Singh-Manoux, 2009). It was found that individuals whose diets consisted mainly of whole foods (that is, foods that are as close to their natural form as possible, including generous intakes of vegetables, fruits, and fish) had a lower rate of depression, as opposed to those who consumed more processed foods.

A study from the Harvard School of Public Health examining the link between diet and depression in 43,685 participants in the Nurses' Health Study found that those consuming a more inflammatory diet showed higher risk for depression (Lucas et al., 2014). Participants were free of depression at the beginning of the study. An inflammatory diet pattern refers to a diet that is associated with greater levels of blood markers of inflammation, including C-reactive protein, interleukin-6, and tumor necrosis factor alpha receptor 2 (Lucas et al., 2014). According to analyses by the research group, an inflammatory dietary pattern is relatively high in sugar-sweetened beverages, refined grains, red meat, diet soft drinks, and margarine, but low in olive oil, green leafy and yellow vegetables, wine, and coffee. The researchers hypothesized that inflammation could increase risk for depression through several mechanisms. Proinflammatory cytokines (immune cell messengers) might have a negative effect on neurotransmitters. The decline in endothelial function (which influences arterial health) associated with inflammatory markers also could influence brain health (Lucas et al., 2014).

Two other epidemiological studies in women have shown associations between a Mediterranean diet and depression, with higher intakes of fruits, vegetables, legumes, fish, poultry, wine, and olive oil predicting lower risk of depression (Rienks, Dobson, & Mishra, 2013; Sanchez-Villegas et al., 2009). A study of 9,272 men and 3,132 women in France found that greater risk for depression was associated with low-fat and high-snack diets in women (Le Port et al., 2013). In men, greater risk for depression was predicted by low-fat, Western, high-snack, and high fat–sweet diets. (A more Western dietary pattern typically is characterized as having relatively greater consumption of red and processed meats, sweets and desserts, french fries, and refined grains.)

Although there probably is not one perfect diet that guarantees no risk of depression, the studies discussed above seem to indicate that greater intakes of plant foods (fruits, vegetables, legumes) and healthful fats along with reduced intakes of refined grains, added sugars, artificial fats, and dessert-type foods are more likely to reduce depression risk.

Depression and Nutrients

Recent studies have shown several links between nutritional deficiencies and risk of depression. Some studies have found a positive relationship between neurotransmitters (such as dopamine, norepinephrine, and serotonin) and amino acids in natural supplements.

A number of nutrients play important roles in the metabolism of neurotransmitters and brain health (*see* Table 1). Research on these individual nutrients is intriguing. Megadosing on individual nutrients, however, is not generally associated with significant improvement for most people with depression. Rather, people should strive to achieve recommended intakes for all vitamins and minerals.

Table 1. Nutrients Linked to Depression

Nutrient	Health Benefits	Effects on Depression	Food Sources	Daily Value
B6	• Essential for the communication of neurotransmitters • Vital for the synthesis of hemoglobin needed to carry oxygen throughout the body • Low hemoglobin levels are associated with depression	Given its role in the tryptophan-serotonin pathway, it has been suggested that a B6 deficiency might contribute to symptoms of depression	Salmon, bananas, avocado, potato	2.0 mg
Folate	• Important for cell growth and the production of DNA	Increasing folate intake has been associated with a decrease in depressive symptoms; deficiencies in people with depression have also been reported	Asparagus, spinach, legumes, broccoli	400 mcg
B12	• Essential for metabolism • Forms new red blood cells and nerve cells • Involved in DNA synthesis	Studies have shown that individuals with a high intake of B12 are less likely to experience depression	Seafood, meat, poultry, dairy, eggs	6 mcg
Magnesium	• Important for nerve and heart function • Reduces blood pressure	Some research has shown magnesium supplements to be beneficial to people with depression; however, excessive calcium intake might alter the bioavailability of magnesium after absorption	Whole grains, broccoli, potato, nuts, legumes	310–400 mg

(continued)

Table 1. Continued

Nutrient	Health Benefits	Effects on Depression	Food Sources	Daily Value
Omega-3	• Important for brain function and cardiovascular health. Research has shown that countries that consume high amounts of fish per capita have lower rates of depression	Although studies remain inconclusive, research shows that omega-3 fatty acids promote cognitive and behavioral function, and ease symptoms of mood swings and depression	Fish, walnuts, flaxseeds	(No daily value set) Nutritionists generally recommend 1.1-1.6 g
Zinc	• Essential for cell growth • Important for the regulation of endocrine, immune, and neuronal systems • Facilitates the development of bones and sexual organs	Individuals with depression have been found to have low concentrations of zinc in the blood	Meat, dairy, whole grains, nuts, legumes	15 mg
Vitamin D	• Important for absorption of calcium from the intestines • Involved in storage of calcium in the bones • Facilitates cell development	Rates of depression have been linked to deficiencies in vitamin D	Milk, salmon, sardines, tuna	400 I.U.

Research generally supports an increased consumption of omega-3 fatty acids from foods and supplements as a possibly helpful dietary change for mild to moderate depression.

Herbs and Natural Supplements

Several herbs and dietary supplements have preliminary support for their beneficial effects in reducing symptoms of depression. Some of the most studied of these include the following.

Inositol

Although not an essential nutrient, inositol is important for muscle and nerve function, as well as for the transmission of serotonin. Inositol can be found in legumes, whole grains, citrus fruits, and cantaloupe. Side effects from supplements can include nausea, fatigue, dizziness, and headache.

Tryptophan

Tryptophan is an amino acid that assists in the production of serotonin. There still are safety concerns regarding contaminants detected in samples of tryptophan. In 1990, after 1,500 individuals developed eosinophilia myalgia syndrome, the FDA temporary recalled L-tryptophan products.

Saffron

Saffron supplements are composed of extracts found in various parts of the saffron plant. Research has shown that saffron and antidepressants are similarly effective in improving symptoms of depression. Although its specific medical properties are unknown, saffron's antioxidant and radical scavenger properties could contribute to its antidepressant effects. Side effects can include headache, nausea, anxiety, and decreased appetite.

Sam-E (an abbreviation for the chemical S-adenosyl methionine, or S-adenosylmethionine)

A natural compound that assists in the transmission of serotonin and dopamine in the brain. Although not a stimulant, Sam-E claims to boost mood and attention levels and is used for the treatment of attention-deficit disorder (ADHD). Side effects can include anxiety and skin rashes.

St. John's Wort

The St. John's Wort supplement is derived from a yellow flower, the Hypericum perforatum. The exact mechanisms of its antidepressant effect remain unclear. It has been suggested that the hypericin and hyperforin extracts found in St. John's Wort interact with the nerve receptors involved in depression. Side effects can include gastrointestinal issues, itching, fatigue, increased sensitivity to sunlight, and headache.

Eating a balanced diet has been shown to be beneficial in decreasing depressive symptoms and promoting overall health and well-being. Some studies have shown that supplements are beneficial to some individuals experiencing mild depression. Severe depression should be treated by a professional health caregiver, such as a psychiatrist, however, and usually requires antidepressants or other psychiatric treatment. People experiencing symptoms of depression should seek help from a professional.

Nicole D. Teitelbaum

See Also: "Brain foods"; Inflammation; Mood and food; S-adenosylmethionine; St. John's wort.

Further Reading

Akbaraly, T. N., Brunner, E. J., Ferrie, J. E., Marmot, M. G., Kivimaki, M., & Singh-Manoux, A. (2009). Dietary pattern and depressive symptoms in middle age. *The British Journal of Psychiatry, 195* (5), 408–413.

American Psychiatric Association. (2013). *Diagnostic and Statistical Manual of Mental Disorders* (5th ed.) (DSM-5). Arlington, VA: American Psychiatric Association.

Depression: out of the shadows—statistics. (2008). PBS.org. Retrieved from http://www-tc.pbs.org/wgbh/takeonestep/depression/pdf/dep_stats.pdf.

Ehrlich, S. D. (2011). Omega-3 fatty acids. University of Maryland Medical Center. Retrieved from http://umm.edu/health/medical/altmed/supplement/omega3-fatty-acids

Le Port, A., Gueguen, A., Kesse-Guyot, E., Melchoir, M. Lemogne, C., Nabi, H., Goldberg, M., Zins, M., & Czernichow, S. (2012). Association between dietary patterns and depressive symptoms in a 10-year follow-up study of the GAZEL Cohort. *PLOS One, 7,* e51593. doi: 10.1371/journal.pone.0051593

Lucas, M., Chocano-Bedoya, P., Shulze, M.B., Mirzaei, F., O'Reilly, E. J., Okereke, O. I., Hu, F. B., Willett, W. C., & Ascherio, A. (2014). Inflammatory diet pattern and risk of depression among women. *Brain Behavior and Immunity, 36,* 46–53. doi: 10.1016/j.bbi.2013.09.014

Rienks, J., Dobson, A. J., & Mishra, G. D. (2013). Mediterranean dietary pattern and prevalence and incidence of depressive symptoms in mid-aged women: Results from a large community-based prospective study. *European Journal of Clinical Nutrition, 67,* 75–82.

Sanchez-Villegas, A., Delgado-Rodriguez, M., Alonso, A., Schlatter, J., Lahortiga, F., Majem, L. S, & Martinez-Gonzalez, M. A. (2009). Association of the Mediterranean dietary pattern with the incidence of depression: The Seguimiento Universidad de Navarra/University of Navarra follow-up (SUN) cohort. *Archives of General Psychiatry, 66,* 1090–1098.

Detoxification

Detoxification refers to the processes by which toxins are removed from the body. The term "detoxification" is used in several different contexts. The human body employs a wide variety of physiological processes to eliminate waste products and potentially toxic substances. Detoxification in this context refers to these physiological processes. The term detoxification also refers to medical treatments designed to remove environmental toxins—particularly heavy metals such as lead or mercury—from the body. The term also is used to describe numerous products and practices thought to promote good health by accelerating or furthering the body's natural detoxification processes. The popularity of "detox" diets, therapies, and products has risen dramatically in recent years, yet there is little empirical evidence substantiating the extensive health claims made by supporters.

Physiological Detoxification Processes

The lungs, colon, kidneys, lymphatic system, and liver all play integral roles in detoxifying the body. Carbon dioxide—a byproduct of respiration—is excreted by the lungs. Without this function, excess carbon dioxide would build up in the bloodstream and eventually result in death. The colon forms feces, allowing undigested materials to be eliminated from the gastrointestinal tract. Microorganisms throughout the body, and especially in the gastrointestinal tract, help to break down some potentially carcinogenic substances. Hydration status and electrolyte balance are maintained by the kidneys, which excrete water, salts, and nitrogen-containing waste. The lymphatic system transports proteins and particulate matter too large to be absorbed into the blood away for removal, preventing these substances from accumulating in the interstitial fluid (the solution surrounding cells). Perhaps the most vital organ in physiological detoxification, the liver, often is referred to as the body's primary filter. It removes toxic chemicals from the blood and neutralizes or breaks them down. The byproducts of these metabolic processes are released either into the bile the liver produces or back into the bloodstream. Thus, the byproducts ultimately leave the body as components of feces or urine. Sweat glands also help reduce the burden of heavy metals in the body by moving toxic elements into the sweat (Sears, Kerr, & Bray, 2012). These physiological detoxification processes continuously remove waste products and help to maintain health.

Medicinal Detoxification for Toxic Metals

Some types of medicinal detoxification treatments have widely recognized therapeutic value for individuals with certain conditions. One such example is chelation therapy for the treatment of heavy metal poisoning, such as lead or mercury poisoning. Heavy metal poisoning occurs when metals are not metabolized by the body and instead accumulate in the soft tissues. Heavy metal poisoning can occur from environmental pollution and from jobs that involve working with metals such as lead, mercury, cadmium, and arsenic. Chelation comes from the Greek word "chele," meaning "claw," and refers to the mechanism by which the chelating chemical binds to the metals. In chelation therapy, a substance such as the synthetic amino acid EDTA (ethylene diamine tetraacetic acid) is intravenously injected. The EDTA and other chelation agents bind to heavy metals, enabling them to be released from the soft tissues and excreted in urine. Chelation has numerous side effects; chelating agents also bind to minerals such as calcium, so chelation therapy can cause bone damage. Chelation therapies also carry a small risk of kidney damage and heart failure.

Chelation Therapy for Chronic Health Problems

Chelation therapy has been promoted as an alternative treatment for many chronic illnesses, including artery disease, cancer, multiple sclerosis, and Alzheimer's disease. Given that the effectiveness of alternative applications of chelation therapy for most of these conditions has not been established through scientific study, it could be associated with more risks than benefits for most patients.

The one possible exception is chelation therapy for artery disease, specifically to prevent subsequent cardiovascular events in people who have already suffered a heart attack. A small study followed about 1,700 such adults in the United States and Canada (Lamas et al., 2013). Subjects were randomly assigned to treatment groups. After one to five years, the group receiving the chelation treatment had somewhat lower rates of cardiovascular events such as heart attacks or strokes than the group receiving a placebo treatment. People with diabetes had even more clinically significant benefits. Researchers caution that larger studies should continue to explore the efficacy of chelation therapy before clinical recommendations can be made.

Detox Products

A multitude of supplements and other items are advertised as at-home methods of medicinal detoxification—ways to remove or enhance the body's ability to remove toxins. Manufacturers often include a feature meant to confirm that their product works as advertised; detox patches and ionic saltwater foot spas, for example, change color after use, which is said to be visual evidence that toxins have been drawn out of the body. In fact, the patches contain water-soluble herbal extracts and simply change color in response to moisture. The footbaths' color change results from iron oxides in the electrodes.

Detox supplements contain a wide range of ingredients. Though their efficacy has not been established, most herbal formulas carry little risk unless the individual using them is allergic to a certain ingredient or is taking a drug that produces a harmful interaction. Some detox teas and tablets contain stimulant laxatives such as senna, however, which can be dangerous in large doses or if used for a prolonged period, and can result in dehydration, electrolyte imbalance, and reduced bowel function.

Intestinal Cleansing

An extension of the idea that laxatives assist the body in eliminating toxins, colonic irrigation is a common detox therapy. In colonic irrigation, low-pressure water pumps and small tubes are used to flush waste from the colon. The underlying belief is that fecal matter lingering in the colon results in a buildup of toxins that are absorbed into the bloodstream, causing fatigue and general poor health. Gastroenterologists, however, argue that the concept of fecal matter adhering to the intestinal walls as "sludge" is inaccurate—bowel transit time varies, but waste does not remain in the body indeterminately (Harvard Medical School, 2008). Colonic irrigation carries risks similar to those of heavy laxative use—dehydration, electrolyte imbalances, and impaired bowel function. Increased fiber and water intake are recommended as safer alternatives for people considering colonics due to constipation.

Detox Diets

Fasting, juicing, and certain eating regimens also are said to detoxify the body and promote weight loss. Some suggestions are far from controversial, including drink more water, eat more leafy green vegetables, and avoid processed foods. It is unclear, however, whether these diets carry any health benefits independent of such suggestions. Weight loss associated with the regimes is unsurprising given that most—if not all—include caloric restriction. Doctors and nutritionists worry that the "detox mentality" will lead individuals to fluctuate between periods of unhealthy eating and fasting or restrictive eating rather than making long-term lifestyle changes (Crowe, 2010).

Psychological Aspects

Enthusiasm for detox diets, therapies, and products could stem from sources other than actual health benefits achieved through enhanced removal of toxins from the body. The placebo effect appears to have a powerful influence: An individual who believes that he or she is engaging in a health-promoting behavior typically feels good about it. In the case of very low-calorie detox diets, restriction can trigger a "starvation high" marked by increased release of endorphins, which further enhances the individual's sense of well-being. Doctors and dietitians warn that associating restriction with positive feelings can contribute to the development of an eating disorder (Iliades, 2011).

Laura C. Keenan

See Also: Lead; The liver; Mercury.

Further Reading

Allen, J. A, Montalto, M., Lovejoy, J., & Weber, W. (2011). Detoxification in naturopathic medicine: A survey. *Journal of Alternative and Complementary Medicine, 17* (12), 1175–1180. doi: 10.1089/acm.2010.0572

Crowe, T. (2010). Diets, weight loss and detox diets. *Nutridate, 21* (1). Retrieved from http://moodle.plc.nsw.edu.au/pluginfile.php/6378/mod_page/content/8/NutriDate_Vol_21_No_1_March_2010.pdf

Harvard Medical School. (2008). The dubious practice of detox. *Harvard Women's Health Watch, 15* (9). Retrieved from http://www.health.harvard.edu/fhg/updates/The-dubious-practice-of-detox.shtml

Iliades, C. (2011). *The truth about detox diets*. Retrieved from http://www.everydayhealth.com/digestive-health/the-truth-about-detox-diets.aspx

Lamas, G. A., Goertz, C., Boineau, R., Mark, D. B., Rozema, T., Nahin, R. L., Lindblad, L., Lewis E. F., Drisko, J., & Lee, K. L. (2013). Effect of disodium EDTA chelation regimen on cardiovascular events in patients with previous myocardial infarction; the TACT randomized trial. *Journal of the American Medical Association, 309* (12), 1241–1250. doi: 10.1001/jama.2013.2107

Sears, M. E., Kerr, K. J., & Bray, R. I. (2012). Arsenic, cadmium, lead, and mercury in sweat: A systematic review. *Journal of Environmental and Public Health,* February 22, 2012, 184745. doi: 10.1155/2012/184745

Diabetes, Type I

Diabetes mellitus, commonly known as diabetes, occurs when a person has high blood glucose (blood sugar) due to inadequate insulin production, or because the body's cells do not respond properly to insulin, or both. There are three main types of diabetes: type 1 diabetes, type 2 diabetes, and gestational diabetes. Type 1 diabetes is less common than type 2 diabetes, representing approximately 5% of all diabetes cases (CDC, 2011). Type 1 diabetes is an autoimmune disease that usually begins in childhood or adolescence but can develop at any age. Type 1 diabetes occurs when a person's immune system mistakenly destroys the insulin-producing beta cells in the pancreas. Insulin is required for normal blood glucose regulation; it signals cell membrane receptors to take up glucose from the blood, allowing glucose to enter cells. Without the release of insulin, glucose stays in the blood, creating a condition known as hyperglycemia, or high blood glucose. Scientists do not yet know what causes the body's immune system to attack insulin-producing cells or why the onset of the disease begins so early in life. People with type 1 diabetes must learn to manage their blood sugar levels with insulin medication and by regulating the factors that can influence blood sugar, such as diet, physical activity, and stress.

Type 1 diabetes was recognized by ancient civilizations around the world. The first use of the word diabetes has been traced to 230 BCE and Greek physician Appollonius of Memphis. Diabetes comes from the Greek word for "to flow through," or "siphon," based on the observation that type 1 diabetes is characterized by excessive urination. Second century Greek physician Aretaeus of Cappadocia was one of the first to write a thorough clinical description of the disease. Seventeenth-century London physician Thomas Willis diagnosed diabetes in his patients by tasting their urine. Sweet urine indicated a positive diagnosis. He called his diagnosis "diabetes mellitus"; the word "mellitus" was derived from "mel," the Latin word for "honey" (Sattley, 2008).

Before the discovery of insulin and the development of medical insulin in the early decades of the 1900s, treatment for type 1 diabetes consisted of various ineffective strategies and restrictive diets that did little to halt the course of the disease, which always ended within a few years of diagnosis with the patient's death. Insulin, isolated from the pancreases of animals, was first used on humans in 1922. Commercial insulin initially was produced from the pancreases of cows or pigs, as this insulin is most similar to human insulin. Since 1983, biotechnology has harnessed bacteria to produce insulin. In this process, the human gene for insulin production is inserted into bacteria, stimulating the organisms to produce human insulin.

Until recently, type 1 diabetes was referred to as juvenile diabetes because it typically strikes during childhood. Because adults also can suffer from the disease, it was later renamed insulin-dependent diabetes mellitus. People with type 2 diabetes, however, also can become insulin dependent. Therefore, several years later, the disease was renamed "type 1 diabetes," to better distinguish between the various types of diabetes.

Although the cause of type 1 diabetes is unknown, researchers suspect genetic factors could be involved, as people with a parent or sibling with type 1 diabetes are at greater risk for developing the disease. Caucasians have a higher risk than other groups, and certain countries—such as Finland and Sweden—have higher rates. Several dietary factors have been associated with increased risk of developing type 1 diabetes, including consumption of cow's milk and cow's milk formula in infancy, and low vitamin D levels.

Symptoms and Diagnosis

Symptoms of type 1 diabetes usually develop over a short period. Some symptoms include excessive thirst, frequent urination, blurred vision, weight loss, constant hunger, and extreme fatigue. If hyperglycemia is not controlled, people with diabetes can develop ketoacidosis and even suffer a life-threatening diabetic coma.

Type 1 diabetes is diagnosed using a variety of blood glucose tests (ADA, 2014a). These tests typically are administered twice to obtain an accurate diagnosis.

- A1C: The glycated hemoglobin (A1C) test measures the percentage of hemoglobin that is bound to glucose. Hemoglobin is the compound that carries oxygen in red blood cells. Higher A1C measures reflect greater exposures of hemoglobin to blood glucose. The A1C measure reflects average blood glucose levels over the previous three months, because that is the average lifespan of red blood cells. Patients are diagnosed with diabetes if their A1C level is 6.5% or more. An advantage of the A1C test is that patients do not need to fast before the blood tests are administered.
- Fasting plasma glucose test: This test checks the blood glucose levels after a person has not eaten for at least eight hours. Diabetes is diagnosed if blood glucose is 126 mg/dl or greater.
- Oral glucose tolerance test: This test measures how the body responds to glucose. At the beginning of the test, the patient gives a blood sample to determine the fasting blood glucose level. Then the patient consumes a sweet drink containing 75 to 100 grams of glucose. After two hours, another sample of blood is collected from the patient to measure the glucose level. Diabetes is diagnosed if the blood glucose level is equal to or greater than 200 mg/dl.
- Casual (or random) or plasma glucose test: A blood sample can be taken at any time that the patient experiences diabetic symptoms. People are diagnosed if their blood glucose reaches 200 mg/dl or more.

Medical and Lifestyle Treatments

Diabetes increases a person's risk for several health problems. Some of the more severe long-term consequences of type 1 diabetes include hypertension, artery disease, kidney disease, blindness, and damage to the nervous system. In some cases, circulatory problems can lead to heart attack, stroke, and lower-limb amputations. Risk of long-term complications decreases with good blood glucose control.

Medication

People diagnosed with type-1 diabetes must take insulin every day. Several different types of insulin are available; these vary by concentration, duration, and speed of action. Insulin is either injected or infused. Common forms of insulin delivery are via syringe (shots), insulin pen (an instrument that is filled with insulin and looks like a pen), and insulin pump. An insulin pump is a small device that releases insulin via a catheter under the skin of the abdomen. Insulin infusions also can be administered under medical supervision through intravenous fluids.

Physical Activity Recommendations

Regular physical activity can help to prevent the long-term complications associated with diabetes. People with type 1 diabetes, however, often fear engaging in physical activities because exercise influences blood sugar regulation. Fortunately, scientists have found that people with type 1 diabetes can exercise safely and effectively. It is critical to develop an understanding of how one's body responds to exercise, and learn to balance insulin, food intake, and physical activity. When planning to exercise, diabetics might have to reduce insulin dosage. For unplanned exercise, people might need to ingest extra carbohydrates. The American Diabetes Association recommends five days of moderate to intense aerobic exercise for 30 minutes per session, and two to three days of strength training per week (ADA, Exercise, 2014b).

Nutrition

A heart-healthy diet is recommended for people with diabetes. A well-planned diet that includes plenty of vegetables, fruits, and whole grains, and limited intake of added fats and sugars helps reduce risk of the chronic health problems associated with diabetes. Additionally, people with type 1 diabetes must follow a regular meal plan that has been developed with a dietitian to ensure that carbohydrate intake and timing accommodates physical activity level and insulin dosage.

People with type 1 diabetes must monitor intake of carbohydrates because carbohydrates increase blood glucose levels. Type 1 diabetics should select foods with low glycemic index. A food's glycemic index indicates how much and how quickly the carbohydrate food elevates blood glucose. Foods high in added sugars—such as soft drinks—generally should be avoided. Consuming meals that include healthful fats and fiber can slow the absorption of carbohydrates from the digestive system, and thus slow the rise in blood glucose following a meal.

Limiting unhealthy fats is part of a healthful diet, especially for diabetics who have an increased risk for cardiovascular diseases. Unhealthy fats consist of saturated and trans fats. These fats can increase blood cholesterol levels, which increases the risk of heart disease. Foods high in saturated fats include butter, cream sauces, high-fat dairy and meats, lard, poultry skin, and salt pork. Foods high in trans fats include processed snacks and baked goods that contain hydrogenated oil, shortening, stick margarines, and various fast-food items. Healthy fats are found in foods high in monounsaturated fats and omega-3 fatty acids. Monounsaturated fats can help lower "bad" LDL cholesterol levels, and are found in avocado, olive oil and olives, sesame seeds, canola oil, and peanut butter. Omega-3 fatty acids reduce inflammation in the arteries and reduce risk of blood clots. Foods containing high amounts of omega-3 fatty acids are salmon, herring, rainbow trout, sardines, walnuts, and ground flaxseed.

Fruits and vegetables are high in antioxidants and other phytochemicals that help to protect the arteries and organs vulnerable to the oxidation caused by high blood glucose levels. People with type 1 diabetes should consume low levels of sodium to avoid hypertension, and use alcohol in moderation, because alcohol exerts a strong influence on blood glucose levels.

Amina Z. Seay and Oksana M. Tsichlis

Research Issues

Researchers are working to develop a cure for type 1 diabetes. A cure for this disease only can be achieved by stopping the autoimmune destruction of pancreatic beta cells, and restoring insulin production (JDRF 2014). Promising areas include the transplantation of pancreatic beta cells to the pancreas or liver of people with type 1 diabetes. Scientists also are trying to develop methods of generating pancreatic beta cells from stem cell precursors.

See Also: Blood sugar regulation; Cardiovascular disease and nutrition; Diabetes, type 2; Hyperglycemia; Hypoglycemia; Insulin.

Further Reading

American Diabetes Association (ADA). (2014a, April 10). *Exercise and type 1 diabetes.* Retrieved from http://www.diabetes.org/food-and-fitness/fitness/exercise-and-type-1-diabetes.html?loc=DropDownFF-exercise-type1

American Diabetes Association (ADA). (2014b, September 22). *Diagnosing diabetes and learning about prediabetes.* Retrieved from http://www.diabetes.org/diabetes-basics/diagnosis/

Centers for Disease Control and Prevention (CDC). (2011). *National diabetes fact sheet.* Retrieved from http://www.cdc.gov/diabetes/pubs/pdf/ndfs_2011.pdf

JDRF. (2014, December 1). *The basic challenges of curing type 1 diabetes.* Retrieved from http://jdrf.org/research/cure/

Mayo Clinic Staff. (2013). *Diabetes.* MayoClinic.com. Retrieved from http://www.mayoclinic.com/health/diabetes/DS01121

National Diabetes Information Clearinghouse (NDIC). (2013). *Diabetes, heart disease, and stroke.* Retrieved from http://diabetes.niddk.nih.gov/dm/pubs/stroke/index.aspx#risk

Sattley, M. (2008). The history of diabetes. *Diabetes Health.* Retrieved from http://diabeteshealth.com/read/2008/12/17/715/the-history-of-diabetes/

Diabetes, Type 2

Diabetes mellitus is a group of disorders characterized by abnormal blood sugar regulation. Blood sugar level is influenced by a number of factors, several of which contribute to the development of type 2 diabetes mellitus (T2D) when disrupted. Problems occur at the cell membrane-receptor level, causing the body's cells to become less responsive to the hormone insulin and sluggish in their uptake of glucose from the blood. Additionally, over time insulin production can decline, further compromising blood-sugar regulation processes. Type 2 diabetes is the most common kind of diabetes; approximately 80% of people with diabetes have type 2. The onset of T2D is gradual and most commonly affects adults and the elderly. In the past 20 years, however, the incidence of children and adolescents diagnosed with type 2 diabetes has increased. People with type 2 diabetes often are overweight or obese and do not exercise regularly. Decreasing caloric intake with or without weight loss surgery; weight loss; and increasing levels of physical activity can restore normal blood glucose regulation for many people with T2D, at least for a number of years.

Type 2 diabetes occurs when the cell membrane receptors do not respond appropriately to insulin, a hormone that is produced by the pancreas beta cells. This condition is called insulin resistance, meaning the receptors "resist" responding to insulin. Insulin resistance requires an increased output of insulin to regulate blood glucose levels. In the early stages of this condition (before an actual diagnosis of T2D), blood glucose levels are normal, but insulin levels are higher than normal. Over time, the severity of insulin resistance can increase to the point where even higher insulin levels cannot achieve adequate glycemic (blood glucose) control; this results in hyperglycemia (high blood glucose). If blood glucose is only slightly elevated (a fasting blood glucose of 100 to 125 mg/dl), the condition is called prediabetes. After some time, unless intervention occurs, insulin resistance typically worsens and blood glucose levels become high enough for a diagnosis of type 2 diabetes (a fasting blood glucose level of 126 mg/dl or higher). People with type 2 diabetes often experience problems with insulin production over time, as the number of pancreatic beta cells appear to decline. Therefore, during the early stages of T2D, insulin levels are normal or even high, but eventually they can decrease, making blood glucose levels even more difficult to control.

Symptoms and Diagnosis

Symptoms of type-2 diabetes might not be detected for several years in the beginning stages of this disease. Regular symptoms that occur in T2D include increased thirst and urination, fatigue, higher incidence of infections and slow healing of sores, increased hunger, weight loss, patches of darkened skin, and blurred vision. Fluids in the body tissues are depleted in response to the increased amounts of glucose in the bloodstream. In T2D, the kidneys excrete the excess glucose in the bloodstream, along with the fluid required

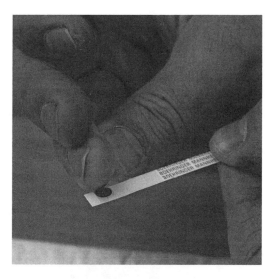

People with diabetes can monitor their blood glucose levels to obtain feedback on the efficacy of their treatment efforts. With one of the most common monitoring methods, people place a drop of blood onto a test strip of paper that is then analyzed by a glucose meter. (National Institutes of Health)

to make extra urine. This causes dehydration, so people become thirstier and start a more frequent cycle of drinking and urination. People sometimes experience fatigue and some irritability because their cells are not getting enough glucose.

All forms of diabetes can lead to several long-term complications, especially if blood glucose levels remain high over a long period. Complications can include poor wound healing that can lead to amputation; heart and blood vessel diseases; Alzheimer's disease; kidney disease resulting in reduced kidney function that can lead to kidney failure and treatment with dialysis; and eye problems, including blindness. People with T2D experience a slower healing process for several reasons, which include poor circulation, nerve damage, and weaker immune system. People with diabetes have a higher risk of artery disease—marked by plaque deposition in the arteries—which causes a decrease in blood circulation and limits the amount of nutrients and oxygen available to heal a wound. Diabetes increases risk for the development of neuropathy (nerve damage). The most common form is peripheral neuropathy, which starts at the foot and can eventually affect the whole leg. As a result, type-2 diabetics with neuropathy might be unaware of an injury, which could lead to an open sore that is vulnerable to infection. In severe cases, when the wound is not treated properly and in time, an infection that won't heal can lead to amputation. Artery damage can affect the arteries supplying the heart with blood, a condition known as coronary artery disease—the leading cause of heart disease. The artery disease and inflammation associated with diabetes

Diabetes in Children and Adolescents

"SEARCH for Diabetes in Youth Study" is a multicenter study funded by the CDC and NIH to examine diabetes (type 1 and type 2) among children and adolescents in the United States. SEARCH findings for the communities studied include the following.

- During 2002–2005, 15,600 youth were newly diagnosed with type 1 diabetes annually, and 3,600 youth were newly diagnosed with type 2 diabetes annually.
- Among youth younger than 10 years of age, the rate of new cases was 19.7 per 100,000 each year for type 1 diabetes, and 0.4 per 100,000 for type 2 diabetes. Among youth 10 years of age and older, the rate of new cases was 18.6 per 100,000 each year for type 1 diabetes, and 8.5 per 100,000 for type 2 diabetes.
- Non-Hispanic White youth had the greatest rate of new cases of type 1 diabetes (24.8 per 100,000 per year among those younger than 10 years of age and 22.6 per 100,000 per year among those ages 10–19 years).
- Type 2 diabetes was extremely rare among youth aged 10 years of age and younger. Although still infrequent, rates were greater among youth aged 10–19 years than in younger children, with higher rates among U.S. minority populations than in non-Hispanic Whites.
- Among non-Hispanic White youth 10–19 years of age, the rate of new cases was greater for type 1 than for type 2 diabetes. For Asian/Pacific Islander and American Indian youth 10–19 years old, the opposite was true—the rate of new cases was greater for type 2 than for type 1 diabetes. Among non-Hispanic Black and Hispanic youth aged 10–19 years, the rates of new cases of type 1 and type 2 diabetes were similar.

A table showing the rates of new cases of diagnosed diabetes among people younger than 20 years of age in the United States is provided in the CDC *National Diabetes Fact Sheet.*

Centers for Disease Control and Prevention (CDC). (2011). *National Diabetes Fact Sheet: National Estimates and General Information on Diabetes and Prediabetes in the United States, 2011.* U.S. Department of Health and Human Services. Retrieved from http://www.cdc.gov/diabetes/pubs/pdf/ndfs_2011.pdf

increases risk of Alzheimer's disease, a type of dementia. Prolonged exposure to high blood glucose levels damage the kidney, causing a gradual decline in kidney function. Diabetes increases risk for several eye diseases, including diabetic retinopathy, cataracts, and glaucoma. Diabetic retinopathy is caused by damage to the blood vessels of the retina, interfering with vision. Cataracts involve a clouding of the eye lens, and glaucoma is characterized by an increase in fluid pressure in the eye that damages the optic nerve.

Some tests used to determine whether a person has type 2 diabetes include measuring fasting blood glucose levels, the glycated hemoglobin (A1C) test, the oral glucose tolerance test (OGTT), and the random/casual plasma glucose test. Doctors usually administer tests twice to ensure an accurate diagnosis. The first test uses a fasting blood sample and measures blood sugar. Diagnosis is made if the results show blood sugar level at 126 mg/dL or greater. The A1C test calculates the percentage of hemoglobin attached to glucose; it reflects average blood sugar levels over previous two to three months. Diagnosis is made if the percentage of hemoglobin attached to sugar is 6.5% or greater. The OGTT measures blood glucose level two hours after a person consumes a sugary drink. Diagnosis is made if blood sugar levels exceed 200 mg/dL. The casual or plasma glucose test is a blood test taken whenever the patient starts to experience any diabetic symptoms. Diagnosis is made if blood sugar levels are 200 mg/dL or more.

Treatment

Treatment for T2D usually begins with monitoring blood sugar levels, and changing eating behaviors and physical activity levels to improve blood glucose regulation. Doctors recommend that patients with type 2 diabetes check their blood sugar levels at least once a day, depending on type of treatment administered. Blood sugar levels vary throughout the day in response to different factors such as eating, alcohol intake, stress level, medication, type and duration of physical activity, and (for women) hormone fluctuations. Testing blood sugar regularly can help people understand the links between blood sugar and these factors, and can indicate whether more aggressive treatment is indicated. In people with excess fat, weight loss (fat loss) usually improves blood glucose regulation.

Weight loss can be achieved through lifestyle change programs or weight-loss surgery. It is important to note that surgery is effective only if it leads to reduced food intake and weight loss, and if these changes are maintained. The benefits of surgery are lost if harmful eating habits are resumed and weight is regained. Many medications can help people with type 2 diabetes achieve better blood sugar control. None reverse the disease, but they can slow the development of long-term complications.

Diet

Healthy eating is a critical component in the treatment of T2D, both for improving glucose levels and for weight control in people who have excess fat. A healthful diet for type 2 diabetics emphasizes a reduced calorie intake, if the person is overweight; a relatively low intake of carbohydrates, focusing primarily on vegetables; increasing intake of dietary fiber; reducing intake of foods with added fats and sugars; and maintaining or increasing intake of healthy fats. People diagnosed with T2D should meet with a dietitian who can help them plan delicious and nutritious meals that follow these recommendations.

Reducing intake of carbohydrates is critical, because these are the source of blood glucose. High-sugar foods such as non-diet sodas and fruit juice should be avoided. The healthiest carbohydrates are found in foods such as fruits, vegetables, low-fat dairy products, legumes, and whole grains. Intake of most starchy foods must still be limited, however. Many people with diabetes learn how to keep track of carbohydrates' glycemic load to reduce the impact of carbohydrates on blood glucose levels. Dietary fiber reduces the rise in blood sugar level following a meal, therefore a diet high in fiber is encouraged for people with T2D. Healthy fats commonly are found in almonds, walnuts, peanut butter, avocados, olives, and canola. Fish with good levels of omega-3 fatty acids, including salmon, bluefish, halibut, and sardines also are recommended.

Because T2D increases a person's risk of cardiovascular disease, people with diabetes usually are advised to follow dietary recommendations for the prevention of artery disease. Type 2 diabetics should avoid foods high in saturated fats, trans fats, and sodium. Saturated fats are found in many meats and high-fat dairy products. Foods rich in these fats include beef, hot dogs, bacon, and sausage. Trans fats should be avoided completely and are found in baked goods, processed snacks, and margarine. Clinicians recommend that people with type 2 diabetes limit sodium intake to less than 2,300 mg per day, because people with T2D often develop hypertension.

Physical Activity

Regular, almost daily, physical activity is recommended to improve glycemic control, reduce cardiovascular diseases, and help maintain a healthy weight for people with diabetes. Several studies have shown that exercise improves insulin sensitivity and blood sugar regulation, even without weight loss. Additionally, exercise stimulates blood glucose uptake by muscle tissue in an insulin-independent molecular pathway (Colberg et al., 2010). This means that glucose uptake by muscle during exercise is normal even in people with diabetes. These effects of physical activity are short lived. The insulin-independent pathway remains active for only a few hours after exercise, but insulin sensitivity remains elevated for up to 72 hours (Colberg et al., 2010). Researchers are exploring the molecular mechanisms through which these effects occur. With exercise, muscles release peptide (protein) molecules. These molecules help the muscles communicate with the nervous, endocrine, and immune systems. They generally have an anti-inflammatory effect on the body and appear to contribute to many exercise benefits, such as better blood sugar regulation and reduced artery disease (Pedersen, 2011). In addition to its effects on insulin sensitivity and blood glucose uptake by skeletal muscle, physical activity can contribute to a negative energy balance, fatty acid oxidation, and weight loss. Physical activity can help normalize high blood pressure and improve blood lipid profile and arterial function.

Recent research suggests that exercise decreases the likelihood that prediabetes will develop into type2 diabetes by 58% when subjects engage in exercise for at least 150 minutes per week (Colberg et al., 2010). The American College of Sports Medicine and the American Diabetes Association recommend at least 150 minutes per week of moderate aerobic exercise, with some amount of physical activity at least five days a week. Some studies suggest that longer periods of exercise are even more effective. A combination of resistance training (at least three times a week) and aerobic activity is even more beneficial for improving blood glucose regulation than aerobic exercise alone (Colberg et al., 2010).

Medical Treatment

A significant number of medications are available to help improve blood glucose control. Drugs often are prescribed in a variety of combinations, depending upon a person's diagnosis. Some drugs enhance the sensitivity of cells to insulin; others increase insulin production and release in the pancreas. Some drugs decrease the amount of glucose the body absorbs from food by inhibiting the breakdown of carbohydrates in the digestive system. Other drugs inhibit the liver's production and release of glucose. Glucose monitoring and diet and exercise records can help patients and health care providers work together to find the medications that work best.

Active Lifestyle Treatment Can Reverse or Delay Type 2 Diabetes for Some People

Type 2 diabetes often can be reversed—or at least postponed—with appropriate lifestyle changes, primarily changes in diet and physical activity. A recent study demonstrated total reversal of type 2 diabetes in 7 of 10 subjects undergoing 8 weeks of intensive dietary intervention. The 10 participants consumed a very low-calorie diet of 600 calories per day for eight weeks. The results showed that 70% of the participants (seven) no longer had symptoms of T2D by the end of the study. This outcome is similar to that seen with bariatric (weight loss) surgeries, following which most people only can eat small portions of food and thus experience dramatic weight loss. Dramatic lifestyle change is difficult for most people, however. Less-stringent lifestyle changes also have been shown to reverse or postpone type 2 diabetes. Research by Wing and colleagues (Wing et al., 2011) found significant improvement in cardiovascular disease risk factors after one year when overweight and obese people with T2D lost 5% to 10% of their body weight through prescribed diet and exercise. This is important because type 2 diabetics who are overweight are more at risk for developing cardiovascular diseases. People diagnosed with diabetes or prediabetes should work with their health care providers to achieve optimal glucose control using a combination of diet, physical activity, weight loss, and, if necessary, medication.

Barbara A. Brehm and Amina Z. Seay

Research Issues

Researchers still are exploring the relationship between type 2 diabetes and obesity. Obesity might contribute to the T2D disease state in several ways, many of which presently are under investigation. Insulin resistance could result from defects in signaling molecule production or function, either inside or outside the cells. The process might be influenced by lipotoxicity, in which fatty acids or their products interfere with cellular response to insulin. Obesity also could interfere with optimal pancreatic beta cell function via the deposition of amyloid in the islet cells, excess fat deposits in the pancreas, oxidative stress, and inflammation, or interfere with signaling molecules that modulate insulin release (Taylor, 2013). An increase in the concentration of fatty acid metabolites is associated with an increased rate of beta cell death via apoptosis.

See Also: Blood sugar regulation; Cardiometabolic syndrome; Diabetes, type 1; Glycemic index and glycemic load; Hyperglycemia; Hypoglycemia; Insulin; Obesity, definition and health effects.

Further Reading

American Diabetes Association. (2013). *Diabetes statistics*. Retrieved from http://www.diabetes.org/diabetes-basics/statistics/

American Diabetes Association. (2014). *Diagnosing diabetes and learning about prediabetes*. Retrieved from: http://www.diabetes.org/diabetes-basics/diagnosis/

Colberg, S. R., Sigal, R. J., Fernhall, B., Regensteiner, J. G., Blissmer, B. J., Rubin, R. R., Chasan-Taber, L., Albright, A. L., & Braun, B. (2010). Exercise and type 2 diabetes. The American College of Sports Medicine and the American Diabetes Association: joint position statement. *Diabetes Care, 33* (12), 2010. Retrieved from http://care.diabetesjournals.org/content/33/12/e147.full. doi: 10.2337/dc10-9990

Mayo Clinic Staff. (2013). *Diabetes diet: Create your healthy-eating plan*. Mayo Clinic. Retrieved from http://www.mayoclinic.com/health/diabetes-diet/DA00027

Mayo Clinic Staff. (2013). *Type 2 Diabetes*. MayoClinic.com. Retrieved from http://www.mayoclinic.com/health/type-2-diabetes/DS00585

Pedersen, B. K. (2011). Muscles and their myokines. *Journal of Experimental Biology, 214*, 337–346.

Taylor, R. (2013). Type 2 diabetes; etiology and reversibility. *Diabetes Care, 36* (4), 1047–1055. Retrieved from http://care.diabetesjournals.org/content/36/4/1047.full

Wing, R. R., Lang, W., Wadden, T. A., Safford, M., Knowler, W. C., Bertoni, A. G., Hill, J. O., Brancati, F. L., Peters, A., & Wagenknecht, L. (2011). Benefits of modest weight loss in improving cardiovascular risk factors in overweight and obese individuals with type 2 diabetes. *Diabetes Care, 34* (7), 1481–1486. Retrieved from http://care.diabetesjournals.org/content/34/7/1481.long. doi: 10.2337/dc10-2415

Diarrhea

Diarrhea is a health problem characterized by loose, frequent, watery stools. For most adults in North America, diarrhea usually is nothing more than an annoyance that quickly passes even with no treatment. Chronic diarrhea can be indicative a serious underlying medical condition, however. If diarrhea is severe and prolonged, it can lead to dehydration—which can be particularly dangerous in infants and children, and in people with health problems. In resource-poor countries, dehydration from diarrhea is a leading cause of death, especially in infants and young children. Globally, diarrheal illnesses are responsible for 1 in 9 child deaths (CDC, 2014). Diarrhea has many causes. Treatment consists of addressing the causes of the illness and giving rehydration medications.

In some cases, diarrhea is a useful physical response. The body develops diarrhea to assist in the elimination of harmful agents from the digestive tract. The rate of peristalsis, the muscular contractions that move food and waste through the digestive system, increases. Additionally, inflammation and some infectious agents sometimes draw more water into the large intestine. (During normal digestive processes, water is absorbed from the material in the large intestine back into the body.) The increased movement of watery stools through the large intestine enhances removal of potentially dangerous microorganisms and chemicals.

Diarrhea can be caused by many factors, including infectious agents such as certain bacteria, viruses, and parasites. Such agents often enter the digestive system from contaminated water and food, or from hands that have come into contact with infectious agents. Diarrhea also can result from food allergies and intolerances, including celiac disease and lactose intolerance. Chronic diarrhea can be a symptom of inflammatory bowel diseases, such as Crohn's disease and ulcerative colitis, and functional bowel disorders, such as irritable bowel syndrome. Some medications, including antibiotics and antacids containing magnesium, can cause diarrhea. Even feelings of stress can lead to bouts of diarrhea.

People experiencing acute episodes of diarrhea should drink plenty of water. Sports beverages that replace electrolytes also can be helpful. Foods high in fiber and fat should be avoided. Bland foods such as bananas, white rice, applesauce, toast, and crackers often are recommended. Adults who have diarrhea should seek medical care when diarrhea does not resolve after several days, or if diarrhea is accompanied by any of the following (Donowitz & Fordtran, 2013).

- Severe abdominal or rectal pain
- Fever of 102 degrees F or higher
- Blood or pus in the stools
- Black or tarry stools

Children should receive medical care for the same symptoms, but earlier in the course of diarrhea, for example, if severe diarrhea persists for longer than 24 hours (Donowitz & Fordtran, 2013). Infants and young children should receive medical care very early as well, especially if they are not taking fluids. Infants and children can die from even just one day of severe dehydration (Donowitz & Fordtran, 2013).

Barbara A. Brehm

See Also: Digestion and the digestive system; Diverticular disease; Foodborne illness and food safety; Inflammatory bowel diseases; Irritable bowel disease; Large intestine.

Further Reading

Centers for Disease Control and Prevention (CDC). (2014, Jan. 24). *Global diarrhea burden.* Retrieved from http://www.cdc.gov/healthywater/global/diarrhea-burden.html

Donowitz, M. & Fordtran, J. S. (2013). *National Digestive Diseases Information Clearinghouse.* Retrieved from http://digestive.niddk.nih.gov/ddiseases/pubs/diarrhea/index.aspx

Mayo Clinic Staff. (2013, June 11). *Diarrhea.* Retrieved from http://www.mayoclinic.org/symptoms/diarrhea/basics/definition/sym-20050926

Dietary Guidelines for Americans

The *Dietary Guidelines for Americans* (DGA) is a document that provides the foundation for all federal nutrition programs. The *Dietary Guidelines* are created by the United States Departments of Agriculture (USDA) and Health and Human Services (HHS) to guide nutrition policy in the United States and are revised every five years. The guidelines will be revised again in the fall of 2105, and they should be reviewed at the USDA's website; currenty there are available at http://www.cnpp.usda.gov/dietaryguidelines.htm.

The DGA are designed to provide a consistent, evidence-based summary of recommendations regarding nutrition advice for generally healthy people older than two years of age. The goals of the advice offered by the DGA are not only to help people to avoid deficiency diseases caused by poor nutrition, but to encourage people to make food choices that will reduce their risk for chronic diseases such as obesity, type 2 diabetes, hypertension, heart disease, and cancer. By law, all federal dietary recommendations, such as the MyPlate nutrition advice, must be consistent with the DGA.

History and Development

The DGA grew out of work that began in 1970s by the U.S. Senate Select Committee on Nutrition and Human Needs, chaired by Senator George McGovern. During this time, epidemiologists were trying to determine the factors that increased a person's risk for heart disease, the leading cause of death in the United States. Reviewing the existing research—much of it focused on the link between high blood lipid levels and heart disease risk—the Committee issued a report, *Dietary Goals for the United States,* in 1977. This landmark document marked the beginning of a shift in federal nutrition policy away from the prevention of nutrient-deficiency diseases, which were becoming increasingly rare in the U.S. population, and toward the prevention of heart disease and other chronic illnesses. The report advised people to reduce the consumption of refined and processed sugars, total fat, saturated fat, cholesterol, and sodium, and to increase the consumption of complex carbohydrates and naturally occurring sugars. At the time, it was believed that higher amounts of fat in the diet translated into higher blood lipid levels, and a low-fat diet was thought to lower blood fat levels. Polyunsaturated fats were believed to be less harmful than saturated fats. These basic recommendations were translated into the following dietary advice that was issued in the 2010 Dietary Guidelines.

- Increase consumption of fruits, vegetables, and whole grains
- Decrease consumption of:
  - refined and processed sugars and foods high in such sugars
  - foods high in total fat and animal fat, and partially replace saturated fats with polyunsaturated fats
  - eggs, butterfat, and other high-cholesterol foods
  - salt and foods with high salt content
- Choose low-fat and non-fat dairy products instead of high-fat dairy products

Although some groups applauded the government's efforts to improve the eating habits of U.S. citizens and stem the rising tide of heart disease, many people questioned the scientific validity of the committee's report. Industry groups, such as those that produced meat and dairy products, challenged the guidelines that could impact their members' interests. In an effort to improve the scientific foundation of government dietary advice, the U.S. Department of Agriculture and the U.S. Department of Health and Human Services formed a group of scientists charged with evaluating and revising the goals into an evidence-based set of dietary guidelines. The committee wrote the first version of the DGA, titled *Nutrition and Your Health: Dietary Guidelines for Americans,* which was released in 1980. Not surprisingly, this report also was met with criticism from both scientists and industry groups. This response prompted Congress to direct the USDA and HHS to establish another committee to gather and review the criticism, and advise on future revisions of the DGA, which were issued in 1985 and 1990. In 1990, the National Nutrition Monitoring and Related Research Act mandated the USDA and HHS to update the DGA every five years, directed by a Dietary Guidelines Advisory Committee. This procedure continues to operate, with the secretaries of the USDA and HHS appointing new advisory committees every revision cycle, and releasing new versions of the DGA every five years.

Over time, the Dietary Guidelines Advisory Committees have tried to make the revision procedures more research based. In 2009, the USDA created a Nutrition Evidence Library (NEL), compiling the scientific research articles related to diet and health. The USDA and HHS also established a public comments database for feedback from the scientific and lay communities as the guidelines were being revised. In these ways, the Advisory Committee has attempted to expand the input that shapes the DGA.

Dietary Guidelines

The DGA consist of 23 key recommendations that are spelled out in a 100-plus-page document available on the Internet (*Dietary Guidelines for Americans,* 2011). Recommendations from the Dietary Guidelines include the following.

Balance Calories to Manage Weight

This guideline encourages people to balance calorie intake with expenditure throughout all the life stages. It encourages people to increase physical activity and reduce sedentary behaviors. Emphasis in this section is on achieving and sustaining a healthy weight.

Consume Nutrient-Dense Foods and Beverages

Nutrient density refers to the nutritive value per calorie of a given food. If one food has a higher nutrient density than another, it means it has more nutrition per calorie. For example, milk has a higher nutrient density than soda, because milk contains more protein, vitamins, and minerals than soda. The dietary guidelines emphasize the observation that people get too many of their calories from solid fats (trans fatty acids and saturated fatty acids), added sugars, and refined grains. These ingredients add calories but have little helpful nutrition. Foods and beverages high in these ingredients often are said to be "empty-calorie" foods, meaning that the calories contribute little toward a person's nutritional needs. The guidelines urge readers to avoid empty-calorie foods and make good food and beverage choices by looking for foods that contribute positively to one's nutritional needs.

Foods and Food Components to Reduce

This section of the *Dietary Guidelines* goes into some depth on several issues. Much of this advice is difficult to translate into food intake and thus is confusing for consumers. The issues addressed include the following.

- Sodium: The guidelines recommend that sodium intake be reduced to less than 2,300 mg per day for healthy young people. The guidelines suggest an even lower limit, 1,500 mg, for about half of the population, including people older than 50, all African-Americans (who have a higher risk of hypertension), and anyone with hypertension, diabetes, or kidney disease.
- Saturated fatty acids: The guidelines recommend reducing these to less than 10% of total daily calories, and replacing them with unsaturated fats.
- Cholesterol: The guidelines recommend less than 300 mg per day.
- Trans fatty acids: The guidelines recommend keeping these as low as possible by limiting consumption of products with hydrogenated oils.
- Refined grains: The guidelines suggest limiting food with refined grains, especially those with added sugars, sodium, and solid fats.
- Alcohol: The guidelines suggest limiting alcoholic beverages to one per day for women and two per day for men, if alcohol is consumed at all.

Foods and Nutrients to Increase

Individuals are cautioned to stay within their calorie needs as they increase the foods listed below.

- Increase vegetable and fruit intake: Health and nutrition professionals have been universally pleased to see this advice take center stage in the *U.S. Dietary Guidelines*.
- Eat a variety of vegetables: This guideline encourages consumers to expand their vegetable choices and to include dark-green, red, and orange vegetables in their diet, as well as beans and peas.
- Consume at least half of all grains as whole grains: This guideline encourages people to replace refined grains with whole grains. For example, the guidelines advise people to replace white rice with brown rice and use whole-wheat products in place of those made with white flour.

- Increase intake of fat-free or low-fat milk and milk products: Consumers are encouraged to look for non-fat or low-fat dairy products such as milk, yogurt, and cheese.
- Choose a variety of protein foods: The protein food group is no longer called the "meat" group. Better sources of protein include seafood, lean meat and poultry, eggs, beans and peas, soy products, and unsalted nuts and seeds.
- Increase the amount and variety of seafood: Consumers are encouraged to consume seafood in place of some other meats, but to consume a variety to avoid high intakes of heavy metals such as mercury.
- Replace protein foods that are higher in solid fats with choices that are lower in solid fats: This guideline encourages people to reduce intake of saturated fat.
- Use oils to replace solid fats: This guideline's goal is similar to the one above.
- Choose foods that provide more potassium, dietary fiber, calcium, and vitamin D: These nutrients are likely to be low in the average diet. The guideline urges consumers to increase consumption of vegetables, fruits, whole grains, milk, and milk products.

Criticisms of the *Dietary Guidelines for Americans*

Many scientists and consumer groups have criticized the DGA. One of the most common points of contention concerns the continuing recommendations for the restriction of saturated fats and promotion of a relatively high intake of grain products. Many experts believe the evidence for a harmful effect of saturated fats on artery disease is not well supported by the research (Malhotra, 2013). Additionally, many researchers now believe that a high intake of carbohydrates, especially added sugars and refined grain products, contributes to obesity, type 2 diabetes, and heart disease (Willett & Ludwig, 2011).

One of the most well-respected critic groups of the DGA is led by Walter Willett and colleagues from the Harvard School of Public Health. In a letter to the Advisory Committee for the 2010 DGA, Willett and colleagues outlined several criticisms of the DGA.

- Evidence to support recommending three servings of milk per day is lacking and could cause harm to some people. Additionally, if everyone consumed this much milk per day, milk production in the United States would need to double, which would exert a serious negative impact on the environment.
- Recommendations for a high intake of lean meat could be problematic, as research has found a link between intake of red meat and risk for colorectal cancers.
- Recommendations for a high intake of folic acid for women of child-bearing age should be stronger.
- Recommendations that half of grain products consumed can be refined grains is not scientifically based, as these foods can contribute to obesity and associated health risks.

Willett and colleagues also have charged that members of the USDA have ties to industries, such as the dairy and cattle industries, that present a conflict of interest with their ability to appoint members to the advisory committee who can provide objective advice. Willett and colleagues have suggested that responsibility for the DGA be shifted to a more science-based organization, such as the Centers for Disease Control and Prevention.

Barbara A. Brehm

Research Issues

Some critics of the *Dietary Guidelines for Americans* (DGA) have charged that the guidelines are too vague and that they should more clearly name the foods to be avoided, such as empty-calorie foods. Read the DGA, and then make a list of foods whose consumption probably should be limited. Soft drinks, for example, generally are considered empty-calorie foods. What other foods and food categories contain food components that should be reduced?

See Also: Public policy on nutrition.

Further Reading

Center for Nutrition Policy and Promotion, U.S. Department of Agriculture. (2013a). *Dietary guidelines for Americans.* Retrieved from http://www.cnpp.usda.gov /dietaryguidelines.htm

Center for Nutrition Policy and Promotion, U.S. Department of Agriculture (2013b). *2010 Dietary guidelines for Americans; backgrounder: History and process.* Retrieved from http://www.cnpp.usda.gov/Publications/DietaryGuidelines/2010/DGAC/Report/E -Appendix-E-4-History.pdf

Malhotra, A. (2013). Saturated fat is not the major issue. *British Medical Journal, 347.* doi: http://dx.doi.org/10.1136/bmj.f6340

U.S. Department of Agriculture & U.S. Department of Health and Human Services. (2011). *Dietary guidelines for Americans 2010.* Retrieved from http://www.health.gov/di-etaryguidelines/dga2010/DietaryGuidelines2010.pdf

Willett, W., Cheung, L., Stampfer, M., and Kalin, S. (2010, July 15). *Commentary on the Report of the Dietary Guidelines Advisory Committee on the Dietary Guidelines for Americans, 2010.* Harvard School of Public Health. Retrieved from http://www.hsph .harvard.edu/nutritionsource/files/2012/10/commentary-hsph-dga-2010-advisory.pdf

Willett, W. C., & Ludwig, D. S. (2011). The 2010 Dietary Guidelines—The best recipe for health? *New England Journal of Medicine, 356,* 1563–1565. doi: 10.1056 /NEJMp1107075

Dietary Reference Intakes

Dietary Standards

Dietary standards are important for the planning and evaluating of individual diets; the planning and evaluating of diets for different groups of individuals; and making nutrition policy decisions. An example of a nutrition policy decision is the amount of foods or vouchers for foods that are to be provided for individuals who are a part of the Special Supplemental Nutrition Program for Women, Infant, and Children (WIC). The WIC program provides supplemental foods, health care referrals, and nutrition education to low-income pregnant, breast-feeding, and non-breast-feeding postpartum women; infants; and nutritional-risk children up to age five. Dietary standards also are useful to nutritionists who plan meals for institutions such as schools and hospitals.

History

In 1938, Health Canada published the Recommended Nutrient Intakes (RNIs) as a dietary standard. Three years later, in 1941, the United States published the Recommended Dietary Allowances (RDAs). In 1989, the tenth and final version of the RDAs was published (Insel et al., 2013). In the mid-1990s, a new framework for dietary standards—the Dietary Reference Intakes (DRIs)—was published as a joint effort between Health Canada and the United States Food and Nutrition Board of the National Academy of Sciences to set dietary standards to replace the RNIs and RDAs. In 1997, the first set of DRIs was published for calcium, phosphorus, magnesium, vitamin D, and fluoride (Insel et al., 2013).

Definitions

The DRIs include: estimated average requirement (EAR); recommended dietary allowance (RDA); adequate intake (AI); and tolerable upper intake levels (UL). The U.S. Department of Agriculture (USDA, 2014b) defines estimated average requirement (EAR) as "the average daily nutrient intake level estimated to meet the requirement of half the healthy individuals in a particular life stage and gender group."

Recommended Dietary Allowance (RDA) is defined as "the average daily dietary nutrient intake level sufficient to meet the nutrient requirement of nearly all (97% to 98%) healthy individuals in a particular life stage and gender group" (USDA, 2014b). The DRI values are derived from the EAR values. There are RDA values for calcium, carbohydrate, copper, folate, iodine, iron, magnesium, molybdenum, niacin, phosphorus, protein, riboflavin, selenium, thiamin, vitamin A, vitamin B6, vitamin B12, vitamin C, vitamin D, vitamin E, and zinc (USDA, 2014d).

Adequate intake (AI) is defined as "the recommended average daily intake level based on observed or experimentally determined approximations or estimates of nutrient intake by a group (or groups) of apparently healthy people that are assumed to be adequate—used when an RDA cannot be determined" (USDA, 2014b). Adequate intake information is available for alpha-linolenic acid, biotin, chloride, choline, chromium, fat (for infants 0 to 12 months old), fluoride, linoleic acid, manganese, pantothenic acid, potassium, sodium, total fiber, vitamin K, and water (USDA, 2014d).

Tolerable upper intake level (UL) is defined as "the highest average daily nutrient intake level that is likely to pose no risk of adverse health effects to almost all individuals in the general population. As intake increases above the UL, the potential risk of adverse effects may increase" (USDA, 2014b). For individuals who are one year old or older there are UL values for boron, calcium, chloride, choline, copper, folate, fluoride, iodine, iron, magnesium, manganese, molybdenum, niacin, nickel, phosphorus, selenium, sodium, vitamin A, vitamin B6, vitamin C, vitamin D, vitamin E, vanadium, and zinc. For infants 0 to 12 months old there is UL information for calcium, fluoride, iron, selenium, vitamin A, vitamin D, and zinc.

Tables

The USDA (2014c) has a website with much useful information (http://fnic.nal .usda.gov/dietary-guidance/dietary-reference-intakes/dri-tables). Information is provided for the different life-stage groups, such as infants, children, male adults, female adults, pregnant women, and lactating women.

- Dietary Reference Intakes: Recommended Intakes for Individuals— Comprehensive DRI tables for vitamins, minerals, and macronutrients such as calcium, carbohydrates, copper, folate, iodine, iron, magnesium, molybdenum, niacin, phosphorus, protein, riboflavin, selenium, thiamin, vitamin A, vitamin B6, vitamin B12, vitamin C, vitamin D, vitamin E, and zinc.
- Dietary Reference Intakes: Recommended Dietary Allowance and Adequate Intake for Vitamins and Elements—Similar to Recommended Intakes for Individuals.
- Dietary Reference Intakes: Upper Intake Levels for Vitamins and Elements— Carbohydrates, cholesterol, polyunsaturated fatty acids, saturated and trans fatty acids, total fat, and total fiber.
- Dietary Reference Intakes: Macronutrients—Carbohydrates, fat, fatty acids, fiber, and protein.
- Dietary Reference Intakes: Estimates Average Requirements—Calcium, carbohydrates, copper, folate, iodine, iron, magnesium, molybdenum, niacin, phosphorus, protein, riboflavin, selenium, vitamin A, vitamin C, vitamin D, vitamin E, thiamin, vitamin B6, vitamin B12, and zinc.
- Dietary Reference Intakes: Electrolytes and Water—Chloride, inorganic sulfate, potassium, sodium, and water.

Online DRI Calculator

The USDA (2014c) has an online calculator called Interactive DRI for Health Care Professionals (http://fnic.nal.usda.gov/fnic/interactiveDRI/). The calculator enables individuals to determine their DRI values for nutrients after entering their sex, age, height, weight, physical activity level. After the user enters the required information, the online calculator is able to determine the individual's body mass index (BMI) and daily calorie needs.

The calculator provides information on:

- Macronutrients in terms of a-linolenic acid, carbohydrates, dietary cholesterol, fat, linoleic acid, protein, saturated fatty acids, total fiber, total water, and trans fatty acids;
- Vitamins in terms of biotin, carotenoids, choline, folate, niacin, pantothenic acid, riboflavin, thiamin, vitamin A, vitamin B6, vitamin B12, vitamin C, vitamin D, vitamin E, and vitamin, K; and
- Minerals (elements) in terms of arsenic, boron, calcium, chromium, copper, chloride, fluoride, iodine, iron, magnesium, manganese, molybdenum, nickel, phosphorus, potassium, selenium, silicon, sodium, sulfate, vanadium, and zinc.

Health care practitioners can help individuals understand the information provided by the online DRI calculator.

Susana Leong

See Also: Daily values; Health Canada; U.S. Department of Agriculture.

Further Reading

Insel, P., Ross, D., McMahon, K., & Bernstein, M. (2013). *Discovering Nutrition* (4th ed.). Burlington, MA: Jones and Bartlett Publishers.

United States Department of Agriculture. Food and Nutrition Information Center. (2014a, May). DRI tables. Retrieved from http://fnic.nal.usda.gov/dietary-guidance/dietary-reference-intakes/dri-tables

United States Department of Agriculture. Food and Nutrition Information Center. (2014b, May). Interactive DRI glossary. Retrieved from http://fnic.nal.usda.gov/interactive-dri-glossary

United States Department of Agriculture. Food and Nutrition Information Center. (2014c, December 2). Interactive DRI for healthcare professionals. Retrieved from http://fnic.nal.usda.gov/fnic/interactiveDRI/

United States Department of Agriculture. Food and Nutrition Information Center. (2014d, May). Learn more about the DRIs. Retrieved from http://fnic.nal.usda.gov/learn-more-about-dris

Dietary Supplements

A dietary supplement is a product manufactured from ingredients that could be found in the diet—components of plants and animals. The ingredients can be concentrated or changed in other ways, however, so that in the end they bear little resemblance to food. Dietary supplements are a multibillion-dollar-a-year industry in the

United States, Canada, and other countries around the world, with new formulations appearing on the market daily. The advertisements and product labels for dietary supplements often are very sophisticated, and the products mimic pharmaceutical preparations. The regulation of dietary supplements, however, is very different from the regulation of drugs. Consumers therefore must be wary when using supplements.

In the United States, the regulation of dietary supplements is described in the Dietary Supplement Health and Education Act (DSHEA), which was enacted by Congress in 1994. This Act allows manufacturers to market many products as "dietary supplements" rather than as drugs. To qualify as a "dietary supplement," the product must contain one or more of the following substances: "a vitamin; a mineral; an herb or other botanical; an amino acid; a dietary substance for use by man to supplement the diet by increasing the total dietary intake (e.g., enzymes or tissues from organs or glands); or a concentrate, metabolite, constituent, or extract" of the above (U.S. Food and Drug Administration, 2009). In the United States, the sale of dietary supplements is regulated by the U.S. Food and Drug Administration (FDA), a division of the Department of Health and Human Services.

The DSHEA mandates that manufacturers of dietary supplements ensure that their products are safe before selling them. Supplements do not require approval before being sold, however, nor must manufacturers submit any studies to the FDA before marketing a new product. Products sometimes contain substances that are not listed, such as caffeine. The FDA is not required to evaluate a product unless it receives enough complaints about the product. When the FDA becomes aware of a questionable dietary supplement, it must show that product is unsafe before it can be removed from the marketplace. An example of such action occurred in 2004, when the FDA declared that ephedrine could no longer be used in dietary supplements. The FDA ruling followed the heat stroke death of Baltimore Orioles pitcher Steve Bechler, a death attributed to ephedrine. (Ephedrine still can be a component of over-the-counter medicines, which are regulated more strictly).

The DSHEA does not mandate that dietary supplements be effective. If a product is shown to be ineffective, then the FDA does not require that the product be removed from shelves. If many complaints are received, however, then the Federal Trade Commission (FTC) can take action by investigating fraudulent advertising.

Some sports-nutrition and weight-loss products—such as sports drinks and energy bars—fall into the category of food, and not supplements. Both foods and supplements are subject to labeling requirements of the Nutrition Labeling Education Act of 1990 (NLEA). A supplement will have a "Supplement Facts" panel on the label. The NLEA prohibits labels from claiming that a product or its ingredients help to treat or prevent disease, except for certain health claims allowed by the FDA. Because sports performance is not a disease, statements claiming to improve performance are allowable without manufacturers providing proof that the claim is true. Many experts have urged reform to require better regulation of dietary supplements (Denham, 2011).

About half of the U.S. population, and approximately 70% of adults age 71 and older, take dietary supplements regularly (Bailey et al., 2011). About one-third of U.S. adults take a multivitamin mineral supplement (Bailey et al., 2011). Health

Canada reports similar use among Canadians. Many people take supplements on the advice of their health care providers. For example, people at risk of osteoporosis might be taking vitamin D and calcium. Supplements to slow the progress of macular degeneration appear to be supported by good research. People with heart disease often are told to take fish oil supplements. The *Dietary Guidelines for Americans* recommends including foods fortified with folate for women during their childbearing years, and vitamin B12 supplementation for people age 50 and older. People with iron-deficiency anemia usually are prescribed iron supplements.

Canadian Regulations

In Canada, dietary supplements are more tightly regulated. A product must be authorized for sale by the Natural Health Products Directorate. The manufacturer must show evidence of safety and efficacy of the product. The Directorate also imposes regulations on good manufacturing practices, labeling and packaging requirements, and the reporting of adverse reactions.

Is Natural Always Safe?

One of the biggest problems with supplement use is that consumers often assume that because the product is "natural," it is harmless. This belief can lead to consuming high levels of compounds that have negative side effects. Even vitamins and minerals can be harmful if people consume too much of them. Most vitamin and mineral supplements contain safe levels, but some consumers could get the same vitamin in different preparations. For example, a consumer might take a multivitamin supplement, an additional supplement for eye health, and a preparation for the immune system. Each of these is likely to contain zinc and vitamin A, both of which can be toxic at high doses. People who take several different preparations should read the labels, and add up the dosage they are getting for each vitamin and mineral. Consumers can check the safe upper limits against the charts for Tolerable Upper Intake Levels produced by the Food and Nutrition Board (Food and Nutrition Board 2005). Consumers also must remember that many foods contain added nutrients, such as calcium. People might consume orange juice, waffles, cereal, and antacids with calcium added, for example. It is easy to exceed the safe upper limit for calcium (2,500 mg) if taking calcium supplements and consuming calcium in the diet.

Supplement-Drug Interactions

People who take supplements should inform their health care providers about their intake. Many supplements interact with drugs, or could have effects on particular health conditions. Vitamin E, fish oil supplements, gingko biloba, and other herbal preparations can act as "blood thinners," for example, reducing the speed at which blood clots. This is beneficial for many people, but patients facing surgery are reminded to stop taking these drugs for several days before surgery to avoid excess blood loss.

Buyers Beware

Many supplement manufacturers are honest and provide helpful products and good information on use of their products. Unfortunately, others stretch the truth, and some are frauds. The Federal Trade Commission can prosecute companies whose advertising is false or misleading, but it could take the FTC years to get a product off the market. In the meantime, consumers must investigate products for themselves.

Consumers should remember that testimonials from users and endorsements by doctors or scientists do not prove that a product is safe or effective. Some people see results simply because they believe that they will—this is called the "placebo effect." Doctors and scientists promoting products might have mail-order degrees, or believe in the product because they are well paid to promote it.

Aside from a basic multivitamin and mineral supplement, children and teens should avoid using supplements unless prescribed by their health care providers, for two reasons. One reason is that little information is available about the long-term safety of these chemicals. The second reason is that most supplements have not been tested in children or adolescents. The effects of supplements could be very different in young people, and the potential for harm rarely is worth the potential health benefits. Similarly, pregnant women and nursing mothers should avoid using most supplements, except for those prescribed by their health care providers.

Barbara A. Brehm

Research Issues

In many countries, herbal medicines and other dietary supplements are widely prescribed by health care providers. Researchers in Germany have produced many good reports on a wide variety of supplements. There are called the Commission E Reports and can be accessed through the American Botanical Council website (http://cms.herbalgram.org/commissione/index.html).

In the United States, not all supplements contain the ingredients in the quantities stated on the label. Some are contaminated with unhealthy ingredients such as lead or mercury. Some do not dissolve quickly enough in the human digestive tract to be absorbed effectively. An independent testing agency, ConsumerLabs, tests products and publishes results. These reports are available online to subscribers (www.consumerlab.com).

See Also: Herbs and herbal medicine; Multivitamin and mineral supplements; U.S. Pharmacopeial Convention and USP-verified mark. Supplement use also is discussed in the entries for many of the individual nutrients (e.g., calcium, iron).

Further Reading

Bailey, R. L., Gahche, J. J., Lentino, C. V., Dwyer, J. T., Engel, J. S., Thomas, P. R., Betz, J. M., Sempos, C. T., Picciano, M. F. (2011). Dietary supplement use in the United States, 2003–2006. *Journal of Nutrition, 141* (2), 261–266.

Brehm, B. A. (2014). *Psychology of health and fitness*. Philadelphia: F.A. Davis.

Denham, B. E. (2011). Dietary supplements: Regulatory issues and implications for public health. *Journal of the American Medical Association, 306* (4), 428–429.

Food and Nutrition Board. (2005). *Tolerable upper intake levels.* Retrieved from http://iom .edu/Activities/Nutrition/SummaryDRIs/~/media/Files/Activity%20Files/Nutrition /DRIs/ULs%20for%20Vitamins%20and%20Elements.pdf

National Institutes of Health. Office of Dietary Supplements. (2014, December 2). [website]. Retrieved from http://ods.od.nih.gov/

National Institutes of Health. Office of Dietary Supplements. (2011). *Dietary supplements: What you need to know.* Retrieved from http://ods.od.nih.gov/HealthInformation/DS _WhatYouNeedToKnow.aspx

U.S. Food and Drug Administration. (2009, May 20). Regulatory Information: Dietary Supplement Health and Education Act of 1994. Retrieved from http://www.fda.gov /RegulatoryInformation/Legislation/FederalFoodDrugandCosmeticActFDCAct /SignificantAmendmentstotheFDCAct/ucm148003.htm#sec3

U.S. Food and Drug Administration. (2014, October 14). *FDA 101: Dietary supplements.* Retrieved from http://www.fda.gov/ForConsumers/ConsumerUpdates/ucm050803.htm

Digestion and the Digestive System

Digestion is the process of breaking down food into its constituent nutrients and into other chemicals to make these molecules available for absorption and utilization in the body. Food is broken into smaller pieces by mechanical processes (e.g., chewing in the mouth, churning in the stomach) and chemical processes. Digestion and nutrient absorption occur in the digestive system. The core of the digestive system is the gastrointestinal (GI) tract, a long hollow tube that begins at the mouth, where food is ingested, and ends at the anus, where the unabsorbed matter is excreted as "stool."

The GI tract includes the mouth, esophagus, stomach, small intestine, large intestine (which includes the colon and the rectum), and the anus. The digestive system also includes a number of accessory organs that contribute digestive fluids that assist with the chemical breakdown of food, including the salivary glands, liver, gallbladder, and pancreas. Digestion is regulated by the nervous and endocrine systems, through the action of nerves and their neurochemicals, and hormones, respectively. Chemical messengers released by the digestive organs themselves, along with the microbiota in the large intestine, contribute to the regulation of digestion.

The Gastrointestinal Tract

The organs of the GI tract share several similarities in their structure. Each organ, from the esophagus to the anus, is composed of several specialized tissue layers. The innermost layer that lines the organ, and through which the digestive matter passes, secretes mucus that protects the organ and eases the passage of contents. The lining of the stomach contains specialized cells that produce hydrochloric acid, which aids the chemical digestion of food; digestive enzymes; and hormones that regulate digestive processes. The cells lining the small intestine are

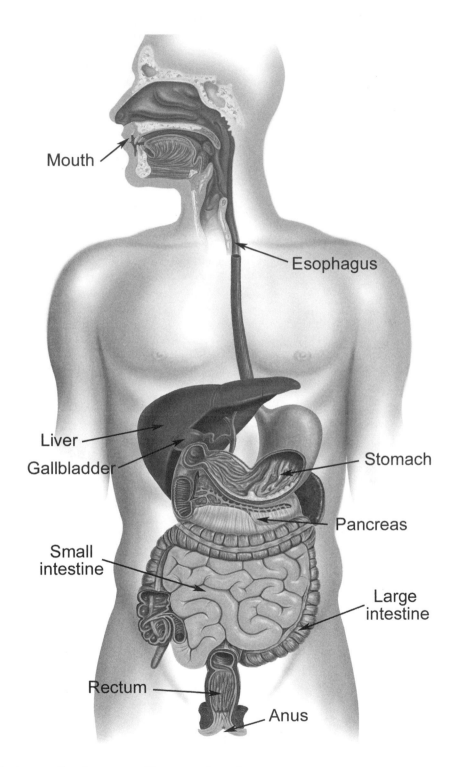

Mouth

Esophagus

Liver

Gallbladder

Stomach

Pancreas

Small
intestine

Large
intestine

Rectum

Anus

The human digestive system. (Shutterstock.com)

responsible for the absorption of most nutrients from the digestive mass; some chemical digestion also occurs in these cells.

The organs of the GI tract contain two or more layers of smooth muscle that work in a coordinated fashion to produce waves of movement that propel food down the GI tract and contribute to the mechanical breakdown of food. This movement is known as "peristalsis." Ring-like bands of muscle, known as "sphincters," prevent the backflow of GI contents. A sphincter located where the esophagus empties into the stomach, for example, prevents stomach contents from flowing back into the esophagus. (When this sphincter does not function properly, heartburn, also known as "gastroesophageal reflux," occurs.)

Steps in the Process of Digestion

Digestion can be broken down into a series of steps by following the path of ingested food.

Mouth

Digestion begins when food is taken into the mouth. The teeth crush the food as is chewed and the salivary glands secrete saliva to moisten the food. Saliva also contains some enzymes that begin the chemical breakdown of food, particularly starch. The tongue moves the food around in the mouth so that it can be thoroughly chewed. Once the food is chewed, it is swallowed into the esophagus.

Esophagus

The esophagus moves the food to the stomach via the smooth muscle contractions of peristalsis. The mucus produced by the lining of the esophagus helps the food to slide easily.

Stomach

The lower esophageal sphincter, located where the esophagus meets the stomach, opens to allow the chewed food to pass into the stomach, then closes to keep the food in the stomach. As food accumulates in the stomach, the stomach secretes hydrochloric acid to create an environment conducive for the chemical breakdown of molecular bonds. This acid environment also kills many microorganisms, which helps prevent the development of foodborne illnesses. The stomach also releases special enzymes to speed the digestion of protein, and releases a substance necessary for the absorption of vitamin B12. The food mass in the stomach is called "chyme." When chyme leaves the stomach, about 10% of fat, 10% to 20% of protein, and 30% to 40% of carbohydrate bonds have been completely broken down (Insel et al., 2014). The chyme gradually leaves the stomach over the course of 1 to 4 hours. The pyloric sphincter, located where the stomach empties into the small intestine, allows small amounts of chyme—about 2 ml per minute—to pass into the small intestine.

Small Intestine

The majority of digestion and absorption occurs in the small intestine. As the chyme enters the small intestine, the pancreas releases a basic fluid containing bicarbonate to neutralize the acidic chyme. The pancreas also releases digestive enzymes into the small intestine to further the chemical breakdown of the molecules in the chyme. The small intestine adds more digestive enzymes to the mix. The presence of fat in the chyme signals the gall bladder to release bile, which is produced by the liver but stored in the gall bladder. Bile helps break large groups of fat molecules into smaller groups, allowing greater exposure of the molecules to digestive enzymes. The absorptive cells lining the small intestine take up small molecules from the chyme. These molecules are further broken down and sent into the circulatory and lymphatic systems to be carried to all parts of the body. The chyme typically moves through the small intestine in about 3 to 10 hours, and then enters the large intestine through a sphincter called the "ileocecal valve."

Large Intestine

The large intestine is comprised of the colon and the rectum. The peristaltic movement of the colon is much slower than that of the small intestine. The chyme passes slowly through the colon, taking about 18 to 24 hours to reach the rectum (Insel, Ross, McMahon, & Bernstein, 2014). The large colonies of bacteria residing in the colon further digest some of the remaining matter, providing the host with a small number of additional calories and vitamin K. The colon absorbs water, sodium, chloride, potassium, some polysaccharides, and vitamin K from the chyme. The remaining mass is composed of dietary fiber, bacteria, and water, and is stored in the rectum until defecation. When a person responds to the urge to pass the stool, the rectal muscles relax and the anus opens, expelling the stool.

Barbara A. Brehm

See Also: Esophagus; Gallbladder and gallbladder disease; Gastroesophageal reflux disease; Large intestine; The liver; Microbiota and microbiome; The mouth; Pancreas; Small intestine; Stomach.

Further Reading

Insel, P., Ross, D., McMahon, K., & Bernstein, M. (2014). *Nutrition*. Burlington, MA: Jones & Bartlett.

Taylor, T. (2014, December 2). *Digestive system*. InnerBody. Retrieved from http://www .innerbody.com/image/digeov.html

Wallace, M. (2013, September 18). *Your digestive system and how it works*. National Institutes of Health. Retrieved from http://digestive.niddk.nih.gov/ddiseases/pubs/yrdd /index.aspx

Diverticular Disease

Diverticular disease refers to disorders associated with the development of diverticula in the colon and the rectum. Diverticula (diverticulum is the singular form) are marble-sized, bulging sacs that form in the inner layers of the colon and rectum, and then push out through weak areas in the wall of the colon. Diverticulosis is a disorder marked by the presence diverticula. Diverticulosis often has no symptoms and is common in countries where people consume diets high in processed foods and low in fiber. Diverticular bleeding can result when one of the small blood vessels in a diverticulum breaks. This condition can require surgery if bleeding continues. Diverticulitis is diagnosed when the diverticula become inflamed and infected. Diverticular disease affects about 40% of people 65 years and older, and 60% of people 80 years and older (McNevin, 2013). Almost everyone older than age 80 have diverticula, although not all go on to develop diverticular disease (McNevin, 2013). Diverticular disease usually can be treated with antibiotics, rest, and a change in diet. Serious cases can require surgery.

Diverticular disease was described as early as the 17th century. Medical research on these disorders, however, did not begin in earnest until the 20th century. Rates of diverticular disease began to increase in North America, England, and Australia at about the same time that the use of refined grains became popular, in the early 1900s. This association has led researchers to suggest that a low-fiber diet increases risk of diverticular disease, but the exact mechanism for the causation of diverticula remains unclear. It is possible that low-fiber diets contribute to constipation, and to increased pressure in the colon during elimination. Stool particles can become trapped inside the diverticula and increase the risk of infection. Low-fiber diets could alter the composition of the bacterial colonies residing in the colon, contributing to the proliferation of harmful bacteria that increase risk of infection in the diverticula.

Most people with diverticulosis do not experience any discomfort or symptoms, although on occasion, they might experience cramping or feel slight abdominal discomfort. Symptoms that arise with diverticulitis include severe abdominal pain, fever, nausea, and a significant change in bowel habits. Abdominal pain often is sharp and sudden, and felt in the lower left side of the abdomen. Diverticular bleeding causes blood to appear in the stool. Bleeding can be severe; therefore if rectal bleeding occurs people should seek medical assistance immediately. Diverticular disease symptoms mimic those of many other digestive system disorders. To diagnose diverticular disease, patients usually undergo medical tests such as a CT scan or a colonoscopy.

Mild cases of diverticular disease are commonly treated with antibiotics, a liquid diet, and rest. In most cases these steps will assist the body in fighting the infection. More serious cases can require the administration of intravenous antibiotics. In a minority of cases surgery is required. In severe cases, infection can create long-term complications. Peritonitis can result if infection spreads from the colon to the lining of the abdominal cavity (the peritoneum). Scar tissue that develops from infection can form blockages in the colon. Sometimes infected diverticula develop abscesses, with the accumulation of pus, which can be drained via medical procedures. In extreme cases, fistulas can form. Fistulas are openings that develop between the colon and other organs, such as the bladder or vagina, or from the colon into the abdominal cavity. Fistulas usually are repaired with surgery.

Epidemiologists have attempted to determine the factors that help to prevent diverticular disease. They are trying to answer the question: Why do diverticula form? And why do some people with diverticulosis never develop diverticulitis, and others progress to serious complications? Answers to these questions are still unclear. Some evidence suggests that lifestyle factors predict risk of diverticular disease. Most—although not all—studies indicate that risk increases with smoking, sedentary lifestyle, obesity, and low fiber intake (Maconi, Barbara, Bosetti, Cuomo, & Annibale, 2011). Risk increases with age, which has led researchers to propose that diverticula might increase with age-related declines in the strength and elasticity of the colon wall.

Debate continues regarding the role of diet in preventing the progression of diverticulosis to diverticulitis. In general, a high-fiber diet is recommended, although some experts advise people with diverticulosis to avoid fibrous foods that can become caught in the diverticula, such as seeds, nuts, and popcorn kernels. People with diverticulosis should prevent constipation by exercising regularly; consuming plenty of fruits, vegetables, legumes, and whole grains; and developing regular bowel habits. Medications such as fiber supplements and stool softeners also might be helpful. Probiotic foods (e.g., yogurt) and supplements could be useful for developing a healthful bacteria balance in the colon.

Barbara A. Brehm and Victoria Brown

See Also: Fiber; Large intestine.

Further Reading

Maconi, G., Barbara, G., Bosetti, C., Cuomo, R., & Annibale, B. (2011). Treatment of diverticular disease of the colon and prevention of acute diverticulitis: A systematic review. *Diseases of the Colon & Rectum, 54* (10), 1326–1338. doi: 10.1097/DCR .0b013e318223cb2b

Mayo Clinic Staff. (2014, August 7). *Diverticulitis.* MayoClinic.com. Retrieved from http://www.mayoclinic.com/health/diverticulitis/DS00070/DSECTION=symptoms

McNevin, M. S. (2013). *Diverticulitis.* American Society of Colon & Rectal Surgeons. Retrieved from http://www.fascrs.org/physicians/education/core_subjects /2009/diverticulitis/

Strate, L. L. (2012). Lifestyle factors and the course of diverticular disease. *Digestive Diseases, 30* (1), 35–45. doi: 10.1159/000335707

U.S. Dept. of Health and Human Services. (2013). *Diverticular disease.* National Digestive Diseases Information Clearinghouse. Retrieved from http://digestive.niddk.nih.gov /ddiseases/pubs/diverticulosis/

E

Eating Disorders

Eating disorders are psychiatric illnesses characterized by extreme disturbances in eating behavior and severe distress concerning body weight or shape. Eating disorders can be chronic, with symptoms lasting years or even decades. The *Diagnostic and Statistical Manual of Mental Disorders* (DSM-V) is the handbook used to classify or diagnose mental disorders. It lists four categories of eating disorders, listed below.

Anorexia Nervosa

The three diagnostic criteria for Anorexia Nervosa (AN) are (1) Restriction of food intake resulting in significant weight loss (or for children and adolescents, resulting in the failure to gain or maintain weight relative to appropriate growth); (2) Intense fear of weight gain or being overweight, regardless of low weight; and (3) Extreme distress concerning body weight or shape, or lack of acknowledgment of the seriousness of the disorder. Individuals with AN usually fall below the normal range in terms of body mass index (BMI less than or equal to 18.5).

Other Symptoms

- Restrictive eating patterns or excessive dieting
- Food preoccupations, such as obsessions with calories and fat contents
- Eliminating entire categories of food (such as fats or carbohydrates) or specific foods from diet
- Food rituals, such as cutting food into small pieces or chewing and spitting
- Excessive exercise, despite injury
- Fear of (or avoiding) eating in public
- Misusing medication to achieve weight loss or prevent weight gain. This is especially true for diabetics, who might restrict insulin doses.

Subtypes

- Restricting type—Achieves significantly low weight by means of starvation and, in some cases, excessive exercise. The individual presents no signs of binge eating or purging.

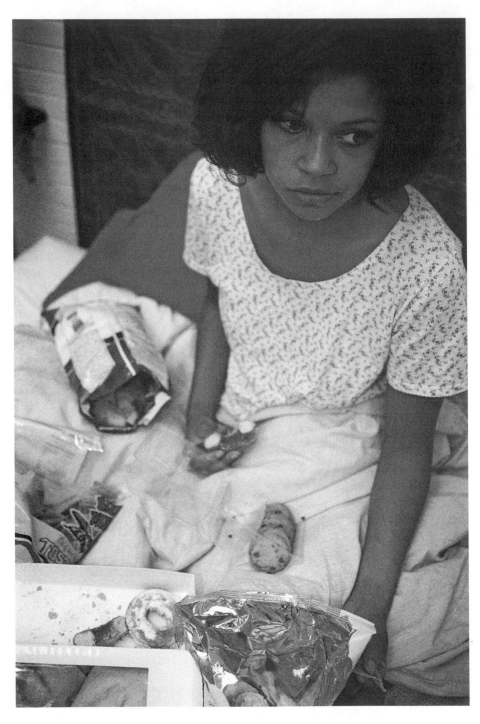

Binge eating is a characteristic of both binge eating disorder and bulimia nervosa. During a food binge, people consume an unusually large amount of food, often "forbidden" foods high in fat, sugar, and/or salt. (PhotoDisc, Inc.)

How to Help a Friend Who Has an Eating Disorder

To get well, people with eating disorders require professional help. If you think that a friend could have an eating disorder, encourage him or her to talk to a trusted adult. Don't make the mistake of thinking that you simply can "talk your friend out of" this serious illness. Following are a few ideas on how you can help your friend get the help he or she needs.

- Reach out. Express your concern about your friend's eating disordered behaviors. Refer to specific instances (i.e., meals, social events, athletic activities) when you felt he or she engaged in disordered eating behaviors.
- Educate yourself. Read books, newspaper articles, and research written by trusted organizations to find helpful information about eating disorders. The list below can get you started.
  - National Eating Disorders Association. Check out their free and confidential online screening for eating disorders at https://www.mentalhealthscreening.org/screening/NEDA
  - National Institute of Mental Health
  - Active Minds, Inc.
  - Eating Disorder Hope
- Be mindful of your language. Refrain from making comments about people's bodies, including your own.
- Encourage your friend to seek help. Remind your friend that this is a serious, life-threatening condition that requires treatment.
- Seek medical attention. If your friend refuses to seek help, then tell an adult that you trust or someone else in authority, such as a school counselor, a medical professional, a parent, or a coach.

- Binge-eating/purging type—In addition to meeting the criteria for AN, the individual presents symptoms of binge eating or purging (i.e., self-induced vomiting or abuse of laxatives, diuretics, or enemas).

Statistics

- Highest mortality rate of any mental illness
- An estimated 10-to-1 female-to-male ratio
- Twelve times the mortality rate of all other causes of death in women 15 to 24 years of age
- Less than half fully recover
- An estimated 4% of affected individuals die

Medical Complications

- Low blood pressure and heart rate
- Dehydration

- Electrolyte disturbances
- Muscle loss and weakness
- Heart failure
- Kidney failure
- Anemia
- Osteopenia or osteoporosis
- Amenorrhea and infertility
- Lanugo (growth of fine hair on the body)
- Edema
- Growth problems
- Gastrointestinal issues

Bulimia Nervosa

There are five diagnostic criteria for Bulimia Nervosa (BN): (1) Regular episodes of binge eating (consuming an unusually large amount of food within a two-hour period accompanied by a sense of lack of control while eating); (2) Engaging in regular inappropriate compensatory behaviors, such as self-induced vomiting, abuse of laxatives or diuretics, restricting, or excessive exercise; (3) Episodes are present at least once a week for three months; (4) Severe distress concerning body weight or shape; and (5) Symptoms are not solely present during episodes of AN. Individuals with BN usually fall between the normal and overweight range in terms of BMI.

Other Symptoms

- Frequent trips to the bathroom after meals
- Restrictive eating patterns between binges
- Eliminating entire categories of food (such as fats or carbohydrates) or specific foods from diet that might trigger a binge
- Swelling of the glands in the neck and jaw
- Weight fluctuations
- Excessive exercise
- Calluses on the knuckles or hands as a result of purging
- Sore throat

Statistics

- Affects one to 1.5% of young women
- An estimated 10-to-1 female-to-male ratio
- An estimated 3.9% of affected individuals will die

Health Risks

- Electrolyte imbalances

- Cardiac arrhythmia (irregular heart beat)
- Gastric rupture
- Inflammation/rupture of the esophagus
- Tooth decay, enamel loss, and tooth staining
- Edema
- Peptic ulcers and pancreatitis
- Acid reflux disorder and other gastrointestinal issues
- Amenorrhea
- Infertility

Binge Eating Disorder

There are five diagnostic criteria for Binge Eating Disorder (BED): (1) Regular episodes of binge eating (consuming an unusually large amount of food within a two-hour period accompanied by a sense of lack of control while eating); (2) Episodes are accompanied by rapid eating, eating until uncomfortably full, eating when not hungry, eating alone because of feeling embarrassed by the behavior, or feelings of disgust or guilt after bingeing; (3) Severe distress associated with binge eating; (4) Episodes are present at least once a week for three months; and (5) Symptoms are not accompanied by compensatory behaviors, nor are they solely present during episodes of AN or BN. Individuals with BED usually fall in the ranges of normal, overweight, and obese in accordance with BMI.

Statistics

- Affects an estimated 1 to 5% of the general population
- An estimated 40% of affected individuals are male

Health Risks

- High blood pressure (hypertension)
- High cholesterol
- Cardiovascular disease
- Heart disease
- Type 2 diabetes
- Gallbladder disease
- Gastrointestinal issues

Eating Disorder Not Otherwise Specified

An Eating Disorder Not Otherwise Specified (EDNOS) is diagnosed when symptoms of eating disorders are present but do not meet the full diagnostic criteria of any specific category. Some examples of EDNOS include the following.

- Atypical anorexia nervosa: All symptoms of AN are present except that the individual's weight does not fall below the normal range.
- Bulimia nervosa (of low frequency/limited duration): The individual does not engage in compensatory behaviors at the minimum frequency or duration listed in the diagnostic criteria.
- Binge-eating disorder (of low frequency/limited duration): The individual does not engage in compensatory behaviors at the minimum frequency or duration listed in the diagnostic criteria.
- Purging disorder: The individual engages in purging behaviors but not binge eating.
- Night eating syndrome: The individual awakens during the night to engage in excessive eating, is aware of such behaviors, and experiences significant distress associated with night eating.

Statistics

- EDNOS is the most commonly diagnosed eating disorder
- An estimated 5.2% of affected individuals die

History

The most credited early physician with regard to eating disorders was Richard Morton, who described the first medical condition in history that is most akin to today's "anorexia nervosa." It wasn't recognized as a true medical condition, however, until 1873, when Sir William Gull devised the name "anorexia nervosa." Ernest-Charles Lasègue, a French physician, also published similar case studies that same year.

In 1952, anorexia nervosa was the first eating disorder to be recognized as a psychiatric illness in the first edition of the *Diagnostic and Statistical Manual* (DSM-I). With the publication of the DSM-III 28 years later, bulimia was added as a separate category.

Although exploration continued in the field of medicine, the majority of cases and discoveries remained hidden from the public eye until the 1970s. Psychoanalyst Hilde Bruch became widely known in the medical field of eating disorders after her publication of *Eating Disorders: Obesity, Anorexia Nervosa, and the Person Within*. Dr. Bruch went on to publish a book aimed at a more secular audience, *The Golden Cage: The Enigma of Anorexia Nervosa*, which is credited today as one of the first publications to spread eating disorders awareness among the general public.

One of the most recent contributions to the field of eating disorders was the publication of the fifth edition of the DSM. Using the criteria listed in the previous edition, DSM-IV-TR, it was found that two-thirds of individuals with eating disorders were diagnosed with EDNOS. Diagnosing patients with such an ambiguous diagnosis as EDNOS often results in providing treatment targeting other types of eating disorders. Additionally, insurance companies are significantly less likely to reimburse patients for medical expenses due to "not otherwise specified" disorders. Physicians and families alike hoped that improving the diagnostic criteria for each category would reduce the high prevalence of diagnoses of unspecified eating disorders. Since the new edition's changes were proposed, evidence has pointed to a significant decrease in the diagnosis of EDNOS. It is anticipated that the new criteria outlined in the DSM-V will promote better treatment and reimbursement, and ultimately better prognoses.

Contributing Factors

Biological Factors

- Family history, having first-degree relatives with an eating disorder, especially with AN or BN
- Obesity, especially for individuals with BN
- Abnormalities in the brain in individuals with AN
- Possible genetic transmission

Environmental Factors

- Pressure to obtain the "perfect body"
- Cultural values of thinness
- Hobbies and careers that encourage thinness, such as athletics, dance, modeling, and acting
- History of childhood abuse, trauma
- Experiences of being teased about size, shape, or weight

Psychological Factors

- High levels of anxiety and/or obsessive traits
- Symptoms of depression
- Low self-esteem
- Feelings of lack of control

Comorbidity

Eating disorders have been found to exist alongside several psychiatric illnesses, including depressive, bipolar, anxiety, and substance-abuse disorders. Furthermore, comorbidity also has been found to exist with eating disorders and physical health conditions. Eating Disorder–Diabetes Mellitus Type 1 (ED-DMT1), a condition commonly known as "diabulimia," represents a dual diagnosis of an eating disorder and type 1 diabetes. Individuals with ED-DMT1 misuse insulin in an attempt to manipulate or lose weight.

Treatment and Outcomes

Eating disorders are multifaceted illnesses and should be treated by a team of professionals. There are three crucial aspects of treatment, medical, nutritional, and therapeutic. A specialist or primary care physician evaluates the individual's physical state of health. Regular weight-checks, vital signs checks, and blood tests usually are administered depending on the patient's status and the severity of symptoms. A nutritionist or dietician works with the individual to provide a meal plan to meet the individual's nutritional needs. There are several successful therapeutic approaches to eating disorders. These include, but are not limited to, those listed below.

Cognitive Behavioral Therapy

In Cognitive Behavioral Therapy (CBT), a therapist works with an individual to identify negative thought patterns and replace them with positive and effective ones. The notion of CBT is that changing a person's thoughts ultimately can change the person's behavior.

Dialectical Behavioral Therapy

In Dialectical Behavioral Therapy (DBT), an individual learns to identify and cope with uncomfortable or distressing thoughts that might be contributing to urges and behaviors. Gradually, the individual learns to tolerate his or her emotions without acting on them. Mindfulness techniques—such as muscle relaxation and deep breathing—are implemented as a way of accepting, rather than resisting, negative emotions.

Maudsley Approach

A relatively new model, the Maudsley Approach is family-based treatment specifically designed for children and adolescents with Anorexia Nervosa. Unlike other models, this treatment takes place at the patient's home. The primary goals are weight restoration, encouraging the children or adolescents to take control over their eating patterns, and providing the patient with familial support.

Medication

Some individuals also respond well to psychiatric medications, but it is important that this be used as a supplement to other means of treatment. Inpatient care is recommended when the individual has regressed or has failed to make any significant progress. Hospitalization also might be necessary if the eating disorder has become dangerous or life-threatening in a physical or psychological way.

Research has shown that earlier medical intervention results in a better prognosis. Many individuals continue to experience symptoms after treatment, however, and require multiple bouts of treatment. Others have symptoms that last a lifetime. The duration and outcome of treatment ultimately depend on the individual's willingness to participate in treatment, the duration of the illness, the existence of co-morbid disorders, and insurance coverage or reimbursement for treatment.

Nicole D. Teitelbaum

See also: Feeding disorders; Food addiction.

Further Reading

American Psychiatric Association. (2013). *Diagnostic and Statistical Manual of Mental Disorders* (5th ed.). Arlington, VA: American Psychiatric Association.

Arcelus, J., Mitchell, A. J., Wales, J., & Nielsen, S. (2011). Mortality rates in patients with anorexia nervosa and other eating disorders: A meta-analysis of 36 studies. *Archives of General Psychiatry, 68* (7), 724–731.

Eating Disorder Hope. (2013). *Eating disorder statistics & research.* Retrieved from http://www.eatingdisorderhope.com/information/statistics-studies#Anorexia-Nervosa-Statistics.

Freidl, E. K., Hoek, H. W., & Attia, E. (2012). Anorexia nervosa in DSM-5. *Psychiatric Annals, 42* (11), 414–417. http://dx.doi.org/10.3928/00485713-20121105-07

National Eating Disorders Association. (2013a) *Factors that may contribute to eating disorders.* Retrieved from https://www.nationaleatingdisorders.org/factors-may-contribute-eating-disorders

National Eating Disorders Association. (2013b) *Health consequences of eating disorders.* Retrieved from https://www.nationaleatingdisorders.org/health-consequences-eating-disorders

Pearce, J. M. S. (2004). Richard Morton: Origins of anorexia. *European Neurology, 52* (4), 191–192.

Echinacea

Echinacea is a genus of flower that is native to the North American Midwest and most often is used to treat the common cold and the flu. Three species of the plant, *Echinacea angustifolia*, *Echinacea pallida*, and *Echinacea purpurea*, commonly are used to create echinacea tablets, capsules, tinctures, ointments, and teas. The roots, leaves, and flower parts of the plant are used in herbal preparations. Due to the variety of methods employed to prepare echinacea supplements, and the multiple varieties of plant that are available for harvest, echinacea products vary widely. The mechanism through which echinacea is thought to impact health is uncertain, but it generally is thought to influence the normal immune response and reduce inflammation.

The word "echinacea" is derived from the Greek word "echinos," meaning "hedgehog"—a name attributed to the plant's large, spiky seed head. Echinacea has been used for centuries to treat diseases such as malaria, syphilis, diphtheria, and scarlet fever. Archaeological evidence indicates that echinacea commonly was used by Native Americans for more than 400 years to treat infections, wounds, and many other ailments, and that settlers adopted the practice. Indeed, echinacea was listed on the U.S. National Formulary—an official list of medications approved for prescription in the United States—from 1916 to 1950. With the increasing development of antibiotics throughout the 1900s, however, therapeutic echinacea use in North America declined. Echinacea has become popular again in the United States, but as an alternative herbal remedy. Echinacea still is the primary treatment for minor respiratory-tract infections in Germany, where 1.3 million prescriptions for echinacea are written each year (EBSCO, 2012). Preparations from the leaves and flowers of *E. purpurea* are thought to be most effective.

Myriad variations in the production process result in different concentrations of echinacea's various chemical compounds in different commercially available products. Therefore, each particular product has different dosing instructions, indicating that vastly different amounts, concentrations, and varieties of the supplement are curative. For these reasons, studies of the restorative effects of echinacea have been difficult to compare to one another. Nevertheless, well-designed human studies suggest that echinacea is possibly effective for reducing the length and severity of respiratory-tract infection symptoms.

General guidelines for using echinacea recommend taking the supplement as soon as respiratory symptoms become apparent, and discontinuing use once symptoms are gone, which usually occurs within one to two weeks. Echinacea seems to be safe for most people. Occasionally, people allergic to plants in the ragweed, marigold, mum, and daisy families develop allergic reactions to echinacea products, including skin rashes, and rarely, anaphylaxis. Additionally, although short-term use of echinacea seems to be harmless, it is important to note that long-term effects of echinacea use have not yet been widely studied.

Elizabeth J. Thompson

See Also: Dietary supplements; Herbs and herbal medicine.

Further Reading

EBSCO CAM Review Board. (2012). *Echinacea. Natural and alternative treatments.* Retrieved from http://www.consumerlab.com/tnp.asp?chunkiid=21677

Ehrlich, S. D. (Ed.). (2012). *Echinacea.* University of Maryland Medical Center. Retrieved from http://www.umm.edu/altmed/articles/echinacea-000239.htm

Linde, K., Barrett, B., Wölkart, K., Bauer, R., & Melchart, D. (2006). *Echinacea for preventing and treating the common cold.* Cochrane Database of Systematic Reviews, 1, CD000530

Therapeutic Research Faculty. (2014, July 7). *Echinacea.* MedlinePlus. Natural Medicines Comprehensive Database. Retrieved from http://www.nlm.nih.gov/medlineplus/druginfo/natural/981.html

Electrolytes

Electrolytes are positively or negatively charged ions that form when salts, acids, or bases dissolve in water. Ions are molecules that carry different amounts of electrons and protons, giving the molecule a net electric charge. This charge can be negative or positive—an ion with a negative charge is called an "anion," and an ion with a positive charge is called a "cation." Electrolytes are essential for water balance, blood pH (acidity), nerve and muscle function, and many other processes. Electrolytes commonly found in the human body include sodium, potassium, chloride, calcium, magnesium, and phosphate.

To maintain electrolyte balance, electrolytes are moved in or out of the cell through specialized ion pumps that are embedded in the cell membrane. These pumps are used by the cell to maintain specific electrochemical gradients and to regulate fluid volumes. The movement of electrolytes influences the movement of water into and out of cells; this is called "osmosis." When electrolytes are more concentrated on one side of the cellular membrane, osmosis moves water to the side with the greater electrolyte concentration so that the same concentration of ions is present both inside and outside of the cell.

Sodium is the primary cation in extracellular fluids, including the blood, and potassium is more highly concentrated inside the cells. Sodium-potassium pumps maintain these concentrations. The kidneys help to maintain correct levels of electrolytes in the body. During electrolyte imbalance—such as when a person is dehydrated—osmosis is disrupted, causing water to move out of the cell to equalize the ionic concentration gradient. When water moves out of the cell, the cell can shrink and eventually could die. Common causes of dehydration include illnesses accompanied by symptoms such as vomiting and diarrhea that lead to excess loss of body water; conditions that cause excessive sweating, such as exercising or working in the heat; and failure to drink enough water. Dehydration commonly is treated by oral ingestion of electrolyte solutions, such as with sports drinks or medicines such as Pedialyte, or by intravenous delivery. Electrolyte imbalances can accompany a number of health problems, such as heart failure and kidney disease.

Paula Sophia Seixas Rocha and Alexandra A. Naranjo

See Also: Calcium; Chloride; Minerals; Phosphorus; Potassium; Sodium and salt; Sports beverages; Water needs, water balance.

Further Reading

Brown, T. E., LeMay, H. E. H., Bursten, B. E., Murphy, C., & Woodward, P. (2011). *Chemistry: The Central Science* (12th ed.). Boston: Prentice Hall.

Dugdale, D. C., & Zieve, D. (2011, September 20). *Electrolytes.* MedlinePlus. Retrieved from http://www.nlm.nih.gov/medlineplus/ency/article/002350.htm

Insel, P. M., Ross, D., McMahon, K., & Bernstein, M. (2014). *Nutrition.* Burlington, MA: Jones & Bartlett Learning.

Ellagic Acid

Ellagic acid is an antioxidant found in many fruits and vegetables that recently has shown promise for medicinal applications in humans. In the mid-1800s, the chemists Henri Braconnot and Michel Eugène Chevreul were the first to isolate ellagic acid from an oak gall-nut, an abnormal growth on plants stimulated by parasitic invasion (Hemingway, 1992). Ellagic acid serves a protective purpose in plants by blocking microbial infections, and also might prevent heavy-metal poisoning and predation by insects. Its highest concentrations are found in red raspberry plants, as well as in strawberries, blackberries, cranberries, pomegranates, walnuts, and pecans. Although ellagic acid is located primarily in leaves, fruits also contain the substance. Humans typically ingest the natural phenol as ellagitannin, or ellagic acid with glucose, a form that is water soluble and easy to digest.

Preliminary research thus far only has shown promise in human cell lines in vitro, and in animal models. For example, research has shown that extracts containing ellagic acid drawn from a selection of these plants alleviate some types of inflammation and serve as antioxidants. Although the mechanism is unknown, fruit extracts containing ellagic acid have reduced colon inflammation in rats (Rosillo, 2012). In an in vitro study of cultured human cells treated with walnut extract, inflammation of aortic lining cells was reduced, and the activity of osteoblasts increased (Papoutsi, 2008) (osteoblasts stimulate the formation of new bone tissue in vivo).

Laboratory research has produced some encouraging studies that illustrate ellagic acid's ability to bind with some carcinogenic—cancer-causing—molecules. Ellagic acid preparations have been shown to inhibit chemical-induced esophageal cancers, as well as skin and lung tumors in laboratory rodents. Preliminary research in this area, however, currently is insufficient to label any product as a viable treatment for cancer or other illnesses. New supplements and other products featuring ellagic acid have been frequent targets of the Food and Drug Administration as being in violation of the Federal Food, Drug and Cosmetics Act. False claims warrant increased awareness from consumers, who should seek professional advice when considering supplementing their diet with ellagic acid. Consuming more foods such as berries, pomegranates, walnuts, and pecans as part of a balanced diet is considered prudent advice.

Patricia M. Cipicchio

See Also: Antioxidants; Cancer and nutrition; Dietary supplements.

Further Reading

American Cancer Society. (2008). *Ellagic acid*. Retrieved from: http://www.cancer.org/treatment/treatmentsandsideeffects/complementaryandalternativemedicine/dietandnutrition/ellagic-acid

Haslam, E. (1992). Gallic acid and its metabolites. In *Plant Polyphenols: Synthesis, Properties, Significance*. Hemingway, R. W., & Laks, P. E. (Eds.). New York: Plenum Press, p. 169.

Memorial Sloan Kettering Cancer Center. (2012). *Ellagic acid*. Retrieved from http://www.mskcc.org/cancer-care/herb/ellagic-acid

Papoutsi, Z., Kassi, E., Chinou, I., Halabalaki, M., Skaltsounis, L. A., Moutsatsou, & P. (2008). Walnut extract (Juglans regia L.) and its component ellagic acid exhibit anti-inflammatory activity in human aorta endothelial cells and osteoblastic activity in the cell line KS483. *British Journal of Nutrition, 99*, 715–722.

Rosillo, M. A., Sanchez-Hidalgo, Cárdeno, A., Aparicio-Soto, M., Sánchez-Fidalgo, S., Villegas, I., & de la Lastra, C. A. (2012). Dietary supplementation of an ellagic acid-enriched pomegranate extract attenuates chronic colonic inflammation in rats. *Pharmacological Research, 66* (3), 235–242. doi: 10.1016/j.phrs.2012.05.006

Energy Balance

Energy balance refers to the relationship between energy taken in, or eaten, and energy expended, or "burned." A negative energy balance means that more energy is expended than is consumed. Over time, a negative energy balance causes the body to use stored energy for fuel. A positive energy balance means that more energy is consumed, or eaten, than expended. A positive energy balance encourages the body to store energy. The body can store a little energy as carbohydrate—in the form of glycogen—primarily in the liver and skeletal muscles. The majority of excess energy from a positive energy balance, however, is stored as adipose tissue. People whose energy intake is similar to their energy expenditure are said to be in energy balance, or energy equilibrium. Researchers and people trying to gain or lose weight are interested in the factors that contribute to energy balance because they influence the status of energy stores, especially adipose tissue. A positive energy balance over time results in excess adipose stores and obesity. A negative energy balance over time results in weight loss. In people who are overweight or obese, about 60% to 80% of this weight loss is composed of fat; lean tissue comprises some of the weight that is lost over a period of negative energy balance (Hill, Wyatt, & Peters, 2012). A negative energy balance also can result in muscle wasting and the use of important body tissues for fuel, as is the case in starvation.

Energy Intake

Energy intake can be measured in terms of kilocalories (kcals). People obtain energy from carbohydrates, fats, and proteins in the foods that they eat. The body is able to extract energy from the chemical bonds found in these molecules. Carbohydrates and proteins deliver 4 kcals per gram, and fats contribute 9 kcals per gram. Alcohol also contains chemical bonds that can be used by people to make energy; alcohol has 7 kcals per gram.

Physiologists used to believe that all kilocalories were equal in terms of influencing body energy stores. Recently, an increased understanding of the way foods and their nutrients behave in the body and the complex biochemical processes in which they participate has overturned the mechanistic view of calories from food all having similar effects on adipose tissue storage. Some studies suggest that foods differ in their metabolic impact in ways that lead to variable effects on energy stores.

One study, for example, compared groups that were limiting calorie intake. One group included only whole-grain foods when consuming grains or grain products, and the other group was asked to avoid whole-grain foods (Katcher et al., 2008). Both groups consumed the same amount of calories and lost the same amount of weight during the 12-week study. The whole-grain group, however, lost more body fat from the abdominal region. Extra fat stores in the abdominal region are associated with negative health effects, including hypertension, type 2 diabetes, and heart disease. At the end of the study, subjects in the whole-grains group also had greater decreases in C-reactive protein (CRP) level, a marker of inflammation, than did the subjects in the other group (Katcher et al., 2008). Lower CRP levels and reduced levels of inflammation are associated with better health.

Some studies have suggested that beverages sweetened with fructose could be more likely to contribute to obesity and obesity-related health disorders than beverages sweetened with glucose. One such study found that fructose-sweetened beverages increased abdominal fat and blood lipids and decreased insulin sensitivity (a marker of good blood sugar regulation) in overweight and obese people more than the same amount of beverages sweetened with glucose (Stanhope et al., 2009).

The types of food kcals consumed throughout the day also have an effect on people's level of hunger and their appetite. Feelings of hunger can increase even though people have consumed "enough" calories if those calories have been stored and blood sugar drops. People seeking to reduce food intake must devise eating strategies that minimize feelings of hunger and do not trigger the body's fat-storage pathways.

Energy Expenditure

Daily energy expenditure refers to the total amount of energy used in a 24-hour period and commonly is measured in kcals. The body expends energy in many different ways. Metabolism refers to the entire collection of biochemical processes that occur in the body, many of which require energy. Most bodily functions—from digesting food to contracting muscles—require energy. Metabolic rate is the energy expenditure required to sustain metabolism in a given period, usually expressed per minute or per hour. Metabolic rate at any given moment depends upon activity level and the biochemical processes occurring in the body. Daily energy expenditure often is divided into several components, including those listed below.

Basal Metabolic Rate or Resting Metabolic Rate

Basal and resting metabolic rate both are terms that refer to the energy required just to stay alive in a resting state. Basal metabolic rate (BMR) is measured while a person is awake but is resting and lying down. Resting metabolic rate (RMR) is measured when a person is in a seated position. For most people, RMR consumes more than half of the calories required in a 24-hour period.

The Thermic Effect of Food

The thermic effect of food (TEF) refers to the energy required for the processes of digestion and absorption. The term "thermic" refers to energy expenditure. This word is used because all of the body's metabolic processes generate heat; by measuring heat (calories), scientists can calculate energy use.

Why does eating take energy? Energy is required to chew food, contract the muscles of the gastrointestinal (GI) system, produce digestive enzymes and fluids, and absorb nutrients from the digestive system into the lymphatic system or bloodstream. The thermic effect of food is proportional to the amount of food consumed, and is about 8% to 10% of the kcals consumed (Hill, Wyatt, & Peters, 2012).

The Thermic Effect of Exercise

By far, the most-significant effect on metabolic rate is achieved with exercise. The thermic effect of exercise (TEE) refers to the calories used during exercise. During moderately vigorous physical activity, metabolic rate increases by a factor of 10 or more, burning hundreds of extra calories. The more vigorous the exercise, the more calories expended. After vigorous activity, metabolic rate remains elevated for a while, as the body returns to its resting level.

Nonexercise Activity Thermogenesis

The term nonexercise activity thermogenesis (NEAT) was coined by James Levine to describe activities that do not fall into the categories of sleeping, eating, or exercise (Levine, 2004). In this context, Levine uses the word exercise to refer to activity performed specifically for the purpose of playing a sport or for physical conditioning. Nonexercise activity thermogenesis includes all other activities, such as climbing stairs, chewing gum, and jiggling around when seated, as well as the activities of daily living, such as grocery shopping, cooking, and cleaning. NEAT can expend hundreds of calories per day and exert a significant effect on energy balance. High levels of NEAT appear to have significant health benefits. Conversely, research has found that long periods of sitting, even for people who exercise regularly, are associated with increased risk of obesity and metabolic syndrome.

Applications

Any condition that influences metabolic rate also influences energy balance. Pregnancy for example, raises metabolic rate as many systems gear up to support the growth of the baby. Many hormones influence metabolic rate, and can send a person into either negative or positive energy balance. Illness that decreases appetite or food intake can lead to a negative energy balance and catabolic state in which body tissues are broken down for energy. Growing children are in positive energy balance, as extra energy is consumed to supply the raw materials and support for growth and development.

Barbara A. Brehm

Research Issues

People trying to lose weight often wonder what types of exercise are best for increasing energy expenditure, not only during the exercise session itself, but during the period of recovery from exercise. High-intensity exercise burns more calories per minute, and can have a somewhat greater recovery energy cost. Calories still count, of course, so one hour of moderately vigorous walking might burn more calories than 20 minutes of interval training, depending upon the nature of the two workouts.

See Also: Calorie; Metabolic rate; Metabolism.

Further Reading

Brehm, B. A. (2014). *Psychology of health and fitness*. Philadelphia: F. A. Davis.

Hill, J. O., Wyatt, H. R., & Peters, J. C. (2012) Energy balance and obesity. *Circulation, 126*, 126–132. doi: 10.1161/ CIRCULATIONAHA.111.087213

Katcher, H. I., Legro, R. S., Kunselman, A. R., Gillies, P. J., Demers, L. M., Bagshaw, D. M., & Kris-Etherton, P. M. (2008). The effects of a whole grain-enriched hypocaloric diet on cardiovascular disease risk factors in men and women with the metabolic syndrome. *American Journal of Clinical Nutrition, 87* (1), 79–90.

Levine, J. (2004). Nonexercise activity thermogenesis (NEAT): Environment and biology. *American Journal of Physiology; Endocrinology and Metabolism, 286* (5), E675–E685.

National Cancer Institute. (2014, December 2). *Energy balance: Weight and obesity, physical activity, diet*. Retrieved from http://www.cancer.gov/cancertopics/prevention /energybalance

National Heart, Lung, and Blood Institute. (2012). *Balance food and activity*. Retrieved from http://www.nhlbi.nih.gov/health/public/heart/obesity/wecan/healthy-weight-basics /balance.htm

Stanhope, K. L., Schwarz, J. M., Keim, N. L., Griffen, S. C., Bremer, A. A., Graham1, J. L., Hatcher, B., Cox, C. L., Dyachenko, A., Zhang, W., McGahan, J. P., Seibert, A. Krauss, R. M., Chiu, S., Schaefer, E. J., Ai, M., Otokozawa, S., Nakajima, K., Nakano11, T., Beysen, C., Hellerstein, M. K., Berglund, L., & Havel, P. J. (2009). Consuming fructose-sweetened, not glucose-sweetened, beverages increases visceral adiposity and lipids and decreases insulin sensitivity in overweight/obese humans. *Journal of Clinical Investigation, 119* (5), 1322–1334. doi: 10.1172/JCI37385

Energy Drinks

Energy drinks are beverages that contain caffeine, often in combination with other ingredients, such as vitamins, sugars, herbal supplements, amino acids, or guarana (a plant product high in caffeine). Energy drinks claim to provide a burst of extra energy to their consumers. The term "energy drink" was created by beverage companies and is not recognized by the U.S. Food and Drug Administration (FDA) or the U.S. Department of Agriculture (USDA). Energy drinks are regulated as dietary supplements.

The most common ingredients in energy drinks are caffeine, taurine, guarana, ginseng, and B vitamins. The primary ingredient is caffeine because of its taste and its potential to improve mental and physical performance. The amount of caffeine in energy drinks can range anywhere from 75 mg to more than 200 mg per serving, and some products contain more than one serving per container. The average moderate consumption of caffeine for most individuals is about 300 mg per day, whether from energy drinks or other sources.

Many people find caffeinated beverages such as energy drinks helpful in moderate amounts in situations requiring increased alertness, such as when driving, studying, or working. It is not known whether improvements experienced are due to the effects of caffeine alone, the herbal ingredients, or a combination of the two. Some people consume energy drinks to improve athletic performance. Caffeine does enhance athletic performance, perhaps by raising blood fat levels and enhancing reaction time. It is probable that improvements in athletic performance experienced with energy drinks primarily are due to the caffeine content. People seeking weight loss also turn to energy drinks in hopes of burning extra calories by increasing metabolic rate, a known effect of caffeine. A small increase in resting metabolic rate, however, is easily offset by the consumption of a few extra calories in the diet, and these drinks have not been shown to be effective for weight loss.

Taurine is an amino acid that the body is able to make from other amino acids. Taurine is plentiful in animal tissues, and in the diet comes from foods such as beef, pork, fish, and other meats. Some evidence has suggested that caffeine and taurine combined might improve mental performance. Other amino acids, such as carnitine, sometimes are added to energy drinks. Carnitine is involved in the metabolism of fat, although adding extra carnitine to the diet does not appear to aid weight-loss efforts.

Guarana is a compound that comes from the seeds of a Brazilian shrub. Guarana often is found in beverages from Brazil. The plant is added to energy drinks because it contains a large amount of caffeine, which increases energy and

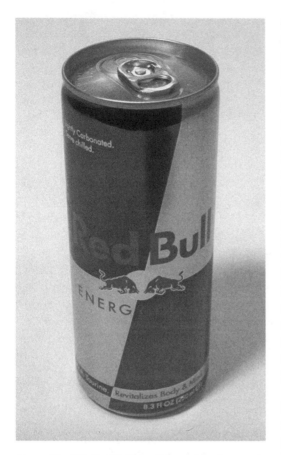

Can of Red Bull, a highly caffeinated carbonated energy drink from Austria. In the United States, energy drinks are regulated as dietary supplements by the U.S. Food and Drug Administration. This means that products are not reviewed or approved by the FDA. Label claims are often exaggerated and misleading. (Photo by Anthony Verde/Time Life Pictures/Getty Images)

improves mental and physical performance, but it is not the main source of caffeine in energy drinks. Despite guarana's high concentration of caffeine (more than that in a coffee bean), in the United States it generally is recognized as safe as a natural flavoring substance. Ginseng is an herb that supposedly increases sense of well-being and stamina and reduces feelings of stress. Its effectiveness as a component of energy drinks has not been established. The B vitamins play many important roles in the production of energy from carbohydrates, fats, and proteins in the diet. Unless a person has a deficiency of a particular B vitamin, however, consuming extra B vitamins does not appear to increase alertness or improve athletic performance.

Energy drinks can be consumed in moderation safely. A moderate consumption of 300 mg caffeine per day is safe for most adults. Children, however, should limit their caffeine intake to less than 100 mg per day because caffeine has been associated with many negative effects in this age group, including behavioral problems and sleep disorders. Some people react negatively to caffeine and experience disturbing symptoms such as irritability, anxiety, irregular heart rhythms, insomnia, and stomach pain. Most energy drinks also contain added sugars, which can increase risk for obesity.

Recently, controversy has arisen over the sale and regulation of energy drinks because many believe they are dangerous to children and teenagers. Some people believe that the intake of excessive amounts of caffeine and the ability for young people to easily access it is a major problem. A common energy drink, 5-Hour Energy, for example, is ingested like a "shot" and claims that users will feel its effect within minutes. Many think that this type marketing toward youth is

Emergency Department Visits Involving Energy Drinks

- The number of emergency department (ED) visits involving energy drinks doubled from 10,068 visits in 2007, to 20,783 visits in 2011.

- Among energy drink–related ED visits, there were more male patients than female patients; visits doubled from 2007 to 2011 for both male and female patients.

- In each year from 2007 to 2011, there were more energy drink–related ED visits by patients who were 18 to 39 years of age than there were for all other age groups. The greatest increase, however, was patients 40 years of age or older, for whom visits increased 279%—from 1,382 visits in 2007, to 5,233 visits in 2011.

- In 2011, more than half of the energy drink–related ED visits involved energy drinks only (58%), and the remaining 42% also involved other drugs.

Substance Abuse and Mental Health Services Administration, Center for Behavioral Health Statistics and Quality. (2013, January 10). *The Drug Abuse Warning Network (DAWN) report: Update on emergency department visits involving energy drinks: a continuing health concern*. Retrieved from http://www.samhsa.gov/data/2k13/DAWN126/sr126-energy-drinks-use.htm

inappropriate, and encourages a reliance on substances for psychological effects. Additionally, health professionals recommend that parents and other caregivers encourage children to develop healthful lifestyles that lay the groundwork for bountiful daily energy. Children and adolescents should achieve feelings of energy by developing regular sleeping habits, consuming a healthful diet, and getting plenty of vigorous exercise (American Academy of Pediatrics, 2011).

The combination of energy drinks and alcohol can be very dangerous because feelings of alertness can mask intoxication and give the impression of being sober, leading users to drive drunk and engage in other risky behaviors (Brache & Stockwell, 2011). One study found that bar patrons who drank energy drinks and alcohol were three times more likely to become highly intoxicated than were other patrons (Thombs, O'Mara, Tsukamoto, Rossheim, Weiler et al., 2010). Energy drink–consuming bar patrons also were also four times more likely to report intending to drive than other drinkers. Because of this, several states and colleges have banned alcoholic energy drinks.

Emily Ohrtman

See Also: Alcohol; Caffeine; Dietary supplements.

Further Reading

American Academy of Pediatrics (2011). Sports drinks and energy drinks for children and adolescents: Are they appropriate? *Pediatrics, 127*, (6), 1182–1189. doi: 10.1542/peds.2011-0965 Retrieved from http://pediatrics.aappublications.org/content/127/6/1182.long

Brache, K., & Stockwell, T. (2011). Drinking patterns and risk behaviors associated with combined alcohol and energy drink consumption in college drinkers. *Addictive Behaviors 36* (12), 1133–1140. doi: 10.1016/j.addbeh.2011.07.003

Heneman, K., & Zidenberg-Cherr, S. (2007). *Nutrition and Health Info Sheet: Energy Drinks*. University of California, Division of Agriculture and Natural Resources. Retrieved from ucanr.org/freepubs/docs/8265.pdf

International Food Information Council Foundation (2011, May 21). *Questions and answers about energy drinks and health*. Food Insight. Retrieved from http://www.foodinsight.org/Resources/Detail.aspx?topic=Questions_and_Answers_About_Energy_Drinks_and_Health_

Substance Abuse and Mental Health Services Administration, Center for Behavioral Health Statistics and Quality. (2013, January 10). *The Drug Abuse Warning Network (DAWN) report: Update on emergency department visits involving energy drinks: a continuing health concern.* Retrieved from http://www.samhsa.gov/data/2k13/DAWN126/sr126-energy-drinks-use.htm

Thombs, D. L., O'Mara, R. J., Tsukamoto, M., Rossheim, M. E., Weiler, R. M., Merves, M. L., & Goldberger, B. A. (2010). Event-level analyses of energy drink consumption and alcohol intoxication in bar patrons. *Addictive Behaviors, 35* (4), 325–330.

Enrichment and Fortification

Enrichment and fortification both refer to the adding of nutrients to food. Enrichment refers to the adding of nutrients normally present in a given food but which have been lost during processing. Fortification is defined as the addition of nutrients beyond those that are naturally present in a given food. Fortification and enrichment are terms often used interchangeably, and fortification is typically used as a general term for the addition of nutrients to foods. Enrichment and fortification began as efforts to prevent malnutrition but have expanded to include the creation of functional foods.

The implementation of food fortification in North America began in response to the prevalence of widespread health conditions that were shown to be directly related to nutrient deficiencies. Increased diagnoses of goiter, pellagra, rickets, beriberi, and scurvy created a public health need for better nutrition. Initially, many food manufacturers believed that nutrient deficiencies were the responsibility of the pharmaceutical companies. Public health agencies began to develop educational programs that were aimed at simultaneously creating a demand for fortified products while also encouraging the food industry to see the benefit of developing such products. Schoolteachers were provided with educational programs for their classrooms. Routine visits to the doctor began to include basic education about drinking milk fortified with vitamin D for the prevention of rickets, particularly in small children. Consumer demand soon was followed by industry competition to produce new and improved products that could make health claims. For instance, dairy manufacturers began adding vitamin D to milk and sought the American

Medical Association seal of approval to draw attention of both health-conscious mothers as well as medical providers.

In 1924, iodized salt became the first fortified food in the United States. In Michigan, iodine was added to salt to help prevent a disease of the thyroid gland called goiter. Soon after the introduction of iodized salt into the food supply, Michigan saw the prevalence of goiter drop from 38.6% to 9% (Backstrand, 2002). Iodized salt soon began to be produced throughout the United States. Iodized salt began a trend that later would be followed by other fortified staple foods, such as milk, flour, and various grain products. That same decade, an estimated 75% of infants in New York City suffered from rickets due to low vitamin D intake (Backstrand, 2002). A pellagra epidemic emerged from niacin deficiency. Health practitioners also were seeing beriberi and night-blindness at an increasing rate due to deficiencies in thiamin and vitamin A, respectively.

By 1941, with the impending possibility of U.S involvement World War II, malnutrition was perceived to be a matter of national security. Accordingly, the first Recommended Dietary Allowances (RDAs) were presented at the National Nutrition Conference for Defense. In addition to energy and protein recommendations, the new RDAs covered eight micronutrients—iron, calcium, thiamin, riboflavin, niacin, ascorbic acid, vitamin A, and vitamin D. The RDAs then were used to guide the fortification of foods that suffered nutrient losses due to refining processes. Corn for instance—which was a major dietary staple for low-income households—lost much of its niacin due to processing in motorized corn mills. Enrichment of corn and grain products with niacin soon eradicated the niacin-deficiency disease pellagra within these lower socioeconomic populations. New guidelines also allowed nutrients to be added above "natural levels" if other ways to correct nutritional deficiencies are not available. By 1958, the FDA established enrichment standards for refined grains products such as white bread, pasta, cornmeal, grits, and white rice.

The Food and Drug Administration (FDA) currently has general guidelines for the addition of nutrients to food. Once a documented need for adding a nutrient is established, the food to be fortified must be confirmed as a suitable vehicle to correct specific dietary insufficiency. Additionally, it's required that the nutrient have sufficient bioavailability and not be present at an excessive level. The nutrient also must be stable in customary storage conditions. In 1992, for example, the Centers for Disease Control and Prevention recommended that women of childbearing age achieve higher intakes of folic acid to prevent infant birth defects known as neural tube defects. Soon after, the FDA permitted the addition of folic acid to grain products.

Another approach to food fortification involves modifying food plants themselves. Biofortification currently allows for selective breeding or genetic modification of organisms to produce nutrient-dense foods. Compared to commercial fortification, biofortification generally requires a one-time investment mostly for research and design; for example, biological engineering has created self-fortifying seeds. Biofortification of staple foods can provide a direct method of ensuring daily consumption of nutrient dense foods. Golden Rice is genetically engineered to synthesize its own beta-carotene, the precursor to vitamin A. Vitamin A deficiency is the leading cause of blindness in many countries around the world.

Biofortification faces numerous technological complications. Developing biofortified varieties leaves farmers concerned about sensory changes to current crops. For instance, increasing provitamin A concentration causes color changes. In addition to breeding plants for selective traits, other agricultural practices such as the use of specific soil fertilizers can aid in increasing nutrient concentration. Although debate about genetically modified foods continues, some scientists maintain that with good seed systems breeding for nutrient density can help to address public health demands related to nutrient insufficiencies.

Ana Maria Moise

Research Issues

The FDA currently has little authority to regulate food-fortification efforts on the part of the food industry. An enormous variety of fortified foods can be found on supermarket shelves. Fortified beverages, breakfast cereals, meal-replacement bars, and many other products offer 100% of the Recommended Dietary Allowance for many nutrients. Many nutritionists are concerned that consumption of fortified food products could contribute to nutrient toxicity, in which consumer intake of certain nutrients can surpass the toxic upper limit for that nutrient. For example, the recommended upper limit for the daily intake of calcium for adults is 2,500 mg. If a person consumes three servings of dairy products, as recommended by nutrition guidelines, but also consumes calcium-fortified waffles and orange juice, and then takes a calcium-based antacid, this limit can be easily exceeded.

See Also: Dietary Reference Intakes; Genetically modified organisms; Iodine; Niacin; U.S. Food and Drug Administration.

Further Reading

Backstrand, J. R. (2002). The history and future of food fortification in the United States: A public health perspective. *Nutrition Reviews, 60* (1):15-26. Retrieved from http://www.idpas.org/pdf/1494TheHistoryandFuture.pdf

Bishai, D., & Nalubola, R. (2002). The history of food fortification in the United States: Its relevance for current fortification efforts in developing countries. *Economic Development and Cultural Change, 51* (1), 37–53.

Guangwen Tang, G., Qin, J., Dolnikowski, G., Russell, R., & Grusak, M. (2009). Golden rice is an effective source of vitamin A. *The American Journal of Clinical Nutrition, 89* (6), 1776–1783.

Nestel, P., Bouis, H. E., Meenakshi, J. V, & Pfeiffer, W. (2006). Biofortification of staple food crops. *The Journal of Nutrition, 136* (4), 1064–1067. Retrieved from http://jn.nutrition.org/content/136/4/1064.long

Enteral Nutrition

Enteral feeding provides nourishment to a person through a surgically placed tube in the gastrointestinal (GI) tract, either through the nose, throat, or abdominal wall. It is designed for individuals with functional digestive systems who are unable or unwilling to receive adequate nutrition by mouth. Enteral nutrition has been shown to decrease postsurgical complications, such as malnutrition, delayed wound healing, and infection, and to reduce the amount of time spent in hospital-care settings. Enteral nutrition can last for a short time or can continue throughout a person's life, depending upon medical conditions. Enteral nutrition can improve the quality of life for people who require nourishment in this manner.

History

Enteral feeding dates back to ancient Greece and Egypt, where solutions were inserted into the rectum to treat bowel disorders. Such solutions consisted of milk, wine, wheat, barley, eggs, and brandy. Gastrostomies were introduced in 1845 and had numerous complications, leading many physicians to use nasogastric tubes instead. The first percutaneous endoscopic gastrostomy was performed on an infant in 1979 by Dr. Michael Gauderer, who later published his method; it became a widely used technique in 1980s.

Feeding Tubes

Enteral nutrition can be administered by cervical pharyngostomy or esophagostomy, gastronomy, jejunostomy, or nasoenteral feedings (*see* Table 1). Several clinical factors exist in the decision-making process regarding the route of administration, such as the individual's medical, nutritional, and behavioral status.

G-tubes and J-tubes can be inserted through the skin with a surgical procedure known as percutaneous endoscopic gastrostomy (PEG). Radiological images can help guide surgery, and laparoscopic and open surgical procedures also can be used. The tube is held in place by a water-inflated balloon against the abdominal wall, as well as an external fixation device. A flat open and closeable "button" lies against the skin to enable easy feedings and prevent tube dislodgment.

Methods of Delivery

- Gravity tube feeding—liquid feeds are poured into a feeding bag and pulled by gravity into a drip chamber and through the tube.
- Bolus—liquid feeds are manually administered by syringe in 5- to 10-minute intervals.
- Continuous–liquid feeds are delivered by a feeding pump at a constant rate throughout the day and are often used overnight.

Table 1. Enteral Nutrition

Type	Route of Administration	Indications for Use	Short-term	Long-term
Cervical Pharyngostomy or Esophagostomy	Inserted through the throat and into the esophagus	Following head and neck surgery; rarely used due to hazardous and inconvenient placement.	✓	
Gastrostomy (G-tube)	Administers feeds directly into the stomach.	Avoids issues with speech and swallowing, as well as nasal and esophageal irritation		✓
Jejunostomy (J-tube)	Inserted through the small intestine, into the lumen of the jejunum.	Tracheal aspiration, reflux esophagitis, gastroparesis, gastric or pancreatic cancer. Decreased risk of reflux and aspiration, since this method bypasses stomach.		✓
Nasoenteral (Nasogastric, nasoduodenal, nasojejunal)	Inserted transnasally	Short-term solution; allows for easy removal	✓	

Potential Reasons for Enteral Feeding

- Anorexia nervosa
- Burns
- Cachexia
- Chemotherapy
- Chronic pancreatitis
- Dysphagia
- Esophageal obstruction
- Gastroparesis
- Head and neck cancer
- Hepatic failure
- Impaired consciousness
- Inadequate oral intake
- Inflammatory bowel diseases
- Intestinal failure
- Parkinson's disease
- Postoperative
- Psychological
- Renal failure
- Respiratory failure
- Sepsis
- Trauma

Enteral Feedings

Liquid feeds can consist of commercially prepared feeds or blenderized food, which is rarely used. Although blenderized feeds are less expensive, formulas are more common and have less potential for blockage. The two most common types of enteral feeds are polymeric and monomeric formulas. Polymeric formulas, which consist of macronutrients in isolate form, contain protein, triglycerides, and carbohydrate polymers, and are the most commonly used formulas in enteral feeding. Monomeric formulas consist of proteins in the form of peptides or amino acids, fat as long-chain triglycerides (LCTs) or a combination of medium-chain triglycerides (MCTs) and LCTs, and carbohydrates in the form as partially hydrolyzed starch maltodextrins and glucose. These formulas most often are suggested for individuals with digestive or absorption issues. Other specially designed formulas are administered to patients with renal failure, pulmonary insufficiency, cirrhosis, or diabetes.

During the first 24 to 48 hours, enteral feeding is monitored closely, especially for ill or injured patients. Meal plans are introduced gradually, beginning at 50% of the patient's total caloric intake and gradually increasing to 100%.

Complications of Enteral Feeding

- Acid reflux
- Aspiration
- Clogged tubes, which require regular cleaning
- Constipation
- Diarrhea
- Dumping syndrome (in cases of jejunostomy) in which hypertonic liquid enters the small intestine, causing severe abdominal pain, weakness, diaphoresis, tachycardia, and electrocardiographic changes.
- Impaired speech and swallowing, in cases of nasoenteric feeding
- Nasal and esophageal irritation, in cases of nasoenteric feeding
- Nausea
- Skin irritation at the gastrostomy or jejunostomy site
- Tube dislodgement

Nicole D. Teitelbaum

See Also: Parenteral nutrition.

Further Reading

American Society for Parenteral and Enteral Nutrition. (2014). *What is enteral nutrition?* Retrieved from http://www.nutritioncare.org/Information_for_Patients/What_is_Enteral _Nutrition_/

Bankhead, R., Boullata, J., Brantley, S., Corkins, M., Guenter, P., Krenitsky, J., Lyman, B., Metheny, N. A., Mueller, C., Robbins, S., & Wessel, J. (2009). Enteral nutrition administration. In: A.S.P.E.N. enteral nutrition practice recommendations. *Journal of Parenteral and Enteral Nutrition, 33* (2), 149–58. Retrieved from http://www.guideline.gov/content.aspx?id=14717

Chernoff, R. (2006). History of tube feeding. *Nutrition in Clinical Practice, 21*, 408–410.

Homes, S. (2012). Enteral nutrition: An overview. *Nursing Standard, 26* (39), 41–46.

Pearce, C. B., & Duncan, H. D. (2012). Enteral Feeding. Nasogastric, nasojejunal, percutaneous endoscip gastrostomy, or jejunostomy: Its indications and limitations. *Postgraduate Medical Journal, 78* (918), 198–204.

Ponsky, J. L. (2011). The development of PEG: How it was. *Journal of Interventional Gastroenterology, 1* (2), 88–89.

Enzymes, Digestive

Enzymes are protein catalysts that serve to speed up biochemical reactions. Digestive enzymes are protein molecules that enable the breakdown of large food particles into fatty acids, peptides, amino acids, simple sugars, and other nutrients that can be absorbed by the body. Digestive enzymes play a major role in the chemical digestion of food. The three basic categories of digestive enzymes include (1) amylases, which assist in the break down of starches, also called "complex carbohydrates"; (2) lipases, which assist in the breakdown of fats; and

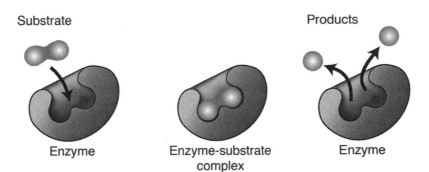

An enzyme is a biological catalyst and is almost always a protein. It speeds up the rate of a specific chemical reaction in the cell. The enzyme is not destroyed during the reaction and is used over and over. A cell contains thousands of different types of enzyme molecules, each specific to a particular chemical reaction. (Darryl Leja/National Human Genome Research Institute)

(3) proteases (also called "proteolytic enzymes"), which assist in the digestion of proteins.

Chemical digestion starts in the mouth where salivary glands secrete the enzyme amylase to break down starch into smaller carbohydrates. In addition to its role as an antibacterial aid in the mouth, lipase also is secreted to initiate the breakdown of fat molecules. Chief cells line the stomach and secrete pepsinogen, which becomes the proteolytic enzyme pepsin when activated by hydrochloric acid. Pepsin speeds the degradation of protein into smaller peptides for further digestion in the small intestine. A majority of the body's digestive enzymes are found in the small intestine, which receives secretions of pancreatic juice. Pancreatic juice contains the enzyme precursors trypsinogen and chymotripsinogen, which are converted into the active digestive enzymes trypsin and chymotrypsin in the small intestine. These proteases assist the breakdown of peptides into amino acids in the small intestine. Pancreatic juice also contains pancreatic amylase and pancreatic lipase. Additional digestive enzymes are present in the absorptive cells that line the villi of the small intestine. Here, disaccharides (small carbohydrate units) are broken down into monosaccharides by the enzymes sucrase, lactase, and maltase. These cells also contain peptidases for digesting peptides into amino acids. Cellulase is a digestive enzyme generated by bacteria in the gut to digest plant materials, such as the cell walls in cellulose.

Supplementing a diet with digestive enzymes typically is beneficial only for those with digestive deficiencies. Many supplements claiming to provide digestive enzymes simply are digested themselves once they reach the acidic environment of the stomach, because enzymes are proteins. There are a few digestive enzyme supplements, however, that have shown some therapeutic benefits. Taking the enzyme lactase enables the digestion of the milk sugar lactose, and enables people with lactose intolerance to consume some dairy products. (People with lactose intolerance do not manufacture enough lactase.) Lactase can be found in over-the-counter preparations, including tablets and drops. Lactase also is added commercially to dairy foods to produce products digestible for those with lactose intolerance.

Some common plant-derived proteolytic supplements include bromelain and papain, which contain enzymes made from pineapples and papaya plants, respectively. Bromelain is the primary ingredient in meat tenderizer, as it speeds the breakdown of the protein components in meat. Both papain and bromelain are thought to contribute to protein digestion in the human digestive tract, and could be helpful for relieving occasional indigestion. Bromelain appears to resist digestion, and can be absorbed into the bloodstream. Small studies have found some therapeutic benefit for bromelain in reducing sinus infections (EBSCO, 2012a). Although other claims have been made for the proteolytic enzyme supplements, significant evidence to support these claims generally is lacking, other than a few small studies.

Digestive enzyme supplements appear to be nontoxic and safe, although high doses might cause mild gastrointestinal discomfort and, occasionally, allergic reactions. Because papain and especially bromelain appear to act as blood thinners, these should not be taken as supplements by people taking warfarin or other anticoagulants, without medical supervision. Bromelain also increases the blood concentration of certain antibiotics and should be avoided by people on antibiotic therapies.

Patricia M. Cipicchio

See Also: Digestion and the digestive system.

Further Reading

EBSCO CAM Review Board. (2012a). *Bromelain.* Natural and alternative treatments. Retrieved from: http://healthlibrary.epnet.com/GetContent.aspx?token=e0498803-7f62 -4563-8d47-5fe33da65dd4&chunkiid=146651#ref38

EBSCO CAM Review Board. (2012b). *Proteolytic enzymes.* Natural and alternative treatments. Retrieved from http://healthlibrary.epnet.com/GetContent.aspx?deliverycontext =&touchurl=&CallbackURL=&token=e0498803-7f62-4563-8d47-5fe33da65dd4&chu nkiid=21671&docid=/tnp/pg000487

List of digestive enzymes and their functions: Digestive enzyme roles. (2011, January 19). Simple Remedies. Retrieved from http://www.simple-remedies.com/health-tips-3/list-of -digestive-enzymes-and-their-functions.html

Roxas, M. (2008). The role of enzyme supplementation in digestive disorders. *Alternative Medicine Review, 13* (4), 307–314.

Esophagus

The esophagus is an organ in the digestive system that creates a tube-like passage from the pharynx (area behind the mouth) to the stomach. There are two sphincters in the esophagus—one at its top and one at its bottom—that regulate the passage of food. The sphincter at the top of the esophagus is called the upper esophageal sphincter. When a person swallows, the upper esophageal sphincter opens to allow the passage of the "bolus"—a chewed ball of food—into the esophagus. Peristalsis, the contraction of muscles, moves the bolus down the esophagus toward the stomach. The lower esophageal sphincter opens to allow the food to move into the stomach. The lower esophageal sphincter prevents stomach contents from moving backward up into the esophagus.

The esophagus lies behind the trachea and the right side of the aorta. The esophagus is approximately 25 cm long and can be visualized as three parts, cervical, thoracic, and abdominal sections. The first section, the cervical esophagus, starts at the pharynx, at the C6 cervical vertebra and continues down to about the T5 thoracic vertebra. The middle section of the esophagus is known as the thoracic section, and starts at the T5 vertebra and extends to the diaphragm. The third part of the esophagus, the abdominal section, runs from the diaphragm to the stomach.

Like the other organs that comprise the gastrointestinal tract, the esophagus is composed of several tissue layers, the mucosa, submucosa, muscularis, and tunica adventitia. The innermost layer of the esophagus is the mucosa. It is named for the mucous glands that secrete mucus to the esophageal lining, helping to promote easy movement of food down the esophagus. The submucosa connects the mucosa to the muscularis. The submucosa is loose connective tissue that contains blood vessels, nerves, and esophageal glands. The muscularis layer is comprised of both circular and longitudinal muscle fibers. These muscles make up the majority of the width of the esophagus. The tunica adventitia is the outermost layer of the esophagus and is composed of dense connective tissue.

The muscles of the esophagus contract and relax in wave-like motions known as peristalsis, and push food down to the stomach. These muscular waves are so powerful that people can swallow, moving food down the esophagus, even when upside down. Other than during swallowing, the esophagus is empty.

Julia Leitermann

See Also: Digestion and the digestive system; Gastroesophageal reflux disease.

Further Reading

The esophagus (human anatomy): Picture, function, conditions, and more. (2014). WebMD. Retrieved from http://www.webmd.com/digestive-disorders/esophagitis-directory

Taylor, T. (2014, December 3). *Esophagus*. InnerBody. Retrieved from http://www.innerbody .com/image_dige01/dige03-new2.html#full-description

Viswanatha, B. (2011). *Esophagus anatomy*. Medscape. Retrieved from http://emedicine .medscape.com/article/1948973-overview#aw2aab6b2

Eye Health

Eye health appears to be strongly influenced by nutrition. Certain nutrient deficiencies can cause damage to eye structure and function, and consuming supplemental doses of other nutrients could slow the progress of two chronic eye problems associated with aging. Good nutrition also can reduce the risk of a vision problem associated with diabetes—diabetic retinopathy. Vitamin A and zinc are essential to healthy eye development and function; vitamin A deficiency is the leading cause of preventable blindness in children around the world. Vitamin A and zinc deficiencies also are associated with reduced visual acuity for both night vision and color vision. Certain antioxidants, including several vitamins, minerals, and phytochemicals, appear to prevent or at least slow the development of degenerative eye diseases, specifically macular degeneration and cataract formation. Long-chain fatty acids could help to prevent diabetic retinopathy. Research suggests that many people fail to obtain the recommended intake levels of these important nutrients (Rasmussen & Johnson, 2013).

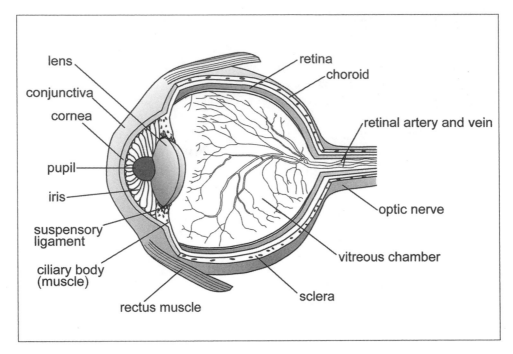

Anatomy of the eye. The health of the eye is influenced by a person's diet. The eye functions by receiving light waves, yet it is also sensitive to damage from these light waves. (Sandy Windelspecht)

Vision and Xerophthalmia

Vitamin A is critical to eye health. It contributes to the reproduction of cells in the cornea and supports the function of the conjunctival membranes, which provide lubrication to the eye's surface. Additionally, a derivative of vitamin A—retinal—is essential for vision. It combines with the protein opsin to form rhodopsin on rod cells in the retina (Insel et al., 2014). When light enters the eye, it splits rhodopsin. This, in turn, sends electric impulses to the brain, which the brain interprets as black-and-white visual images. Rhodopsin then is regenerated, allowing for more light to be registered. If vitamin A levels are low, rhodopsin cannot be re-formed, leading to night blindness, which is the inability of the eyes to adjust to dim light or to regain vision quickly after bright light exposure. Similarly, vitamin A is found in iodopsin, a color-sensitive pigment on cone cells in the retina. Thus, low levels of vitamin A also can impair color vision. Vitamin A deficiency affects rod cells before cone cells, and therefore night blindness occurs before color vision is impaired (Insel et al., 2014).

Vitamin A is only found as retinol in foods of animal origin, with liver being the richest source. Vitamin A can be obtained indirectly from plant foods, however. The cartotenoids found in plants act as precursors to vitamin A. Of the carotenoids, beta-carotene supplies the most vitamin A. The richest plant sources of provitamin A cartotenoids include orange and deep-yellow vegetables and dark-green leafy vegetables.

Vitamin A deficiency can lead to numerous health conditions. One of the first signs of vitamin A deficiency is night blindness. This can be corrected with early treatment, the administration of vitamin A. Failure to treat vitamin A deficiency, however, can lead to total blindness. Without an adequate supply of vitamin A, the cells in the cornea stop reproducing, as do the cells responsible for mucus production and secretion. The conjunctival membranes gradually lose the ability to lubricate the eye's surface. As the eye dries out and the cornea deteriorates, the eye becomes unable to wash away dirt and microbes, and becomes vulnerable to infection. White spots (Bitot's spots) can appear on the eye's surface, and in more severe cases the cornea can harden and scar. This condition is called "Xerophthalmia" and results in permanent blindness.

Although vitamin A deficiency is uncommon in North America and Western Europe, it is the leading cause of preventable blindness in malnourished children in more than half of all countries, especially countries in Africa and Southeast Asia (WHO, 2014). It is estimated that 250,000 to 500,000 vitamin A–deficient children become blind every year, and half of them die within 12 months of losing their sight (WHO, 2014). These statistics illustrate how vital vitamin A is to both eye health and to the human body in general.

The mineral zinc also plays an important role in eye health. Zinc is required for the optimal function of melanin-producing cells. Melanin is a pigment found in the iris and choroid of the eye that provides protection from ultraviolet and high-frequency visible light. (The choroid is the vascular layer of the eye, containing blood vessels and connective tissue.) Zinc also is a component of retinol-binding protein, a protein necessary for transporting vitamin A from the liver to the retina (Higdon et al., 2013). Additionally, it is required for the operation of the enzyme that converts retinol to retinal, the vitamin A form needed for rhodopsin. Zinc deficiency is associated with a decreased discharge of vitamin A from the liver to the eyes and therefore can lead to health issues similar to those which arise from vitamin A deficiency. Thus, people experiencing eye problems, such as night blindness, often are given zinc supplements along with vitamin A supplements. In the diet, zinc is found in shellfish, especially oysters, meats, and wheat bran.

Cataracts and Macular Degeneration

The two most common eye diseases in North America that have been linked with nutrition are cataracts and macular degeneration. Cataract formations are one of the leading causes of visual impairment around the world. Cataracts occur when proteins in the eye are damaged, often from oxidation processes (NEI, 2009). These proteins clump together, causing clouding in the lens. Most cataracts are related to aging, though other forms also can occur.

Macular degeneration, a chronic eye disease that typically occurs in older adults, causes vision loss due to the deterioration of the macula, a part of the retina responsible for clear sharp vision (AOA, 2014b). Age-related macular degeneration (AMD) is the leading cause of blindness in people age 60 and older.

In addition to vitamin A and zinc, several other nutrients and antioxidant phytochemicals have been linked to eye health over the life span, including prevention of cataracts and macular degeneration. These include vitamin C, vitamin E, and the carotenoid antioxidants lutein and zeaxanthin. Vitamin C supports the health of the eyes' connective tissues, including the ocular blood vessels. High concentrations of vitamin C are present in the aqueous humor (the fluid found in the eye ball), the cornea, and the focusing lens of the eye. These high concentrations are believed to be an indication of the importance of vitamin C to eyesight. Vitamin C and vitamin E both exhibit antioxidant activity throughout the body, neutralizing harmful chemicals called free radicals. Free radicals can damage proteins and other cellular structures. Lutein and zeaxanthin are carotenoids found in high concentrations in the eye (AOA, 2014a). They are most concentrated in the macula, which is the central part of the retina. Lutein and zeaxanthin help to filter harmful light wavelengths to prevent eye damage. They also appear to behave as antioxidants in the eye, preventing oxidative damage. Dark leafy vegetables, such as spinach, collard greens, and kale, are good sources of lutein and zeaxanthin.

Multiple studies have shown that higher intakes of vitamin C and E are associated with a reduced risk for cataracts. The Nutrition and Vision Project, for instance, found that higher intakes of vitamin C and vitamin E lowered the risk for cortical and nuclear cataracts, and the Nurses' Health Study found that the need for cataract surgery was lower among women who used vitamin C supplements for 10 years or longer (AOA, 2014c). Similar results were found with lutein and zeaxanthin. The Health Professional's Follow-Up Study and the Nurses' Health Study both found that higher intakes of lutein and zeaxanthin were associated with a reduced need for cataract surgery (AOA, 2014c).

The Age-Related Eye Disease Study (AREDS) was one of the first studies to examine the relationship between nutrition and eye health. Beginning in 1997, the innovative longitudinal study sponsored by the National Institutes of Health lasted for approximately seven years. The focus of the clinical trial was to analyze the effects of antioxidant and zinc supplementation on the progression of macular degeneration and cataract formation in people at high risk for these diseases. The research found that the risk of progressing to advanced macular degeneration for people in earlier stages of AMD decreased by approximately 25% after taking high levels of vitamins C and E, beta-carotene, and zinc. A second trial, the Age-Related Eye Disease Study 2, replaced beta-carotene in the supplement formulation with two other carotenoids, lutein and zeaxanthin, and found this formulation to be equally effective (National Eye Institute, 2013). The replacement was recommended because beta-carotene supplementation has been associated with increased risk of lung cancer in smokers.

Treatment with the supplements used in the AREDS 2 has become the standard of care for people diagnosed with early-stage AMD or found to be at high risk for the disease. The supplements might not be helpful for others, however, and it should be noted that risks could be associated with use of dietary supplements.

Dietary supplements for eye health generally contain vitamin C, vitamin E, lutein, zeaxanthin, zinc, and copper. Copper is added because high doses of zinc prevent the absorption of copper, which can cause negative health effects.

Diabetic Retinopathy and Retinitis Pigmentosa

The most common types of diabetic retinopathy are marked by abnormal blood vessel growth in the retina. These blood vessels leak blood and can produce swelling in the retina, blurry vision, and blindness. Diabetic retinopathy is one of the negative long-term consequences of diabetes, and a leading cause of blindness. More than 4 million adults in the United States have some degree of diabetic retinopathy (Thomas & Chander, 2011). Optimal treatment for diabetes that helps maintain healthful glucose levels can help prevent or delay the development of diabetic retinopathy. Additionally, animal research suggests that the omega-3 fatty acids eicosapentaenoic acid (EPA) and docosahexaenoic acid (DHA) might help to prevent retinopathies. This evidence underscores the importance of including food sources of these fatty acids in the diet. Good sources include cold-water fish such as salmon, sardines, and mackerel. Omega-3 fatty acids supplements also could be recommended for individuals at high risk for diabetic retinopathy.

Retinitis pigmentosa (RP) is a group of eye diseases characterized by damage to the light sensitive cones and rods in the retina. Retinitis pigmentosa generally progresses slowly over time. Research suggests that high intakes of vitamin A, lutein, and DHA might help to slow vision loss somewhat (Berson et al., 2012).

Alexandra M. Gatsios and Hee Jae Lee

See Also: Antioxidants; Beta-carotene; Carotenoids; Diabetes, type 1; Diabetes, type 2; Dietary supplements; Lutein; Marine omega-3 fatty acids; Phytochemicals; Vitamin A; Vitamin C; Zeaxanthin; Zinc.

Further Reading

American Optometric Association (AOA). (2014a). *Lutein and zeaxanthin—eye-friendly nutrients*. Retrieved from http://www.aoa.org/patients-and-public/caring-for-your-vision/nutrition/lutein-and-zeaxanthin?sso=y

American Optometric Association (AOA). (2014b) *Nutrients and age-related macular degeneration*. Retrieved from http://www.aoa.org/patients-and-public/caring-for-your-vision/nutrition/nutrition-and-age-related-macular-degeneration?sso=y

American Optometric Association (AOA). (2014c). *Nutrition and cataracts*. Retrieved from http://www.aoa.org/patients-and-public/caring-for-your-vision/nutrition/nutrition-and-cataracts

Berson, E. L., Rosner, B., Sandberg, M. A., Weigel-DiFranco, C., & Willett, W. C. (2012). Omega-3 intake and visual acuity in patients with retinitis pigmentosa receiving vitamin A. *Archives of Ophthalmology, 130* (6), 707–711. doi: 10.1001/archophthalmol.2011.2580

Higdon, J., Drake, V. J., & Ho, E. (2013). *Zinc*. Linus Pauling Institute, Oregon State University. Retrieved from http://lpi.oregonstate.edu/infocenter/minerals/zinc/

Insel, P., Ross, D., McMahon, K., & Bernstein, M. (2014). *Nutrition*. Burlington, MA: Jones and Bartlett.

National Eye Institute (NEI). (2009). *Facts about cataracts*. Retrieved from http://www .nei.nih.gov/health/cataract/cataract_facts.asp#2a

National Eye Institute (NEI). (2013). *Age-related eye disease study—results*. Retrieved from http://www.nei.nih.gov/amd/

Rasmussen, H. M., & Johnson, E. J. (2013). Nutrients for the aging eye. *Clinical Interventions in Aging, 2013* (8), 741–748. Retrieved from https://www.dovepress.com /nutrients-for-the-aging-eye-peer-reviewed-article-CIA-recommendation1. doi: http:// dx.doi.org/10.2147/CIA.S45399

Thomas, C. G., & Chander, P. (2011). *Researchers learn how certain omega-3 fatty acids may halt vision-robbing blood growth in the retina*. National Eye Institute. Retrieved from https://www.nei.nih.gov/news/scienceadvances/advances/omega.asp

World Health Organization (WHO). (2014). *Micronutrient deficiencies: Vitamin A deficiency*. Retrieved from http://www.who.int/nutrition/topics/vad/en/

F

Fad Diets

The term "fad diet" refers to a temporary eating plan employed to reduce body weight. The word "fad" implies something that is very popular for a short period, often without good reason for its popularity. Fad diets usually promise unrealistic weight loss results in a short time. They generally require followers to only eat certain foods or drink liquid concoctions and, in the process, severely limit calorie intake. Although people generally lose weight on fad diets, the weight usually is regained soon after the diet ends. Fad diets are thought to fail because they do not address the reasons a person is overweight; they do not teach lifelong healthful eating behaviors required to maintain a reduced body weight; and, in some cases, they even can lead to weight gain when frustrated dieters develop uncontrollable food cravings and overeat in response to food restriction. Characteristics of fad diets include the following.

Limited Food Choices

Fad diets often encourage individuals to consume a diet that might completely eliminate a major food group, such as carbohydrates. Some fad diets only permit a few specific foods to be consumed. A diet might only include eating fruit, for example, or even only a few specific fruits. The limited food choices result in a very low calorie intake, and thus, weight loss.

Incomplete or False Explanations for Weight Loss

Many fad diets offer unsupported explanations for why the diet causes weight loss. These diets often suggest that some sort of special component or ingredient in a particular food item contributes to increased weight loss. Some say that the food takes more calories to digest than are in the actual food itself. (No known food has this property.) Others claim that some combination of foods leads to extra "fat burning." Some foods are said to "rev up" the body's metabolic rate. Although some foods (such as spicy foods) can slightly elevate metabolic rate for a brief period, such elevations alone have not been shown to produce weight loss.

Proponents of detox diets have advised dieters to fast and rely on a liquid concoction to rid their body of harmful toxins. It often is promised that once the body

286 | Fad Diets

Very Low-Calorie Diets

The following information—taken from the Weight Control Information Network, an information service of the federal government's National Institute of Diabetes and Gastrointestinal and Kidney Diseases—defines a very low-calorie diet (VLCD) as a special type of diet that replaces all of your meals with prepared formulas, often in the form of liquid shakes. A VLCD can be used for a short time to promote quick weight loss among some people who are considered to be obese. People should not undertake a VLCD on their own. People who need to lose weight should talk to a health care provider about the approaches that might work best.

What Is a Very Low-Calorie Diet?

A VLCD is a special diet that provides up to 800 calories per day. Very low-calorie diets use commercial formulas, typically liquid shakes, soups, or bars, which replace all of the dieter's regular meals. These formulas are not the same as the meal replacements sold at grocery stores or pharmacies, which are meant to replace one or two meals a day.

- Depending on a number of factors, healthy adults require different amounts of calories to meet daily energy needs. A standard amount is about 2,000 calories.
- A VLCD only should be used for a short time—usually about 12 weeks.
- In general, VLCDs are not appropriate for children. In a few cases, they could be used with some adolescents who are being treated for obesity.
- Some people 50 years of age and older could have medical issues that might not make them good candidates for this type of diet.

What Are the Health Risks of a Very Low-Calorie Diet?

Doctors must monitor all VLCD patients regularly—ideally every 2 weeks in the initial period of rapid weight loss—to be sure patients are not experiencing serious side effects. Many patients on a VLCD for 4 to 16 weeks report minor side effects, such as fatigue, constipation, nausea, and diarrhea. These conditions usually improve within a few weeks and rarely prevent patients from completing the program.

National Institutes of Health. National Institute of Diabetes and Digestive and Kidney Diseases. *Very low-calorie diets*. (2012). Weight-Control Information Network. Retrieved from http://win.niddk.nih.gov/publications/low_calorie.htm

---

has cleansed itself of toxins, metabolic processes will be more efficient and result in weight loss. This statement has no scientific foundation. Weight lost on detox programs is likely attributable to the fact that few calories are consumed over the course of the program.

Celebrity and Success Story Advertisements

Advertisements for fad diets often feature a (paid) celebrity who has lost weight on the diet, or stories of individuals who have achieved success with the diet. As stated above, it is not uncommon for weight loss to occur when people consume very few calories, so most fad diets can achieve results for a limited period.

Exaggerated Claims

Fad diets often promise unrealistic weight-loss results. Although initial weight loss on very restrictive diets can be quite significant (several pounds in the first week or two), most of this weight loss is water loss. Water loss occurs as the body uses stored glycogen. Glycogen is a starch that the body uses for energy and stores in the liver and muscles. Water is stored with glycogen therefore, as glycogen is used, water is lost. Fad diets also might promise other results, such as improved sexual function, athletic performance, and mood.

Special Products Could Be Required

Fad diets sometimes require individuals to purchase specific products to reach their weight-loss goals. Many detox diets, for example, rely on a certain drink regimen that is sold to consumers. Most fad diets that feature meal-replacement plans include specific liquid or powdered products that must be consumed daily.

Health Risks Associated with Fad Diets and Rapid Weight-Loss Plans

Fad diets occasionally do jump-start successful weight loss. Sometimes eating programs that initially might have been considered to be fad diets—such as the Pritikin Program—develop into successful behavior change programs with scientific support. The majority of people, however, regain any weight they lost.

Fad diets, and rapid weight loss in general, should occur with medical monitoring if diets are followed for more than a few days. Such diets can result in electrolyte imbalances and dehydration. Side effects also can include fatigue, dizziness, nausea, lightheadedness, and muscle aches.

Many overweight clients have a long history of dieting. In fact, many blame their dieting history for their problems with weight and food. Very restrictive eating can interfere with metabolism, hunger, appetite, and psychological relationships with food. Unsuccessful weight-loss attempts can lead to feelings of guilt and failure, food cravings, and—ironically—obesity, as food becomes too much of a focus in a person's life. Instead of following short-term, restrictive diets, it is more effective to develop healthful eating behaviors that an individual can follow for a lifetime.

Barbara A. Brehm and Mia Copeland-Brock

See Also: The Atkins Diet; Body composition; National Weight Control Registry; Obesity, treatment.

Further Reading

Hensrud, D. (2011). *When it comes to weight loss, there's no magic bullet.* MayoClinic
.com. Retrieved from http://www.mayoclinic.org/healthy-living/weight-loss/expert-blog
/fad-diets/bgp-20056460

Jacobsen, M. T. (2013). *The truth about detox diets.* WebMD. Retrieved from http://www
.webmd.com/diet/detox-diets

Zelman, K. M. (2007). *Top 10 ways to spot a fad diet.* WebMD. Retrieved from http://www
.webmd.com/diet/features/top-10-ways-to-spot-a-fad-diet.

Fast Food

"Fast food" refers to inexpensive food that is prepared and served quickly and easily and is sold in restaurants and at snack bars. The food often contains precooked or preheated ingredients that then are assembled into a meal by employees. There currently are 160,000 fast-food restaurants in the United States, and—according to a July 2013 Gallup poll—47% of people in the United States consume fast food at least once a week (Dugan, 2013). Fast food consumption is associated with higher energy, fat, and sodium intake, and lower intake of dietary fiber and some vitamins. Health problems associated with frequently eating fast food include obesity, type 2 diabetes, cardiovascular disease, asthma, rhinoconjunctivitis, eczema, and metabolic syndrome. In response to criticism, some fast-food companies have worked to create healthier meal options, but progress has been slow. Another controversial aspect of the fast-food industry is the aggressive marketing of its products to children.

A Brief History of Fast Food

White Castle, founded in 1921, generally is recognized as the first fast-food establishment. It initially sold mainly hamburgers, which many people in the United States were suspicious of due to concerns about sanitation and contamination of the meat (Smith, 2006). White Castle convinced its customers of the purity of its products and enjoyed great success, however, encouraging the creation of many other hamburger chains.

During the Great Depression, fast-food outlets flourished, providing motorists with cheap meals that were conveniently located in proximity to major highways. Most of the fast-food outlets were franchises, for which a businessperson looking to establish a new restaurant would pay a fee and purchase goods from the franchisor and then benefit from the recognizable name and marketing power of franchises.

In the 1940s and 1950s, fast-food restaurants that sold food other than the standard hamburgers, hot dogs, and french fries were created. Dunkin Donuts (1948), Dairy Queen ice cream (1940), and Baskin Robbins ice cream (1948)

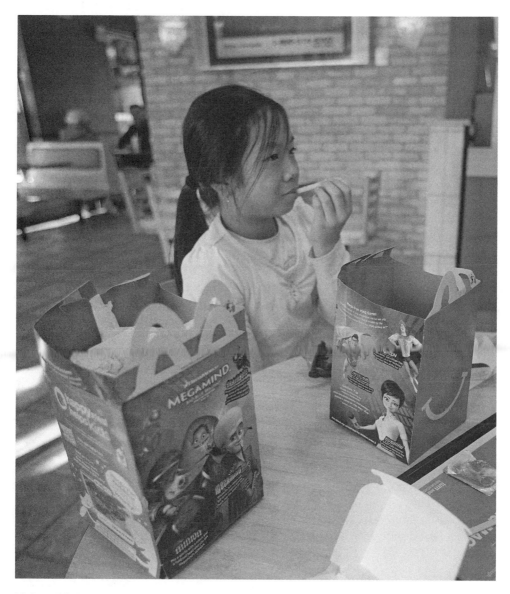

McDonald's Happy Meal. Fast-food meals for children often feature collectable toys, as well as foods that appeal to children, such as french fries, fried chicken, and soft drinks. However, many fast food chains, including McDonalds, also serve salads, fruit snacks, yogurt, and other healthful options. (AP/Wide World Photos)

became popular and rapidly expanded, and restaurants that served chicken—such as Kentucky Fried Chicken (now KFC) and Church's Chicken—became popular in the early 1950s. Hamburger chains, however, still were the most popular franchises, and McDonald's, originally established in 1940 as a barbeque restaurant, would go on the become the most popular fast-food restaurant of all, eventually opening more than 34,000 locations worldwide by 2013 (McDonald's, 2013; Smith, 2006). "Ethnic" fast food such as pizza and Mexican-style food started being served by restaurants like Pizza Hut (1958) and Taco Bell (1962).

Over time, fast-food outlets added more space for seating inside restaurants, as the number of families who preferred to eat in their cars decreased, and added a wider variety of menu options. McDonald's, for example, started serving chicken sandwiches as well as hamburgers, and pizza places started selling pasta dishes and sandwiches. Today, many fast-food chains have locations all over the globe, and their menus vary based on local tastes.

Nutrition and Health Effects

In general, most fast food is high in calories, fat, saturated fat, and sodium, and low in fiber, beta-carotene, and vitamins A and C (Paeratakul et al., 2003). The best-selling fast-food meals are high in red meat, fried potatoes, and refined grains, and low in milk, nuts, seeds, fruits, and vegetables (Paeratakul et al., 2003). For example, there are almost 600 calories and 35 grams of fat in a large hamburger, and there are 650 calories, 96 grams of sugar, and 14 grams of fat in a small Wendy's Caramel Frosty shake (Wendy's International, Inc., 2013).

One cause of the high caloric content of fast food meals is their increasingly larger portion sizes. In 1955, the largest amount of hamburger meat that McDonald's served weighed 1.6 ounces, and now the largest option contains 8 ounces of hamburger meat (Young & Nestle, 2007). By comparison, the 2010 *Dietary Guidelines for Americans* recommends that 5.5 ounces of protein foods be consumed per day by those on a 2,000 calorie food pattern (U.S. Department of Agriculture & U.S. Department of Health and Human Services, 2011). Soda (pop) serving sizes have dramatically increased as well. McDonald's originally served 7-ounce portions of soda, but now the largest serving size offered is 30 ounces (Young & Nestle, 2007).

Some common negative health effects associated with the consumption of fast food are listed below.

Weight Gain and Obesity

Weight gain is caused by consuming more calories than a body uses, and fast food promotes this positive energy balance for several reasons. Fast food often is served in extremely large portions, encouraging consumers to overeat. One meal can contain as many calories and grams of fat as an average person should consume in an entire day (U.S. Department of Agriculture & U.S. Department of Health and Human Services, 2011). The most popular fast-food options also contain large amounts of sugar, salt, and fat, which are the taste preferences that humans evolved thousands of years ago when nourishment was difficult to find; this can cause people to desire to consume large quantities of fast food. When someone has a positive energy balance, extra calories are converted to triglycerides that are stored in fat cells called adipocytes. Excessive weight gain and fat storage can lead to obesity. The Coronary Artery Risk Development in Young Adults (CARDIA) study found that, over 15 years, frequent (greater than twice per week) fast-food consumption was associated with weight gain of 4.5 kg (9.9 lbs) more than infrequent (less than once per week) fast-food consumption (Pereira et al., 2005).

Insulin Resistance and Type 2 Diabetes

Type 2 diabetes occurs when the body becomes resistant to insulin. Insulin is a hormone that is released when blood glucose levels become too high (hyperglycemia). Risk of developing insulin resistance and type 2 diabetes increases with obesity, low levels of physical activity, and poor diet quality. The CARDIA study found that the frequency of fast-food consumption was directly correlated with insulin resistance, and that participants who consumed fast food more than twice a week had an increase in insulin resistance twice the rate of those who consumed fast food less than once a week (Pereira et al., 2005).

Metabolic Syndrome

Metabolic syndrome is defined as having three or more of the following conditions: excess abdominal fat, high blood glucose, high serum triglycerides, low HDL cholesterol, and high blood pressure. Many fast foods have a high glycemic load, which means that they cause blood glucose to quickly rise to very high levels. High triglycerides in the blood also are associated with frequent fast-food consumption because of the tendency for those who frequently consume fast food to eat more calories than they use, which results in higher levels of triglyceride production. Low HDL cholesterol is also connected to increased fast-food consumption, because elevated blood triglyceride levels are associated with low HDL cholesterol. High blood pressure can be caused by high blood glucose levels, which stimulate the release of the neurotransmitter epinephrine and hormone insulin into the bloodstream and an increase in blood pressure as part of the fight-or-flight response. The high sodium levels in the most popular fast-food meals also could contribute to high blood pressure.

Cardiovascular Disease

High LDL cholesterol levels, especially high levels of lipoprotein a—a substance containing LDL and the protein apoprotein a—can contribute to atherosclerosis. High levels of triglycerides also appear to contribute to greater amounts of plaque buildup. Atherosclerosis occurs when arteries progressively become hardened and narrowed due to a buildup of plaque formed from fatty material. It can cause heart attacks and strokes.

Asthma, Rhinoconjunctivitis, and Eczema

The International Study of Asthma and Allergies in Childhood (ISAAC) found that eating fast food more than three times per week was associated with an increased risk of severe asthma, severe rhinoconjunctivitis, and severe eczema (Ellwood et al., 2013). These disorders are associated with inflammation.

Fast-Food Restaurants' Healthier Options

In response to widespread criticism of their products' nutritional values, some fast-food chains have introduced new, healthier menu options and attempted to improve upon old products. McDonald's, Wendy's, and Burger King now offer apple slices and side salads as a substitute for french fries and fruit juices, and these chains offer low-fat and fat-free milk as substitutes for soft drinks. Subway offers 17 different sandwiches and 7 different salads containing less than six grams of fat (Subway, 2013). According to a study analyzing trends in nutritional quality of fast-food meals over a period of 14 years, meals at eight of the most popular fast-food chains have experienced a slight increase in nutrition quality. The chains were rated on a scale of 1 to 100 according to the amount of fruits, vegetables, grains, milk, meat and beans, oils, saturated fat, sodium, and calories from solid fat and added sugars their meals contained, with a score of 100 being the healthiest. The average score increased by three points (45 to 48 points) between 1997/1998 and 2009/2010, and the scores for meat, saturated fat, and calories from solid fats and added sugars improved over this period. In contrast, the scores for sodium levels and milk/dairy decreased, and none of the restaurants had scores near 100 (Hearst et al., 2013).

Katherine A. Blackford

See Also: Adolescence and nutrition; Childhood nutrition; Obesity, causes; Portion size.

Further Reading

Dugan, A. (2013, August 6). *Fast food still major part of U.S. diet*. Retrieved October 27, 2013, from http://www.gallup.com/poll/163868/fast-food-major-part-diet.aspx

Ellwood, P., Asher, M. I., Garcia-Marcos, L., Williams, H., Keil, U., Robertson, C., & ISAAC Phase III Study Group. (2013). Do fast foods cause asthma, rhinoconjunctivitis and eczema? Global findings from the International Study of Asthma and Allergies in Childhood (ISAAC) phase three. *Thorax, 68* (4), 351–360. doi:10.1136/thoraxjnl -2012-202285

Hearst, M. O., Harnack, L. J., Bauer, K. W., Earnest, A. E., French, S. A., & Oakes, J. M. (2013). Nutritional quality at eight U.S. fast-food chains: 14-year trends. *American Journal of Preventive Medicine, 44* (6), 589–594. doi:10.1016/j.amepre.2013.01.028

McDonald's. (2013). *Getting to know us*. Retrieved November 18, 2013, from http://www .aboutmcdonalds.com/mcd/our_company.htm

Paeratakul, S., Ferdinand, D. P., Champagne, C. M., Ryan, D. H., & Bray, G. A. (2003). Fast-food consumption among US adults and children: Dietary and nutrient intake profile. *Journal of the American Dietetic Association, 103* (10), 1332–1338. doi:10.1016/ S0002-8223(03)01086-1

Pereira, M. A., Kartashov, A. I., Ebbeling, C. B., Van Horn, L., Slattery, M. L., Jacobs, D. R., Jr., & Ludwig, D. S. (2005). Fast-food habits, weight gain, and insulin resistance (the CARDIA study): 15-year prospective analysis. *The Lancet, 365* (9453), 36–42. doi:10.1016/S0140-6736(04)17663-0

Schlosser, E. (2001). *Fast food nation: The dark side of the all-American meal.* Boston, MA: Houghton Mifflin.

Smith, A. F. (2006). Fast Food. In *Encyclopedia of Junk Food and Fast Food,* 97–105. Westport, CT: Greenwood Press.

Subway. (2013, September). Official Subway restaurants' nutrition information. Retrieved October 28, 2013, from http://www.subway.com/nutrition/nutritionlist.aspx

U.S. Department of Agriculture, & U.S. Department of Health and Human Services. (2011, January). Building healthy eating patterns. In *Dietary Guidelines for Americans, 2010* (7th ed., p. 53). Retrieved from http://www.health.gov/dietaryguidelines/2010.asp

Wendy's International, Inc. (2013, October 27). *Wendy's nutrition.* Retrieved from http:// www.wendys.com/en-us/nutrition-info

Young, L. R., & Nestle, M. (2007). Portion sizes and obesity: Responses of fast-food companies. *Journal of Public Health Policy, 28* (2), 238–248. doi:10.1057/palgrave .jphp.3200127

Fasting

Fasting is a broad term that can refer to complete abstinence from all foods and beverages, drinking only water, drinking only fresh fruit and vegetable juices, or severely limiting the foods one consumes. The purpose of fasting varies as widely as the definition. Common goals are losing weight, increasing lifespan, enhancing general health, and complying with religious traditions. Safety and recommended duration depend on the form of fasting performed and the condition of the person undertaking the fast.

Total Fasting

Dry fasting, or abstaining from all foods and beverages, and water fasting, or consuming only noncaloric drinks, both represent forms of total fasting. Dry fasting rarely appears outside of religious contexts. Conversely, inpatient water fasting— termed "therapeutic starvation"—was a prevalent treatment for morbid obesity throughout the 1950s and 1960s. Significant weight loss occurred under medical supervision, but follow-up studies showed that the majority of patients regained weight. The risk of micronutrient deficiencies and refeeding syndrome—potentially lethal abnormalities in electrolyte and fluid balance—can be reduced by the intravenous or oral administration of electrolytes, vitamins, and minerals during a fast and the gradual reintroduction to an unrestricted diet following the termination of a prolonged fast.

Nonetheless, numerous other health concerns exist. Weight loss resulting from prolonged fasting tends to lead to a greater loss of lean body mass as compared to more moderate diets. The physiology of fasting accounts for this phenomenon. After 12 to 24 hours of water fasting, circulating amino acids and the liver's glycogen stores become depleted, forcing the body to switch to breaking down fat and using ketone bodies, rather than glucose, as the primary energy source. Red blood cells lack mitochondria, however, which contain enzymes necessary for ketone utilization. Furthermore, ketones can provide up to 70% of the brain's energy requirements, but some level of glucose utilization is obligatory, triggering protein catabolism for glucose production. In the absence of dietary protein intake, the body resorts to breaking down muscle tissue to obtain amino acids for gluconeogenesis. Studies on calorie restriction as well as fasting have identified additional complications that can arise due to prolonged water fasting, including fatigue, irritability, apathy, depression, obsessive thoughts about food, and decreased physical activity and sex drive. Individuals on a long-term fast also can experience headaches, dizziness, low blood pressure, and cardiac arrhythmias. These adverse side effects suggest that total fasting could be difficult to maintain when unsupervised and can reduce overall quality of life.

Intermittent Fasting

Much of the current research on fasting focuses on intermittent fasting (IF): cycling between periods of unrestricted feeding and periods of fasting. Alternate-day fasting (ADF)—fasting every other day—is a popular iteration of IF. It garnered interest as another possible way to achieve the health benefits of daily calorie restriction (CR) in rodent models, which include increased longevity, reduced inflammation, increased insulin sensitivity, improved cognitive function, and decreased risk of cardiovascular disease, neurodegenerative disease, and cancer (Young, 2012). Whether these findings can be applied to humans is a topic of controversy.

Studies of IF of humans are far less numerous than those of mice and rats, but several show a significant effect on biomarkers of cardiovascular disease and diabetes, lowering LDL cholesterol, triglycerides, and levels of insulin and glucose in the blood (Collier, 2013). In contrast, evidence of increased longevity or reduced inflammation has not been established. Even in rodents, it is unclear whether decreased levels of circulating tumor necrosis factor-alpha (TNF-α) and C-reactive protein (CRP)—markers of inflammation—result from IF itself or merely the reduced body weight it causes (Rothschild, Hoddy, Jambazian, & Varady, 2014).

Intermittent fasting is thought to exert its anticancer effects by decreasing levels of insulin-like growth factor 1 (IGF-1) and to defend against Alzheimer's disease and Parkinson's disease by increasing the release of brain-derived neurotrophic factor (BDNF), a protein that heightens neurons' resistance to excitotoxic stress, thereby reducing neuronal cell death (Stipp, 2012). Intermittent fasting–induced increases in neurogenesis and autophagy, a process that involves the breakdown of damaged organelles and other intracellular waste products, might play a role as well. These mechanisms have not been verified in humans, however.

Similarly, a review of the existing literature exploring the impact of IF on cognitive function found that results were mixed, but impairment was more common than improvement (Benau, Orloff, Janke, Serpell, & Timko, 2014).

Intermittent fasting also has been investigated as a potential weight-loss strategy for humans. A 22-day trial of ADF in non-obese subjects recorded weight loss, but reports of irritability and persistently elevated hunger led the researchers to doubt that long-term compliance was likely (Heilbronn, Smith, Martin, Anton, & Ravussin, 2005). Growing attention has been directed at a variant of ADF—sometimes referred to as alternate-day modified fasting (ADMF)—that allows dieters to consume about 25% of their baseline energy needs, usually 500 calories for women and 600 calories for men, rather than eating nothing on fast days. In one study, obese subjects maintained their normal eating habits for two weeks to establish a baseline, and then practiced ADMF for four weeks with fast-day meals provided to them, and finally followed the diet for four weeks and made their own food choices on fast days. Weight loss and adherence to the diet remained consistent throughout the second and third phases, and cardioprotective effects—decreased total cholesterol, LDL cholesterol, and triglycerides—were found (Varady, Bhutani, Church, & Klempel, 2009).

A subsequent study showed habituation to ADMF by the second week of the diet, with obese subjects reporting reduced feelings of hunger and increased satisfaction with the diet. The lack of a hyperphagic response (abnormally increased appetite) on feed days appeared to contradict predictions that ADMF would trigger binge eating (Klempel, Bhutani, Fitzgibbon, Freels, & Varady, 2010). Each of these studies, however, was small and provided no long-term follow-up, indicating the need for large clinical trials to better establish the safety and effectiveness of ADMF.

Juice Fasting

Abstaining from solid food and consuming only fresh fruit and vegetable juices for anywhere from one day to one month, a practice known as "juice fasting," has grown in popularity as a "detox diet." Notwithstanding, the claim that it enhances the body's ability to remove toxins remains scientifically unsupported. Anecdotal reports of an improved sense of well-being could be attributable to the "starvation high"—caloric restriction increases the release of endorphins—and to the psychological appeal of purification. Although juices can serve as a helpful way to incorporate more servings of fruits and vegetables into one's diet, the juicing process removes the fiber and increases the glycemic index. Short-term juice fasts might not be harmful for healthy adults, but the high sugar and mineral content make them inadvisable for diabetics and people with hyperkalemia caused by kidney disease.

Religious Fasting

Most major religions share periods of fasting as a common feature, although the rules differ. Rather than losing weight or achieving other physical effects, religious fasting often is intended to cultivate self-discipline, direct focus toward the spiritual, demonstrate devotion to a deity, purify the soul, or recognize sacred events. Fasting in Hinduism frequently coincides with religious festivals, and fasting in Buddhism is more prevalent among ascetics than laypeople. Prominent religious occasions accompanied by fasting include Ramadan in Islam, Yom Kippur in Judaism, and Lent in both Catholicism and Eastern Orthodox Christianity.

Ramadan fasting—which takes place from sunrise to sunset for one month—could be classified as intermittent fasting. Ramadan fasting also excludes beverages of any kind, however, whereas most IF protocols allow water and sometimes tea. Observing Yom Kippur, or The Day of Atonement, also involves forgoing eating and drinking of any kind, but lasts 25 hours (BBC, 2011). In the Catholic tradition, Lenten fasting means restricting oneself to a single meal per day on Ash Wednesday and Good Friday, as well as avoiding meat on all Fridays during the 40 days preceding Easter Sunday (United States Conference of Catholic Bishops, 2014). Eastern Orthodox guidelines are more stringent, requiring water fasting for short periods and excluding meat, eggs, and dairy products for the full duration. Consumption of oil and wine also might be limited (Public Broadcasting Service, 2010).

Ramadan and Eastern Orthodox Lenten fasting have been studied empirically in terms of their effects on nutrient intake, body mass index, and blood lipid profile. Results largely have been conflicting for Ramadan fasting. Lenten fasting and other Eastern Orthodox fasts were associated with increased fiber and carbohydrate intake, decreased fat, riboflavin, and calcium intake, reduced BMI, and lower levels of total and LDL cholesterol (Trepanowski & Bloomer, 2010). Excessive weight loss and vitamin and mineral deficiencies were not observed, indicating that these fasts are relatively safe for most people.

Notably, potentially at-risk groups such as children, pregnant or nursing women, and the ill are exempt from both Ramadan and Lenten fasting. Most Ramadan observers also can tolerate the negative water balance that results from daytime dry fasting without adverse health effects, but those who are especially vulnerable to extreme dehydration and heat stroke—such as industrial laborers—would need to take special precautions, request a reduced workload, or seek exemption from the fast.

Laura C. Keenan

See Also: Inflammation; Ketosis and ketogenic diets; Obesity, treatment.

Further Reading

Benau, E. M., Orloff, N. C., Janke, E. A., Serpell, L., & Timko, C. A. (2014). A systematic review of the effects of experimental fasting on cognition. *Appetite, 77* (1), 52–61. http://dx.doi.org/10.1016/j.appet.2014.02.014

British Broadcasting Corporation (BBC). (2011). *Yom Kippur—The day of atonement.* Retrieved from http://www.bbc.co.uk/religion/religions/judaism/holydays/yomkippur .shtml

Collier, R. (2013). Intermittent fasting: The science of going without. *Canadian Medical Association Journal, 185* (9), E363–E364. Retrieved from http://www.cmaj.ca/content/early/2013/04/08/cmaj.109-4451.full.pdf

Heilbronn, L. K., Smith, S. R., Martin, C. K., Anton, S. D., & Ravussin, E. (2005). Alternate-day fasting in nonobese subjects: Effects on body weight, body composition, and energy metabolism. *American Journal of Clinical Nutrition, 81* (1), 69–73. Retrieved from http://ajcn.nutrition.org/content/81/1/69.full

Klempel, M. C., Bhutani, S., Fitzgibbon, M., Freels, S., & Varady, K. A. (2010). Dietary and physical activity adaptations to alternate day modified fasting: Implications for optimal weight loss. *Nutrition Journal, 9,* 35–42. http://dx.doi.org/10.1186/1475-2891-9-35

Public Broadcasting Service (2010). *Orthodox fasting.* Retrieved from http://www.pbs.org/wnet/religionandethics/2010/02/19/february-19-2010-orthodox-fasting/5723/

Rothschild, J., Hoddy, K., Jambazian, P., & Varady, K. (2014). Time-restricted feeding and risk of metabolic disease: A review of human and animal studies. *Nutrition Reviews, 72* (5), 308–318. http://dx.doi.org/10.1111/nure.12104

Stipp, D. (2012). How intermittent fasting might help you live a longer and healthier life. *Scientific American, 308* (1). Retrieved from http://www.scientificamerican.com/article/how-intermittent-fasting-might-help-you-live-longer-healthier-life/

Trepanowski, J. F., & Bloomer, R. J. (2010). The impact of religious fasting on human health. *Nutrition Journal, 9,* 57–65. http://dx.doi.org/10.1186/1475-2891-9-57

United States Conference of Catholic Bishops (2014). *Fast & abstinence.* Retrieved from http://www.usccb.org/prayer-and-worship/liturgical-resources/lent/catholic-information-on-lenten-fast-and-abstinence.cfm

Varady, K. A., Bhutani, S., Church, E. C., & Klempel, M. C. (2009). Short-term modified alternate-day fasting: A novel dietary strategy for weight loss and cardioprotection in obese adults. *The American Journal of Clinical Nutrition, 90* (5), 1138–1143. http://dx.doi.org/10.3945/ajcn.2009.28380

Young, E. (2012). *Fasting may protect against disease; some say it may even be good for the brain.* Retrieved from http://www.washingtonpost.com/national/health-science/fasting-may-protect-against-disease-some-say-it-may-even-be-good-for-the-brain/2012/12/24/6e521ee8-3588-11e2-bb9b-288a310849ee_story.html

Fatty Acids

Fatty acids are organic compounds composed of hydrocarbon chains with an organic acid (carboxyl) group at one end and a methyl (CH_3) group at the other end. In the context of human nutrition, fatty acids are found in foods and in the body. Fatty acids often are found as components of triglycerides and other larger structures, but they also can occur unbound, in which case they are often referred to as "free fatty acids." There are many types of fatty acids, and their function in the body varies with their structure. Many fatty acids, such as the long-chain polyunsaturated fatty acids (PUFAs) are beneficial to health. Ingestion of large amounts of saturated fatty acids from animal products is thought to increase risk of artery disease. Some types of fatty acids must come from the diet. These are called essential fatty acids, and they include alpha-linolenic acid (ALA) and linoleic acid.

Fatty acids vary in the length of their hydrocarbon chains and in the types of bonds between the carbon atoms in these chains. Fatty acids found in foods usually have an even number of carbons, with a chain length of 4 to 24 carbons. Fatty acids with a chain length of fewer than 6 carbons are called "short-chain fatty acids"; medium-chain and long-chain fatty acids have 6 to 10, and 12 or more carbons, respectively. Some nutritionists use the term "very long-chain fatty acids" to refer to fatty acids with 20 or more carbons.

The carbon atoms in the fatty acid hydrocarbon chain can form single or double bonds with each other. Saturated fatty acids refer to fatty acids in which the bonds between carbon atoms all are single. Single carbon-carbon bonds are more stable than double bonds and affect the behavior of these fatty acids. Saturated fats tend to be more stable at higher temperatures, for example. This explains why butter (higher in saturated fatty acids) is a solid at room temperature, and plant oils (lower in saturated fatty acids) are not.

Unsaturated fatty acids have at least one carbon-carbon double bond. Monounsaturated fatty acids have one carbon-carbon double bond, and polyunsaturated fatty acids have more than one. The location of this carbon-carbon double bond helps to name the fatty acid, and affects the fatty acid's structure and behavior in the body. Omega-3 fatty acids have the carbon-carbon double bond at the third carbon from the methyl end of the fatty acid. Dietary sources of omega-3s include fish oils and some plant and nut oils. Fish oils contain special long-chain omega-3 fatty acids, including docosahexaenoic acid (DHA) and eicosapentaenoic acid (EPA), which have been associated with beneficial health effects, including reduced levels of inflammation and slower rates of blood clotting. This is why many public-health recommendations suggest that people increase their consumption of fish. Oily fish such as salmon, tuna, sardines, mackerel, and herring have the highest concentrations of these fatty acids. Alpha-linolenic acid is another type of omega-3, although its effects on the health variables mentioned above do not appear to be as strong as those of DHA and EPA. Conversely, omega-6 fatty acids—found primarily in plant oils—have been associated with higher levels of inflammation and increased rates of blood clotting.

Trans fatty acids, (trans fats, or TFAs) usually are created by hydrogenation, a process used by food-product manufacturers to make fatty acids in foods more saturated, thus more stable and with a longer shelf life. Although TFAs technically have a carbon-carbon double bond, the arrangement of other atoms around the bond lead to a shape of the fatty acid that is more similar to saturated fatty acids. Greater intake of trans fats in the diet has been linked to higher rates of artery disease. Trans fats could increase this risk through effects on blood lipid levels (raising LDL cholesterol levels and lowering HDL cholesterol levels), effects on the function of the artery lining, and by making the blood more likely to form blood clots.

Barbara A. Brehm

See Also: Alpha-linolenic acid, Cardiovascular disease and nutrition; Cholesterol; Hydrogenation; Linoleic acid; Lipids; Marine omega-3 fatty acids; The Paleolithic diet; Trans fatty acids; Triglycerides.

Further Reading

Harvard School of Public Health. (2014). *Fats and cholesterol: Out with the bad, in with the good.* http://www.hsph.harvard.edu/nutritionsource/fats-full-story/

Insel, P., Ross, D., McMahon, K., & Bernstein. (2014). *Nutrition.* Burlington, MA: Jones & Bartlett.

Feeding Disorders

Feeding disorders are characterized by patterns of severe disturbances in eating behavior. Individuals with feeding disorders have a high risk for poor social or physical development, as well as for learning disabilities. Some people experience social withdrawal and avoid eating in public. The *Diagnostic and Statistical Manual of Mental Disorders* (DSM-5) is the handbook used to classify or diagnose mental disorders. It lists feeding and eating disorders in the same chapter due to their shared disturbances in eating behavior. Unlike eating disorders, individuals with feeding disorders do not experience severe distress concerning body weight or shape. The DSM-5 lists three categories of feeding disorders.

Pica

The diagnostic criteria for pica include recurrent eating of nonfood items for at least one month; the eating behavior is abnormal for the individual's stage of development; the eating behavior is not accepted as a component of the individual's cultural practices; and the eating behavior is not a direct result of a mental disorder or medical condition. There are three main categories of substances: earth (geophagy), starch (amylophagy), and ice (pagophagy). Other common items include chalk, plaster, paper, charcoal, and baby powder.

Prevalence

- Between 1999 and 2009, the number of inpatient hospital stays for reasons related to pica nearly doubled (Zhao & Encinosa, 2011).
- Pregnant women have the highest rate of pica worldwide.
- Those who develop pica in childhood are more likely to outgrow their behaviors than those who develop it as adults.
- In 2009, 31% of children with pica who underwent inpatient treatment had autism spectrum disorders (Zhao & Encinosa, 2011).

History

Hippocrates documented the first case of pica-related behaviors in 400 BCE (Young, Wilson, Miller, & Hillier, 2008). It was not termed "pica," however, until 1542. As cases continued to surface in the 17th century, it became apparent that the disorder was most prevalent in pregnant women and children. In the 19th century, slaves in the United States were brutally punished if they engaged in pica-related behaviors. In contrast, other cultures condoned and even fostered these habits, making it difficult to identify pica as a true medical condition. Clay eating in particular currently is practiced in more than 200 cultures, and often is used to treat maladies such as diarrhea or morning sickness in pregnant women. Today, the condition is not classified as pica in the DSM-5 if the associated behaviors are a part of one's cultural habits or traditions.

Causes

There are several hypotheses about the etiology of pica and cravings associated with pica.

- Hunger—Food shortages and famine can trigger cravings of nonfood substances.
- Micronutrient deficiencies—Micronutrient deficiencies can disrupt enzymes in the brain associated with taste and appetite and result in pica-related behaviors, especially during pregnancy. Furthermore, pica substances inhibit absorption or bind micronutrients, leading to other health conditions (i.e., anemia).
- Protection against toxins and pathogens—Typical pica substances might absorb harmful chemicals in the gut, which protects the body from toxins and pathogens.
- Psychological stress—Eating behavior might serve as a self-soothing response to external stressors.
- Dyspepsia—Some individuals report a reduction in the discomfort associated with dyspepsia. This might be attributed to the alkalinity in typical pica substances, which can help with gastric acidity.

Comorbidity

- Mental retardation
- Developmental disabilities
- Autism spectrum disorders
- Schizophrenia
- Obsessive-compulsive disorder
- Medical complications
- Intestinal blockage
- Airway obstruction

- Anemia
- Lead or mercury poisoning, which can lead to kidney failure, cognitive deficits, seizures, coma, and death
- Absorption impairment, which can lead to nutritional deficiencies
- Acute weight loss
- Parasites due to the consumption of dirt or feces
- Birth complications in pregnant women
- High blood pressure
- Obesity, due to the consumption of highly caloric substances (e.g., laundry starch)

Treatment

Behavior modification has been shown to be effective in treating individuals with pica—especially children on the autism spectrum (Ferreri, Tamm, & Wier, 2006). This is especially relevant in food-aversion therapy, in which clinicians pair patients' aversive foods with an undesirable behavior or punishment for them to associate less pleasure upon consuming pica substances. The individual then is given positive reinforcement when choosing normative behaviors instead of pica-related behaviors.

Rumination Disorder

Rumination disorder is marked by the following symptoms: for at least one month, regurgitating food and then re-chewing, re-swallowing, or spitting out the food; the behavior is not a direct result of a gastrointestinal condition; the behavior is not a direct result of anorexia nervosa, bulimia nervosa, binge-eating disorder, or avoidant/restrictive food-intake disorder, or another mental disorder. It can develop during infancy, childhood, adolescence, or adulthood. Regurgitation behaviors can be especially self-soothing and self-stimulating for infants and those with neurodevelopmental disorders.

Prevalence

Little is known about the prevalence of rumination disorder. It is seen, however, in up to 10% of institutionalized patients with severe mental retardation (Fredricks, Carr & Williams, 1998).

History

The first case was documented in 1618 (Fredericks, Carr, & Williams, 1998). During the 18th century and 19th century, rumination disorder gained popularity in the entertainment and circus industry. People flocked to freak shows to watch individuals "perform" acts of rumination. Possible treatments did not surface until the 1950s, in which clinicians took a psychodynamic approach. They thought ruminating behaviors to be a result of insufficient progress during the oral and ego phases of development. Behavioral treatments emerged 10 years later, and have been the source of extensive research ever since.

Causes

- Lack of stimulation
- Neglect
- History of abuse
- Stressful life events

Comorbidity

- Mental retardation
- Intellectual disability
- Generalized anxiety disorder

Medical Complications

- Malnutrition
- Weight loss (or failure to gain weight, as seen in infants, children, and adolescents)
- Gastrointestinal issues
- Upper-respiratory distress
- Dental problems
- Aspiration
- Pneumonia
- Primary cause of death in 5% to 10% of individuals who ruminate

Treatment

Both aversive and nonaversive behavioral treatments have been used to target rumination disorder.

- Aversive—Electric shock, withdrawal of positive reinforcement, and noxious tastes. For example, a clinician might decide to spray a patient's mouth with a bitter formula when she gags. These treatments were common until the late 1980s, when they became criticized for their poor ethical standards.
- Nonaversive—Satiation, in which large amounts of food are given to the individual in hopes of increasing oral stimulation and decreasing the desire to consume regurgitated materials; and differential reinforcement, in which positive reinforcement is given for desired behaviors and interfering behaviors are ignored.

Avoidant/Restrictive Food Intake Disorder

Avoidant/Restrictive Food Intake Disorder (ARFID) is characterized by severe disturbances in eating or feeding resulting in at least one of the following: weight loss (or failure to gain weight, as seen in infants, children, and adolescents), nutritional deficiency, poor psychosocial functioning, and relying on tube feeding or oral supplements in an attempt to meet nutritional needs. Examples of eating disturbances might be the avoidance of or disinterest in food, or distress about the consequences of eating. Some individuals might avoid a specific food because of its smell, color, or texture. Infants can exhibit irritability or apathy, especially during feeding. Diagnostic criteria for ARFID also include that the eating behavior is not accepted as a component of the individual's cultural practices; and it is not a direct result of anorexia nervosa, bulimia nervosa, binge-eating disorder, other mental disorder or medical condition.

Prevalence

Avoidant/Restrictive Food Intake Disorder most commonly is seen in infants and children. Those who develop food avoidance or restriction in infancy or childhood could present similar or identical eating disturbances in adulthood.

History

Before the DSM-5, ARFID was previously referred to Feeding Disorder of Infancy and Early Childhood. This new category was devised in part to reduce the number of diagnoses of Eating Disorder Not Otherwise Specified (EDNOS), ultimately improving the prognosis of affected individuals.

Causes

- Developmental impairments
- History of abuse or neglect
- Family history of eating disorders
- History of gastrointestinal issues

Comorbidity

- Anxiety disorders
- Obsessive-compulsive disorders
- Attention deficit hyperactivity disorder
- Autism spectrum disorders

Medical Complications

- Malnutrition

- Growth problems
- Weight loss (or failure to gain weight, as seen in infants, children, and adolescents)

Treatment

Possible treatment for ARFID remains inconclusive, but exposure therapy and cognitive-behavioral therapy have been suggested as a means of targeting avoidance behaviors.

Nicole D. Teitelbaum

Research Issues

The Avoidant/Restrictive Food Intake Disorder (ARFID) classification grew out of a diagnosis known as "Feeding Disorder of Infancy and Early Childhood." Many infants, children, and adolescents have odd eating behaviors, and parents often have difficulty distinguishing between normal picky-eating and ARFID. To help understand how ARFID develops, reading case histories of people with this disorder can be helpful. An example is cited below, but you also might be able to find other descriptions by entering the term "Avoidant/Restrictive Food Intake Disorder" into a search engine.

Bryant-Waugh, R. (2013). Avoidant restrictive food intake disorder: An illustrative case example. *International Journal of Eating Disorders, 46*, 420–423. Retrieved from http://onlinelibrary.wiley.com/store/10.1002/eat.22093/asset/22093_ftp.pdf?v=1&t=hpphzx0v&s=182eefda4ef460e6a93156212152800 22e3a46ca

See Also: Eating disorders.

Further Reading

American Psychiatric Association. (2013*). Diagnostic and Statistic Manual of Mental Disorders* (5th ed.) (DSM-5). Arlington, VA: American Psychiatric Association.

Ferreri, S. J., Tamm, L., & Wier, K. G. (2006). Using food aversion to decrease severe pica by a child with autism. *Behavior Modification, 30*, 456–471.

Fredericks, D. W, Carr, J. E., & Williams, W. L. (1998). Overview of the treatment of rumination disorder for adults in a residential setting. *Journal of Behavior Therapy and Experimental Psychiatry, 29*, 31–40.

Kenney, L., Walsh, T. B. (2013). Avoidant/restrictive food intake disorder (ARFID) Defining ARFID. *Eating Disorders Review, 24* (3).

Young, S. L. (2011). *Craving earth: Understanding pica—the urge to eat clay, starch, ice, and chalk*. Chichester, NY: Columbia University Press.

Young, S. L., Wilson, M. J, Miller, D., & Hillier, S. (2008). Toward a comprehensive approach to the collection and analysis of pica substances, with emphasis on geophagic materials. *PLoS One 3* (9), e3147.

Zhao, Y. & Encinosa, W. (2011). *An update on hospitalizations for eating disorders, 1999 to 2009*. (HCUP Statistical Brief #120). Rockville, MD: Agency for Healthcare Research and Quality. http://www.hcup-us.ahrq.gov/reports/statbriefs/sb120.pdf

Female Athlete Triad

The female athlete triad (the triad) refers to a syndrome composed of three components: low energy availability (not consuming enough calories), disruption of the menstrual cycle, and low bone density. The triad typically begins when an athlete embarks on a weight-loss program to improve her sport performance, limiting calorie intake and increasing exercise volume. For athletes who develop the triad, these measures lead to disruption of the menstrual cycle, and in some cases to amenorrhea, or absence of the menstrual cycle. This disruption in turn causes very low levels of estrogen, the primary female sex hormone. Over time, low estrogen levels accompanied by an inadequate diet result in negative effects on bone growth and maintenance, and bone disorders such as stress fractures, low bone density, and osteoporosis. Girls and women who develop osteoporosis as part of the triad rarely achieve normal bone density, even with a good diet and medical treatment.

The term "female athlete triad" was first coined in 1992 by sports medicine researcher Barbara Drinkwater. She and her colleagues had observed symptoms of osteoporosis in several young female runners. Especially alarming were the presence of vertebral compression fractures, fractures of the spinal vertebral bones, which result in spinal curvature and pain and are difficult to treat. Upon examining these young runners, the researchers found an association between menstrual irregularity and bone density: fewer menstrual cycles per year was associated with reduced bone density. It should be noted, however, that the triad can develop in girls and women who do not consider themselves athletes, but instead exercise recreationally. The triad also can develop in females with eating disorders who might or might not exercise excessively.

Statistics on the prevalence of the triad do not exist, although a number of studies have estimated how frequently the individual components of the triad occur (Gottschlich, 2012). Testing of various groups of female athletes have found rates of osteoporosis to be anywhere from 0% to 13%, compared to about 2% for the general population of young women. Somewhere between 22% and 50% of athletes show lower bone-density scores, versus about 12% of nonathletes. Menstrual dysfunction shows up in anywhere from 6% to 79% of female athletes, depending upon the group studied. Disordered eating patterns have been demonstrated in large numbers of women, including athletes, with rates of up to 62%.

Insufficient calorie intake or calorie restriction, sometimes accompanied by extreme dieting behaviors, appear to be the precipitating factors for the triad. A mismatch between calorie intake and energy expenditure creates an energy deficit: athletes are burning more calories than they are eating. This mismatch is not always intentional. In some cases, athletes might simply fail to ingest a sufficient number of calories to meet the needs of their energy expenditure, even if their caloric intake is normal for a nonathlete of the same age. For example, a distance runner training at a high weekly mileage can burn hundreds of extra calories a day, and can fail to increase her intake to keep up with this level of energy expenditure. Other athletes practice some form of food restriction, intentionally eating less than they need to burn extra body fat. Some athletes might begin trying to burn extra fat with high levels of exercise training and food restriction, and go on to develop disordered eating and excessive exercise behaviors. Athletes participating in sports that emphasize or require a thin physique are most likely to develop the triad.

The body responds to energy deficits by suppressing the bodily functions necessary for growth and development, such as the menstrual cycle. Loss of the menstrual cycle and the resulting low estrogen levels lead to the skeletal problems observed with the female athlete triad. The most common problem observed in these athletes is a stress fracture—a small fracture that is caused by repetitive use. Low bone density, as measured by tests of bone mineral content, is seen in girls and women who have developed the triad. Maximum growth of bone mass occurs during puberty, especially between the ages of 11 and 14 in girls (Nazem, 2012). If an adolescent athlete develops the triad, she might never reach her potential optimal level of bone mass formation, and will begin adulthood with low bone density. (Although exercise is known to improve bone density in general, this is not the case for girls with amenorrhea, and the lack of estrogen interferes with the otherwise positive effects of exercise on bone development.)

Early identification of triad symptoms in young athletes is important so that long-term damage can be prevented. Education programs for coaches, parents, and athletes have been developed by sports medicine organizations to encourage awareness and early intervention when the triad symptoms of inadequate energy intake and menstrual disruption are suspected. Athletes experiencing repeated stress fractures should be assessed for osteoporosis and other triad symptoms. Treatment for athletes who have developed the triad consists of increasing calorie intake, decreasing exercise volume, and, in some cases, hormone therapy to treat low bone density. Many athletes, however, have difficulty reducing training schedules or altering their diets. In these cases, the triad is best managed with a team of experts that includes a mental health practitioner along with a physician and a dietician.

Allison M. Felix and Barbara A. Brehm

Research Issues

Is sport participation generally helpful or harmful to health? What factors influence the answer to this question? Low calorie intakes and energy deficits are more common in some sports than others. Research indicates that sports favoring low body weight (distance running, cheerleading, some forms of dance) or a thin appearance for aesthetic reasons (ballet, figure skating, diving, gymnastics) can create a drive for thinness. Other sports, including team sports such as soccer, ice hockey, and basketball, actually might be protective—if they favor strength and larger size. It is interesting to look at the female athlete triad in the context of the entire sports experience for young women.

See Also: Eating disorders; Osteoporosis.

Further Reading

Ducher, G., Turner, A. I., Kukuljan, S., Pantano, K. J., Carlson, J. L., Williams, N. I., & De Souza, M. J. (2011). Obstacles in the optimization of bone health outcomes in the female athlete triad. *Sports Medicine, 41* (7), 587–607. doi: 10.2165/11588770 -000000000-00000

Gibbs, J. C., Williams, N. I., Scheid, J. L., Toombs, R. J., & De Souza, M. (2011). The association of a high drive for thinness with energy deficiency and severe menstrual disturbances: Confirmation in a large population of exercising women. *International Journal of Sport Nutrition & Exercise Metabolism, 21* (4), 280–290. Retrieved from http:// journals.humankinetics.com/AcuCustom/SiteName/Documents/DocumentItem/02 _J3609_IJSNEM_Gibbs%20280-290.pdf

Gottschlich, L. M. (2012). Female athlete triad. Medscape Reference. WebMD. Retrieved from http://emedicine.medscape.com/article/89260-overview#aw2aab6b2b5

Loucks, A. B., Manore, M., Nattiv, A., Sanborn, C., Sundgot-Borgen, J., & Warren, M. (2007). American College of Sports Medicine position stand: The female athlete triad. *Medicine and Science in Sports and Exercise, 39* (10), 1867–1882. doi: 10.1249/ mss.0b013c318149f111

Nazem, T. G., & Ackerman, K. E. (2012). The female athlete triad. *Sports Health: A Multidisciplinary Approach, 4* (4), 302–311. doi: 10.1177/1941738112439685

Sangenis, P. & International Olympic Committee (IOC) (2009). *Medical Commission Position Stand on the Female Athlete Triad.* 1–46. Retrieved from http://www .femaleathletetriad.org/for-professionals/position-stands/

Fermentation and Fermented Foods

Fermentation is a metabolic process through which certain organisms, including yeast and some types of mold and bacteria, obtain energy. During fermentation, organisms break down a compound such as sugar into simpler molecules, capturing energy from the substance's chemical bonds in the process. Fermentation reactions are anaerobic, which means they do not require oxygen. People have used fermentation to produce foods and beverages since prehistoric times. Fermentation also is used to produce biofuels, medicines, and other substances, and used in sewage treatment. Foods produced with fermentation reactions include beer, wine, bread, yogurt, cheese, sauerkraut, and pepperoni. The food product produced by fermentation depends upon the initial food undergoing fermentation and the organism used to produce the fermentation process. Some fermented foods, such as fermented vegetables and dairy products, contain significant numbers of probiotics—microorganisms that live in the human gastrointestinal tract and contribute to good health.

Although people have used fermentation to produce food and beverages for thousands of years, scientific study of fermentation biochemistry developed in the

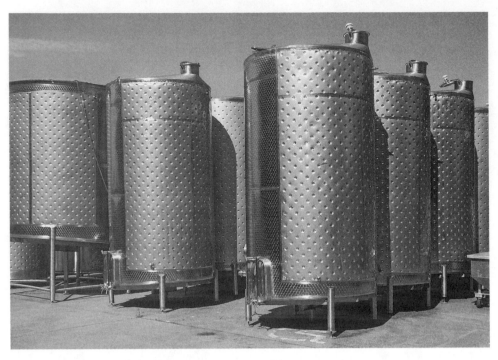

Wine is made from crushed fruit and other tasty ingredients. Yeast is added to the fruit mixture and is responsible for the fermentation process. The fermentation process may occur in stainless steel tanks, as pictured here, or in other containers such as wine barrels and bottles. (Dreamstime.com)

early 20th century. Eduard Buchner, a German biochemist, received the Nobel Prize for Chemistry in 1907 in recognition of his work demonstrating that fermentation results from the action of enzymes produced by yeast. French scientist Louis Pasteur also studied the action of yeast in the fermentation process. Sir Arthur Harden, a biochemist from Great Britain, further clarified the enzymes and chemical processes of fermentation, receiving the 1929 Nobel Prize in Chemistry for this work.

The two main types of fermentation processes used to produce food are ethanol fermentation and lactic acid fermentation. In ethanol fermentation, sugars are broken down for energy, creating ethanol and carbon dioxide in the process. Ethanol fermentation occurs in bacteria and fungi, especially yeast. Ethanol fermentation is used to produce wine, beer, and bread. The carbon dioxide released in ethanol fermentation is what makes bread rise. (The ethanol evaporates when the bread is baked.) In lactic acid fermentation, sugar breakdown by bacteria produces lactic acid. (Human muscle cells use the same process for generating energy at high levels of exercise intensity, a process known as anaerobic energy production.) Foods produced using lactic acid fermentation include cheese, yogurt, vinegar, and soy sauce.

What Is Miso?

"Miso" is a seasoning made from fermented grains and legumes. It most commonly is used to flavor soups, salad dressings, and sauces. Like other fermented food products, miso contains helpful microorganisms that are thought to aid digestion and contribute to other health benefits. In modern-day Japan, most of the population still continues the very old custom of beginning their day with a warm bowl of miso soup. Miso soup is believed to stimulate digestion and energize the body.

Although rice and barley are the primary grains used in making miso, other grains such as millet can be used. Yellow soybeans are the primary beans used, although black soybeans, azuki beans, and chickpeas often also are part of a batch of miso. Generally, a type of bean, a grain, salt, and a culture are the only ingredients needed to make miso. Some people include a small amount of sea vegetables in their recipe to aid in the digestibility of the finished product.

Miso making is a double-fermentation process. The first fermentation is growing a culture using grain. The grain is inoculated with the spores of the *aspergillus* mold. In this fermentation, the inoculated grain is transformed into "koji" as the culture transforms the starches of the grain into simple sugars and creates an abundance of digestive enzymes. The second fermentation begins when the beans, koji, and salt are mixed and placed in large vats for a period that can range from three weeks to three years or more. The result is a salty paste that essentially is darker and more savory the longer it ages.

Robin Cole

Fermentation is used around the world to produce alcoholic beverages and to preserve food. In eastern and southeastern Asian countries, cabbage, vegetables, and sometimes seafood are fermented to make products such as pickles and kimchi. Pork and beef are fermented in southern and central Europe to produce cured sausages, such as prosciutto and chorizo. In West Africa, cassava root is fermented to make gari, a type of flour. Wheat flour is fermented to produce naan and other types of bread in south Asian countries. People around the world enjoy yogurt beverages such as kefir and lassi.

Fermentation is used with many different types of plant and animal products. Dairy products are made into yogurt, cheese, kefir, and other cultured-milk products. Honey can be fermented into the beverage called "mead." Fermented tea produces a drink called "kombucha." Fermented fish produces fish sauce; meat is made into sausages; fruit and vegetables are made into pickled products; and grains are used to produce alcoholic beverages and breads. Grains and legumes, such as soybeans, can be fermented to produce miso, a flavoring paste used in soups and many other dishes. Fermented soybeans are made into natto and tempeh.

Fermented food can offer many benefits. Fermentation can help to preserve foods, increasing food availability and dietary variety for consumers. Because fermentation organisms help to break down starches and fibers, they improve a food's digestibility and reduce cooking time and cooking fuel use. Sometimes fermentation organisms increase nutrient content of a food. For example, the fermentation of some grains increases a food's content of amino acids and certain B vitamins. Fermentation can reduce the concentration of substances such as phytate that interfere with people's absorption of certain minerals, such as iron and calcium, in the digestive tract. In some cases fermentation can reduce the concentration of certain toxins in food. For example, cassava root, a basic food in the West African diet, exhibits lower total cyanide levels after fermentation.

Fermented foods contain a high concentration of probiotics and other microbiological content, for as fermentation organisms metabolize fuel substrates, they reproduce and thrive. Helpful intestinal bacteria and other microorganisms appear to improve the health of the gastrointestinal tract. They might have other health-promoting benefits as well, although research in this area still is preliminary.

Fermented foods tend to have high level of antioxidant activity. For example, a comparative study on garlic found that both fresh and aged garlic displayed strong antioxidant concentrations. Fermented black garlic, however, was discovered to have significantly higher phenolic content and antioxidant activity than fresh garlic (Kim, Nam, Rico, & Kang, 2012). In another study, kimchi demonstrated notably higher antioxidant activity compared to the same vegetables that did not undergo fermentation. The study concluded that fermentation helped to bring out antioxidant compounds in kimchi (Lee, Kim, Kang, Lim, Kim et al., 2010). Red wines fermented in oak barrels showed stronger concentrations of phenolic compounds after the 14 months of fermentation than before fermentation (Hernández, Estrella, Carlavilla, Martín-Álvarez, Moreno-Arribas, 2006).

Unfortunately, certain fermented foods have been associated with increased risk of esophageal and stomach cancers, particularly in countries where large amounts of pickled foods are consumed (WHO, 2013). It is possible that certain organisms used for fermentation, especially fungi, could be carcinogenic, although more research is needed to explain this association. Botulism is a toxic bacterium that thrives in an anaerobic environment, and has been found to occasionally contaminate fermented products, most notably fermented seafood products. Sanitary food production methods usually prevent contamination and food-borne illness from fermented foods.

Barbara A. Brehm and Breanna A. Lindo

See Also: Microbiota and microbiome; Prebiotics; Probiotics.

Further Reading

Haard, N. F., Odunfa, S. A., Lee, C.-H., Auintero-Ramirez, R., Lorence-Quinones, A., & Wacher-Radarte, C. (1999). Fermented cereals: A global perspective. *Food and Agriculture Organization of the United Nations.* Retrieved from http://www.fao.org /docrep/x2184e/x2184e00.htm#con

Helmenstine, A. M. (2013) *What is fermentation?* About.com Chemistry. Retrieved from http://chemistry.about.com/od/lecturenoteslab1/f/What-Is-Fermentation.htm

Hernández, T., Estrella, I., Carlavilla, D., Martín-Álvarez, P. J., & Moreno-Arribas, M. V. (2006). Phenolic compounds in red wine subjected to industrial malolactic fermentation and ageing on lees. *Analytica Chimica Acta, 563* (1–2), 116–125. doi:10.1016/j.aca.2005.10.061

Kim, J. H., Nam, S. H., Rico, C. W., & Kang, M. Y. (2012). A comparative study on the antioxidative and anti-allergic activities of fresh and aged black garlic extracts. *International Journal of Food Science & Technology, 47* (6), 1176–1182. doi:10.1111/j.1365-2621.2012.02957.x

Lee, B.-J., Kim, J.-S., Kang, Y. M., Lim, J.-H., Kim, Y.-M. et al. (2010). Antioxidant activity and γ-aminobutyric acid (GABA) content in sea tangle fermented by Lactobacillus brevis BJ20 isolated from traditional fermented foods. *Food Chemistry, 122* (1), 271–276. doi:10.1016/j.foodchem.2010.02.071

World Health Organization (WHO). (2013). *Agents classified by the IARC Monographs, Volumes 1–105*. International Agency for Research on Cancer. Retrieved from http://monographs.iarc.fr/ENG/Classification/ClassificationsAlphaOrder.pdf

Fetal Alcohol Syndrome and Disorders

Fetal Alcohol Syndrome (FAS) is an irreversible condition caused by heavy consumption of alcohol during pregnancy. This syndrome is marked by pre- and postnatal growth retardation, certain characteristic facial abnormalities, and central nervous system deficits, including problems with memory and impulse control. Fetal Alcohol Syndrome falls under a grouping of disorders known as "Fetal Alcohol Spectrum Disorders" (FASD). This term refers to a wide range of conditions that can develop in people exposed to alcohol during prenatal development, with FAS representing the most severe extreme of the spectrum. These conditions include both physical and psychological problems. Although there are certain trademark characteristics that can be seen in many children who exhibit FASD, symptoms range from mild to severe. Presently, there is no known cure, although treatments for physical, cognitive, and behavioral problems can be helpful. Controversy exists regarding how much alcohol consumption leads to FAS and FASD, and public health recommendations regarding alcohol consumption during pregnancy vary among organizations and from country to country.

The connection between maternal alcohol consumption and the occurrence of mental, behavioral, and learning disabilities in children has been noted by various physicians throughout history. In 1973, the term "Fetal Alcohol Syndrome" was coined by physicians Kenneth L. Jones and David W. Smith who described the "tell-tale" signs of alcohol exposure in infants at birth and in young children. Children of mothers who drank daily and heavily appeared to be at greatest risk. Further research over the years confirmed the notion that alcohol acts as a teratogen, causing birth defects in the fetuses of laboratory animals.

Symptoms

Symptoms of FASD include growth retardation, facial malformation, and central nervous system disorders. Growth retardation is characterized by a child or infant whose weight/length/height is less than the tenth percentile. Common facial malformations include a very thin upper lip, small eyes, a short upturned nose, and a smooth skin surface between the nose and upper lip. Central nervous system (primarily brain) abnormalities include attention deficits, increased activity, intelligence and learning deficits, sleep disturbances, and poor motor skills. Although it is possible for a child to meet many of these criteria at once, a child does not need to exhibit all of these abnormalities to be classified as affected with FASD. There also are less common, but significant symptoms of FAS such as heart defects, eye and ear problems, and deformities of limbs, joints, and fingers.

Some children show some symptoms of milder FAS-type symptoms. These cases previously were categorized as fetal alcohol effects (FAE). In 1996, the U.S. Institute of Medicine (IOM) replaced the ambiguous FAE diagnosis with new terms. Alcohol-related neurodevelopmental disorder (ARND) refers to people with problems of behavior and learning, and alcohol-related birth defects (ARBD) refer to physical abnormalities (CDC, 2013). It often is difficult to diagnose ARND, ARBD, and FASD, because symptoms can be common to many other disorders.

Because Fetal Alcohol Spectrum Disorders are irreversible, affected infants will grow to become affected adolescents and adults. As children, those with FASD could face poor impulse control, poor attention span, and irritability, among other symptoms. This can make school and other daily tasks more difficult for them than for a child without FASD. During adolescence, symptoms can escalate into anxiety, depression, and difficulty controlling emotions. Adults who suffer from many of the symptoms of FASD often face hardships due to poor judgment and poor social skills as a result of the condition. Even everyday tasks such as grocery shopping, keeping clean, using public transportation, and cooking meals can present huge challenges for adults with FASD. They often have difficulty finding and keeping jobs, thus requiring lifelong community support (NOFAS, n.d.).

Causation

When alcohol is consumed during pregnancy, it enters the mother's bloodstream and then reaches the bloodstream of the developing fetus by crossing the placenta. A fetus metabolizes alcohol much more slowly than an adult, and therefore the fetus will have a higher blood alcohol concentration than the mother. Researchers do not know exactly how alcohol exerts its teratogenic effects. It might interfere with the delivery of oxygen and nutrients to developing tissues and organs. The variation in symptoms of FASD could be explained at least partially by the timing of alcohol exposure, as the influence of alcohol on the many processes of fetal development could vary. The effect of heavy alcohol exposure could be especially strong during the first trimester of pregnancy, when cells are differentiating and forming the fetus's organs. This is unfortunate, because at this stage, many women do not yet know that they are pregnant.

What Level of Alcohol Intake Is Harmful?

Experts cannot say with certainty what level of alcohol intake during pregnancy is harmful. Researchers studying babies diagnosed with FAS often have been unable to ascertain degree of alcohol exposure in utero. Women might not accurately recall or report alcohol consumption during pregnancy, and heavy alcohol intake often occurs together with the use of other drugs, poor nutrition, and other factors that influence fetal development. Making the matter more complex is the fact that many babies born to mothers who drank heavily throughout pregnancy show no symptoms of FASD.

Because FAS is a serious and irreversible disorder, public health recommendations have generally erred on the side of caution, advising women to abstain from alcohol during pregnancy. In the United States, alcoholic beverages must carry a warning label stating, "According to the Surgeon General, women should not drink alcoholic beverages during pregnancy because of the risk of birth defects." Warning labels are also mandated in the United Kingdom, France, and Japan. In Canada, labeling regulations vary from province to province.

Evidence supporting such extreme caution is lacking. Recent well-designed epidemiological studies that have recorded how much alcohol women drink while pregnant (rather than asking women to remember what they drank months or years earlier) suggest that one or two drinks a day might not be harmful. Studies have examined not only alcohol consumption and FAS, but also alcohol consumption and milder symptoms such as behavioral problems and cognitive deficits of children at 3 years of age (Kelly, Sacker, Gray, Kelly, Wolke, & Quigley, 2008) and selective and sustained attention in 5-year-old children (Underbjerg et al., 2012). Nevertheless, most professional organizations continue to urge women to abstain or limit alcohol consumption during pregnancy.

Barbara A. Brehm and Kristen A. Estes

Research Issues

Public health authorities do not agree on how much alcohol is safe to consume during pregnancy. How can a woman decide what to do during her pregnancy? Although light drinking (a few drinks a week) appears to be relatively safe, might future research uncover as yet unidentified problems associated with even light alcohol consumption (Hanson, 2013)? How much risk is acceptable?

What should alcohol educators and medical professionals say to their pregnant patients? If public-health statements and health care providers contend that light drinking is probably safe, might some women take this to mean that any level of alcohol consumption is safe? Could these statements serve as a license to drink heavily? How would you counsel a friend who is wondering if she should drink during her pregnancy?

See Also: Alcohol.

Further Reading

Centers for Disease Control and Prevention (CDC). (2013). *Fetal alcohol spectrum disorders (FASDs)*. Retrieved from http://www.cdc.gov/ncbddd/fasd/index.html

Hanson, D. J. (2013). *Fetal Alcohol Syndrome*. Alcohol Problems and Solutions. Retrieved from http://www2.potsdam.edu/hansondj/FetalAlcoholSyndrome.html

Kelly, Y., Sacker, A., Gray, R., Kelly, J., Wolke, D. & Quigley, M. A. (2008). Light drinking in pregnancy, a risk for? *International Journal of Epidemiology, 38* (1), 129–140. doi: 10.1093/ije/dyn230

National Organization on Fetal Alcohol Syndrome (NOFAS). (2014, December 3). *Living with FASD*. Retrieved from http://www.nofas.org/living-with-fasd/

PubMed Health. (2013). *Fetal Alcohol Syndrome*. Retrieved from http://www.ncbi.nlm.nih.gov/pubmedhealth/PMH0001909/

Underbjerg, M., Kesmodel, U. S., Landro, N. I., Bakketeig, L., Grove, J. Wimberley T., Kilburn T. R., Sværke, C., Thorsen, P., & Mortensen, E. L. (2012). The effects of low to moderate alcohol consumption and binge drinking in early pregnancy on selective and sustained attention in 5-year-old children. *British Journal of Obstetrics and Gynaecology, 119* (10), 1211–1221. doi: 10.1111/j.1471-0528.2012.03396.x

Fiber

Fiber refers to the components of food that cannot be digested. Fiber can be found in whole grains, legumes, fruits and vegetables, and foods made from these ingredients. Dietary fiber is the fiber the body gets from the diet. Functional fiber refers to the fiber that is added to foods, as is done in many breakfast cereals, or fiber that is made into a dietary supplement. In the gastrointestinal (GI) tract, fiber increases feelings of fullness during meal consumption, delays gastric emptying, slows blood glucose absorption, and binds bile acids, which could help remove cholesterol (a major component of bile) from the body. Many types of fiber serve as prebiotics, providing food and a healthful environment for helpful microorganisms in the GI tract. An adequate fiber intake has been associated with many positive health effects, including the prevention of constipation, diverticulosis, and cardiovascular disease. A high fiber intake can result in bloating, however, from the fermentation of fiber in the large intestine, and also can cause constipation if an inadequate amount of water is consumed.

Cultures around the world and throughout time have noted the beneficial effects of high-fiber foods on GI function. In 430 BCE, for example, Hippocrates noted that coarse wheat produced bulkier stools than refined wheat (Slavin, 2013). In the United States in the 1920s, physician J. H. Kellogg and other entrepreneurs promoted the use of wheat fiber as a cure to multiple health—and even social—problems. Scientific interest in the health benefits of dietary fiber grew in the 1950s as Irish missionary surgeon Denis Burkitt published his observations that GI diseases common in Western countries were rare in most African groups. He attributed these differences to diet fiber content (Slavin, 2013). Although not all of Burkitt's ideas have withstood the test of time, his work stimulated increased research into the health effects of dietary fiber.

Types of Fiber

Dietary fiber comes primarily from plants. Most types of dietary fiber, such as cellulose, are composed of carbohydrates. Humans lack the necessary digestive enzymes for breaking down these structures, so they pass through the digestive system, adding bulk to the stools. There are many kinds of dietary fiber. Dietary fibers are classified as water soluble and water insoluble, and both groups have beneficial effects on health.

In general, water-soluble fiber attracts water and forms a gel-like mix in the digestive system. This mixture slows stomach emptying, helping a person to feel full longer. Delayed stomach emptying also means that glucose is absorbed from the digestive mass more slowly, thus preventing a rapid rise in blood glucose. A rapid rise in blood glucose can lead to high blood insulin levels. Water-soluble fiber tends to bind bile acids found in the small intestine. Bile acids are high in cholesterol. When the bile acids are bound to the fibrous mixture, their cholesterol is not available for reabsorption; thus, soluble fiber appears to be beneficial for people trying to reduce blood cholesterol levels. Water-insoluble fiber provides bulk to the feces and speeds its passage through the GI tract. Water-insoluble fiber reduces risk of constipation. It should be noted that the functions of water-soluble and water-insoluble fibers as described above often overlap. Psyllium fiber, for example, is primarily water soluble, yet still increases stool bulk. Some of the most common types of fiber in the diet include the following (Insel et al., 2014).

- Cellulose—Cellulose is composed of long, straight chains of glucose molecules. It is a component of the fibrous structures of plants and is found in fruits, vegetables, grains, and nuts.
- Hemicelluloses—Hemicelluloses generally are mixed with celluloses in plant structures and consist of monosaccharides with branching side chains. They are found in wheat bran, legumes, nuts, and vegetables.
- Lignins—Lignins contribute to the tough, fibrous portions of vegetables such as carrots. Unlike other dietary fibers, lignans are not carbohydrates.
- Pectins—Pectins are water-soluble, gel-forming carbohydrates found in all plants, especially fruits. Pectin is used to give texture to jellies and other food products.
- Gums and mucilages—These water-soluble fibers are found in most plants and are used in food products to improve texture and to thicken. The husk of the psyllium seed, known as "psyllium," is a mucilage and the primary component of many laxative products.

- Beta-glucans—This carbohydrate, water-soluble fiber is found in oats and barley and has been found to help lower blood cholesterol levels in some studies.
- Chitan and chitosan—These fibers are extracted from the shells of crabs and lobsters and sold as dietary supplements. They are marketed as being effective for weight loss, but evidence to support this claim is lacking.
- Inulin, oligofructose, and other oligosaccharides—These carbohydrates are found in many plants and resist digestion in the human GI tract, but serve as prebiotics for helpful microorganisms. They are smaller structures than the polysaccharide structures such as cellulose.

Adequate Intake of Fiber

Currently, adults in the United States consume only half of the recommended amount of fiber. The recommended adequate intake (AI) value for fiber is 14 g dietary fiber per 1,000 kcals, or for men ages 19 to 50, 38 grams per day; the value for men age 50 and older is 30 grams per day (Slavin, 2008). For women

Table 1. Examples of Foods That Have Fiber

Food	Amount of Fiber
½ cup of beans (navy, pinto, kidney), cooked	6.2–9.6 grams
½ cup of shredded wheat, ready-to-eat cereal	2.7–3.8 grams
⅓ cup of 100% bran, ready-to-eat cereal	9.1 grams
1 small oat bran muffin	3.0 grams
1 whole-wheat English muffin	4.4 grams
1 small apple, with skin	3.6 grams
1 medium pear, with skin	5.5 grams
½ cup of raspberries	4.0 grams
½ cup of stewed prunes	3.8 grams
½ cup of winter squash, cooked	2.9 grams
1 medium sweet potato, baked in skin	3.8 grams
½ cup of green peas, cooked	3.5–4.4 grams
1 small potato, baked, with skin	3.0 grams
½ cup of mixed vegetables, cooked	4.0 grams
½ cup of broccoli, cooked	2.6–2.8 grams
½ cup of greens (spinach, collards, turnip greens), cooked	2.5–3.5 grams

The recommended adequate intake value for fiber is 14 grams of dietary fiber per 1,000 kcals, or for men ages 19 to 50, 38 grams per day; the value for men age 50 and older is 30 grams per day. For women ages 19 to 50, the AI value is 25 grams per day, and for women age 50 and older it is 21 grams per day.

Source: U.S. Department of Agriculture and U.S. Department of Health and Human Services, *Dietary Guidelines for Americans,* 2010.

ages 19 to 50, the AI value is 25 grams per day, and for women age 50 and older it is 21 grams per day. (Older adults continue to need adequate fiber, but recommendations are lower because older adults need fewer calories to maintain their current weight.) Most dietary guidelines encourage people to consume adequate amounts of vegetables, fruits, legumes, and whole grains to promote a healthy intake of dietary fiber. See the table for a representative group of high-fiber foods.

As is the case for most dietary components, too much fiber, especially in the form of fiber supplements or concentrated sources of fiber such as wheat bran, can be problematic, causing diarrhea and intestinal discomfort. People trying to increase their fiber intake are advised to do so gradually so that their bodies have time to adjust to the new levels.

Health Benefits of Adequate Fiber Intake

Constipation refers to the production of hard, dry, and infrequent stool that is difficult to eliminate from the body. Fiber helps to prevent and treat constipation because it increases fecal bulk and helps waste pass more quickly through the gastrointestinal tract. Water-soluble fiber draws water into the fecal mass; thus, an adequate fluid intake is also important for the prevention and treatment of constipation.

Diverticulosis is a condition that occurs when pouches form along the walls of the colon. Low-fiber diets are associated with diverticulosis. Constipation is thought to contribute to diverticulosis as the muscles along the gastrointestinal tract become strained from pushing the hard stools, which increases the pressure on the colon and causes pouches to form. Conversely, diets rich in fiber allow for the easy passage and removal of the stools, which puts less pressure on the walls of the colon. Similarly, constipation increases risk for the development of hemorrhoids, a condition in which swollen and inflamed veins bulge into the rectum and anus. Straining during elimination is thought to worsen this condition.

Obesity is the condition of having excess body fat that often is a precursor to several negative health effects. The relationship between fiber intake and obesity is complex. Although dietary fiber intake is associated with lower risk of obesity, people with high-fiber diets often have diets that are more healthful in other ways. They also might exercise more. Nevertheless, high-fiber diets are thought to help reduce the chances of becoming overweight and to promote weight loss. Foods rich in soluble fiber make the body feel full because they take longer than other food sources to move from the stomach to the small intestine. Soluble fiber also attracts water molecules, which adds to the feeling of being sated. Along with giving the body a feeling of fullness, these fiber-rich foods often are low in calories and fats, making the body feel full and at the same time, allowing for a lower-calorie diet.

Type 2 diabetes occurs when the cells in the body become resistant to insulin, causing high blood glucose levels. Diets high in fiber are recommended for people with type 2 diabetes for two reasons. Fiber does not increase blood glucose levels because most of it cannot be digested. The second reason is that research has shown that certain fibers slow the release of glucose from the digestive mass into the bloodstream.

The leading cause of cardiovascular disease is artery disease, in which the lining of the arteries becomes thickened by the presence of plaque. High levels of LDL-cholesterol increase the risk of artery disease. Experiments have shown that increasing fiber intake reduces blood LDL-cholesterol; and people who have high-fiber diets are less likely to develop artery disease than people with low-fiber diets. The body uses cholesterol to make bile, and because high intakes of fiber can bind with bile, removing it from the body in the feces, the body can take excess cholesterol from the blood to make more bile, reducing the overall amount of cholesterol in the bloodstream.

Healthful populations of microbiota in the gastrointestinal tract are associated with better health, including the reduced risk of infectious diarrhea, inflammatory bowel conditions, and even certain types of cancer. The relationship between dietary fiber and colorectal cancer is currently unclear, as short-term studies have failed to find a relationship.

Fiber Supplements

Most fiber supplements contain only soluble fiber because they can be dissolved in water, although some supplements contain a mixture of both soluble and insoluble fiber. Although fiber supplements should not be used to replace dietary fiber, they could be effective in lowering low-density lipoprotein (LDL) levels and blood glucose levels. Psyllium is one of the most popular fiber supplements. Because soluble fiber slows down digestion, fiber supplements can increase the amount of time it takes the body to absorb certain medications. It is recommended that medications and fiber supplements be taken at least one hour apart.

Julie M. Voorhes and Barbara A. Brehm

See Also: Cardiovascular disease and nutrition; Cholesterol; Diverticular disease; Glycemic index and glycemic load; Grains; Large intestine; Lipoproteins; The liver; Microbiota and microbiome; Prebiotics; Probiotics.

Further Reading

Insel, P., Ross, D., McMahon, K., & Bernstein, M. (2014). *Nutrition* (4th ed.). Burlington, MA: Jones & Bartlett Learning.

Slavin, J. (2013). Fiber and prebiotics: Mechanisms and health benefits. *Nutrients, 5* (4), 1417–1435. doi: 10.3390/nu5041417

Slavin, J. L. (2008). Position of the American Dietetic Association: Health implications of dietary fiber. *Journal of the American Dietetic Association, 108* (10), 1716–1731.

Vorvick, L. J. (2012, Aug 14). *Fiber*. MedlinePlus. Retrieved from http://www.nlm.nih .gov/medlineplus/ency/article/002470.htm

Fluoride

Fluoride is a naturally occurring mineral made from the element fluorine, which is the seventeenth most abundant element in the earth's crust. Fluorine is never naturally found in a free state. It only is encountered in combinations with other elements as a fluoride compound. The fluoride ion is found in all water sources including the oceans. Since its discovery, elemental fluorine has been used in a multitude of ways, primarily in the form of fluoride compounds which are used in the dental industry and for the purpose of public health. Although fluoride is not an essential nutrient and is not necessary for biological functioning, its effect in the body can have both positive and negative impacts on the health of an individual.

Discovery and Use of Fluoride

Karl W. Scheele was the first to identify the element fluorine in 1771. More than a century later, fluorine was first isolated by the French chemist F. Henri Moissan, who subsequently was awarded the Nobel Prize for Chemistry in 1906

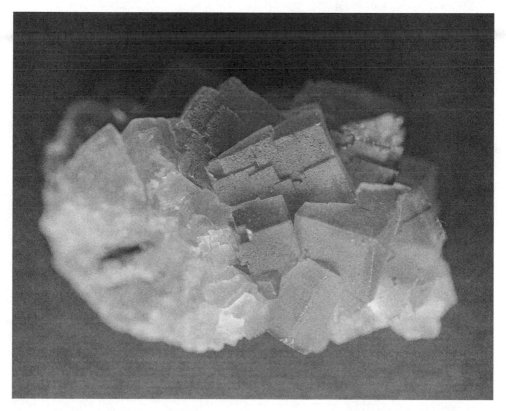

Fluorite is the mineral form of calcium fluoride. It is used to make the forms of fluoride found in toothpaste and other dental care products. (Catalina Zaharescu Tiensuu/Dreamstime.com)

Dental Fluorosis in Children

The U.S. Centers for Disease Control and Prevention offer the following advice on preventing dental fluorosis in babies and young children.

What Is Dental Fluorosis?

Dental fluorosis is a change in the appearance of the tooth's enamel. These changes can vary from barely noticeable white spots in mild forms to staining and pitting in the more severe forms. Dental fluorosis only occurs when younger children consume too much fluoride—from any source—over long periods when teeth are developing under the gums.

Who Develops Dental Fluorosis?

Only children ages 8 years old and younger can develop dental fluorosis, because this is when permanent teeth are developing under the gums. The teeth of children older than 8 years, adolescents, and adults cannot develop dental fluorosis.

What Does Dental Fluorosis Look Like?

- Very mild and mild forms of dental fluorosis—Teeth have scattered white flecks, some white spots; "frosty" edges; or fine, lacy chalk-like lines. These changes are barely noticeable and are difficult to see except by a dental health care professional.
- Moderate and severe forms of dental fluorosis—Teeth have larger white spots and—in the rare severe form—rough, pitted surfaces.

Common sources of fluoride include the following.

- Toothpaste (if swallowed by young children)
- Drinking water in communities which fluoridate municipal sources
- Beverages and food processed with fluoridated water
- Dietary prescription supplements that include fluoride (e.g., tablets, drops)
- Other professional dental products (e.g., mouth rinses, gels, foams)

In the United States, water and processed beverages (e.g., soft drinks, fruit juices) can provide approximately 75% of a person's fluoride intake. Inadvertent swallowing of toothpaste and the inappropriate use of other dental products containing fluoride can result in greater intake than desired. For this reason the CDC recommends that parents supervise the use of fluoride toothpaste by children younger than 6 years of age to encourage them to spit out excess toothpaste. Children younger than 6 years old should not use fluoride mouth rinses because the mouth rinse could be repeatedly swallowed.

Centers for Disease Control and Prevention (CDC). (2013). *Dental fluorosis*. Retrieved from http://www.cdc.gov/fluoridation/faqs/dental_fluorosis/index.htm

(Dicciani, 2003). Varying forms of fluorochemicals have been used widely throughout history, most notably in health care. Fluorocarbons were used heavily in the refrigeration and air conditioning industries, as well as in fire extinguishers. Fluoropolymers and fluoroelastomers are used in the construction of homes, buildings, motor vehicles, and in aerospace for the purpose of thermal, flame, chemical, and solvent resistance. One out of every five active pharmaceutical products is fluorinated, and fluorocarbons are used in synthetic blood substitutes and inhalation drug-delivery systems. The use of fluoride compounds for the prevention of tooth decay first was recognized by dental scientists in the 1930s and continues to this day (Centers for Disease Control, 2013). In the past, fluorine was used in the clinical setting to treat patients with hyperthyroidism (Galletti & Joyet, 1958).

Physiological Effect of Fluoride

Fluoride is absorbed systemically by the stomach and small intestine. In the bloodstream, fluoride enters mineralized tissues such as bones and developing teeth. It reacts with hydroxyapatite crystals in mineralized tissue, forming fluoroapatite, which hardens tooth enamel and bone mineral.

Although most food sources contain low levels of fluoride, there are several foods that are fluoride rich. These include marine fish that are consumed along with their bones and foods made with mechanically separated chicken. Elevated concentrations of fluoride are found in tea leaves, fruit juice, bottled water, and packaged food products made using fluoridated water.

An inadequate intake of fluoride can potentially lead to an increase in dental caries (cavities). Although there currently is little data to suggest the need for a Recommended Dietary Allowance (RDA), the Food and Nutrition Board (FNB) of the U.S. Institute of Medicine has established an Adequate Intake (AI) level based upon the desire to reduce dental caries effectively without creating the unwanted side effects associated with fluoride overexposure. The daily AI is 4.0 mg/day for adult men and 3.0 mg/day for adult women.

The effort to decrease dental caries has led to an increase in the use of fluoride in many consumable products. The use of fluoride to prevent tooth decay exists in topical and systemic forms. Topical fluorides strengthen existing teeth and prevent acid-producing bacteria from causing caries. Topical fluorides include toothpaste, mouthwash, and professional fluoride treatments performed in a dentist's office.

Systemic fluorides are ingested and absorbed by the body to become incorporated into developing tooth structures. Systemic fluorides give topical protection through their presence in saliva, which continually bathes the teeth and gives protection. Systemic fluorides are delivered through water fluoridation or dietary fluoride supplements such as tablets, drops, or lozenges. Through its interactions with calcium and phosphate, fluoride enhances the remineralization of tooth enamel that can be demineralized by acid-producing bacteria. Remineralized enamel is more resistant to bacterial acid and prevents further demineralization that might otherwise lead to dental caries.

The effects of fluoride absorption, however, can be harmful as well as helpful. Consuming fluoride in excessive amounts leads to acute fluoride poisoning, which is particularly dangerous for children. Signs of fluoride toxicity include abdominal pain, nausea, and vomiting. Over long periods, overexposure to fluoride can lead to changes in bone structure known as skeletal fluorosis. The most severe form, "crippling skeletal fluorosis," also negatively affects ligaments and leads to muscle wasting, immobility, and neurological problems. A related problem of excessive fluoride use, though less severe, is dental fluorosis. The presentation of dental fluorosis can range anywhere from white spots on the enamel of teeth to marked staining and pitting, which causes serious cosmetic concerns. The increase in the use of fluoride in consumer products has led to an increased incidence of dental fluorosis over the past decades. According to a 1999–2004 U.S. national survey, 23% of people ages 6 to 49 years had some degree of dental fluorosis (Higdon & Delage, 2013).

Water Fluoridation

Although the use of fluoride spans many facets of life, significant controversy exists over the addition of fluoride to the public water supply. According to the Centers for Disease Control and Prevention, community water fluoridation is a safe, effective, and inexpensive way of delivering the benefits of fluoride to residents of a community. Fluoridating the public water supply allows all members of a community to benefit from the treatment, regardless of age, income, education, or socioeconomic status. The reduction in social barriers affords those with limited access to dental care the opportunity to reduce their risk of dental carries at no cost. Water fluoridation has been subject to public opposition and, in some instances, has been discontinued. In addition to concerns about the harmful effects of fluoride toxicity, many individuals and organizations oppose water fluoridation on the premise that the public is being medicated without consent (Fluoride Action Network, 2012). Nevertheless, studies have shown that over the course of a person's lifetime water fluoridation reduces tooth decay by about 25% (Centers for Disease Control, 2013).

Fluoride Supplements for Children

If children are living in an area without community water fluoridation, or they are at increased risk of developing tooth decay, then daily fluoride supplementation is recommended. The benefit of fluoride supplementation for at-risk children is to give them the protection against dental caries that they might not otherwise have due to location or socioeconomic status. Dentists and physicians, however, must use caution when prescribing fluoride supplements to children to avoid the negative effects of overexposure. Careful attention is required to ensure that a child is not consuming fluoride from other sources, such as bottled water or foods that are rich in fluoride. Misjudging a child's consumption of fluoride when prescribing supplementation could lead to dental fluorosis and other negative side effects. Due to the need for a child to take these supplements for an extended period, fluoride supplementation is less cost effective than community water fluoridation (American Dental Association, 2014).

Timothy Potter

Research Issues

Infants and young children are at the highest risk for consuming too much fluoride. During the first 4 to 6 months of life, infants consume breast milk and infant formula almost exclusively. Infant formula contains fluoride, to ensure that infants meet their adequate intake levels for this nutrient. Formula comes in three forms—ready-to-serve liquid, powder, and concentrated liquids. The powder and concentrated liquid forms must be mixed with water. If the water used in mixing the formula is high in fluoride, then over time an infant's fluoride intake can be too high. People using infant formula should check with their pediatricians to be sure that infant fluoride intake is optimal.

Centers for Disease Control and Prevention (CDC). (2013). *Overview: Infant formula and fluorosis.* Retrieved from http://www.cdc.gov/fluoridation/safety/infant_formula.htm

See Also: Dental caries (cavities).

Further Reading

American Dental Association. (2014, December 4). *Fluoride Supplements: Facts about fluoride.* Retrieved from http://www.ada.org/2684.aspx

Centers for Disease Control (2013, July 25). *Fluoridation basics.* Retrieved from http://www.cdc.gov/fluoridation/basics/

Dicciani, N. (2003). *Fluorine.* American Chemical Society. Retrieved from http://pubs.acs.org/cen/80th/fluorine.html

Fluoride Action Network. (2012). *Water fluoridation.* Retrieved from http://fluoridealert.org/issues/water/

Galletti, P.-M. & Joyet, G. (1958). Effect of fluorine on thyroidal iodine metabolism in hyperthyroidism. *Journal of Clinical Endocrinology & Metabolism,* 18 (10).

Higdon, J., & Delage, B. (2014). *Fluoride.* Oregon State University, Linus Pauling Institute. Retrieved from http://lpi.oregonstate.edu/infocenter/minerals/fluoride/

Folate and Folic Acid

Folate is a B vitamin. It is one of several compounds that the body converts to a family of coenzymes called "tetrahydrofolic acid." Folic acid is a similar compound. Folate and folic acid are also known as vitamin B9. Like all vitamins, folate is an organic compound that is necessary for normal growth, development, and maintenance of basic functions in the body. Folate is water soluble, which means that the body does not store it, so it must be consumed regularly. The terms folate and folic acid are often used interchangeably, but folate specifically refers to the form of the vitamin found naturally in food, whereas folic acid is its synthetic form. Folic acid is absorbed by the body more readily than folate because its structure is simpler.

Folate plays an important role in DNA and RNA production and maintenance in cells; it is particularly important for the synthesis of red blood cells. Consuming folate is essential for the human body to maintain proper cell development, but it is especially important for women of child-bearing age. Adequate folate intake significantly reduces the risk of neural tube birth defects (e.g., spina bifida, anencephaly). An embryo's neural tube closes within the first 28 days of pregnancy, which is before a woman might know she is pregnant; therefore, women should have adequate folate in their diets not only while pregnant, but also before they become pregnant. Folate could play a role in preventing other diseases, such as certain forms of cancer and cardiovascular disease, but further research is necessary to make any significant claims about these effects.

History

In the early 1930s, folate was identified as a substance found in green, leafy vegetables that helped prevent anemia during pregnancy. It is named after the Latin word for leaf, "folium," which is the same root for the English word "foliage." The connection between inadequate folate intake and neural tube birth defects was hypothesized in the 1960s and confirmed by the early 1990s through several randomized research studies. By 1992, the U.S. Public Health Service recommended that all women of child-bearing age consume 400 micrograms (mcg) of folic acid per day (U.S. Department of Agriculture and U.S. Department of Health and Human Services, 2014). By 1998, both the United States and Canada mandated that grain products, such as breads, pastas, and cereals, be fortified with folic acid. Since 1998, the average daily intake folic acid has increased by about 200 mcg per day, and neural tube defects in infants have decreased substantially, by about 36% in the United States and 46% in Canada (CDC, 2013).

Physiological Functions and Deficiency Symptoms

Folate, like all B vitamins, is a coenzyme (coenzymes help enzymes function). As a coenzyme, folate supplies and accepts single carbon compounds. This enables DNA to form. Folate also helps metabolize amino acids into derivative forms. Folate is critical for proper cell division throughout the body; without folate, new cells cannot divide because they cannot form new DNA. Red blood cells are particularly affected. If someone is deficient in folate, then red blood cells have enough protein to synthesize new cell parts, but they do not have enough DNA to form a second nucleus. The result is called a megaloblast, which is a large, immature cell. These cells cannot carry oxygen like mature red blood cells, and this results in anemia.

Anemia is the primary indicator of folate deficiency, but other symptoms include fatigue, depression, tongue inflammation, hair loss, diarrhea, mental confusion, nerve dysfunction, and cognitive problems. Individuals who are more prone to folate deficiency include those who consume large amounts of alcohol, as alcohol inhibits the absorption of folate. People with celiac disease, irritable bowel syndrome, or other disorders that limit the body's ability to absorb nutrients also have an increased risk of folate deficiency.

Folate deficiency in pregnant women can lead to neural tube defects in the developing brain and spinal cord of the embryo, such as spina bifida (when the vertebrae do not form properly around the spinal cord) and anencephaly (when part or all of the brain is missing). Babies born with spina bifida can exhibit paralysis, learning disabilities, and other complications. Those born with anencephaly die shortly after birth. Researchers recommend that women of child-bearing age consume 400 mcg of folic acid per day.

Some studies have found a link between reduced intake of folic acid and increased rates of some kinds of cancers. Other studies have found that people who had higher folic acid intake have a reduced risk for cancers of the colon, breast, ovaries, pancreas, stomach, and esophagus. Other studies suggest that the effect of folic acid on cancer growth depends on when the folic acid is ingested. For example, because folic acid promotes cell division, taking folic acid could be harmful if cancerous or precancerous cells already are present (American Cancer Society, 2011). Some chemotherapy agents block the action of folic acid to limit cell replication in rapidly dividing cells, such as cancer cells. Until clearer evidence becomes available, the American Cancer Society recommends eating a varied diet, limiting alcohol consumption, and only taking a folic acid supplement when it is recommended by a doctor.

Food Sources and Supplements

Food sources of folate include dark, leafy greens such as spinach, lettuce, and broccoli; orange juice, melons, and bananas; legumes, mushrooms, and asparagus; and organ meats such as liver and kidney (*see* Table 1). Cooking and processing can destroy 50% to 90% of folate in food, thus the highest levels of folate are found in raw or lightly cooked (in minimal water) vegetables and fruits. Folic acid is more durable than folate and is used to fortify many grain-based foods, including cereals, breads, and pastas. Folic acid also can be consumed in the form of a supplement; it often is included in multivitamins. The Dietary Reference Intake (DRI) for folate for both male and female adults is 400 mcg per day; for pregnant women, the DRI is 600 mcg per day; and for lactating women is 500 mcg per day.

Tolerable Upper Intake Level

Folate from food sources can be absorbed by the body only in limited amounts, therefore there is no Tolerable Upper Intake Level (UL) for folate. Folic acid (from supplements or fortified foods), however, should not be consumed above the UL unless under the supervision of a doctor. The UL for folic acid is 1,000 mcg per day for adult males and females, as well as for pregnant and lactating women.

Excess folic acid can interact with some drugs, such as those used to treat some cancers (including methotrexate), epilepsy, and ulcerative colitis (National Institutes of Health, Office of Dietary Supplements, 2012). Additionally, folic acid

Table 1. Selected Food Sources of Folate and Folic Acid

Food	mcg DFE per serving	Percent DV*
Beef liver, braised, 3 ounces	215	54
Spinach, boiled, ½ cup	131	33
Black-eyed peas (cowpeas), boiled, ½ cup	105	26
Breakfast cereals, fortified with 25% of the DV†	100	25
Rice, white, medium-grain, cooked, ½ cup†	90	23
Asparagus, boiled, 4 spears	89	22
Spaghetti, cooked, enriched, ½ cup†	83	21
Brussels sprouts, frozen, boiled, ½ cup	78	20
Lettuce, romaine, shredded, 1 cup	64	16
Avocado, raw, sliced, ½ cup	59	15
Spinach, raw, 1 cup	58	15
Broccoli, chopped, frozen, cooked, ½ cup	52	13
Mustard greens, chopped, frozen, boiled, ½ cup	52	13
Green peas, frozen, boiled, ½ cup	47	12
Kidney beans, canned, ½ cup	46	12
Bread, white, 1 slice†	43	11
Peanuts, dry roasted, 1 ounce	41	10
Wheat germ, 2 tablespoons	40	10
Tomato juice, canned, ¾ cup	36	9
Crab, Dungeness, 3 ounces	36	9
Orange juice, ¾ cup	35	9
Turnip greens, frozen, boiled, ½ cup	32	8
Orange, fresh, 1 small	29	7
Papaya, raw, cubed, ½ cup	27	7
Banana, 1 medium	24	6
Yeast, baker's, ¼ teaspoon	23	6
Egg, whole, hard-boiled, 1 large	22	6
Vegetarian baked beans, canned, ½ cup	15	4
Cantaloupe, raw, 1 wedge	14	4
Fish, halibut, cooked, 3 ounces	12	3
Milk, 1% fat, 1 cup	12	3
Ground beef, 85% lean, cooked, 3 ounces	7	2
Chicken breast, roasted, ½ breast	3	1

Notes: * DV = Daily Value. The FDA developed DVs to help consumers compare the nutrient contents of products within the context of a total diet. The DV for folate is 400 mcg for adults and children aged 4 and older. The FDA, however, does not require food labels to list folate content unless a food has been fortified with this nutrient. Foods providing 20% or more of the DV are considered to be high sources of a nutrient.

† Fortified with folic acid as part of the folate fortification program.

The U.S. Department of Agriculture's Nutrient Database website lists the nutrient content of many foods and provides a comprehensive list of foods containing folate arranged by nutrient content and by food name. U.S. Department of Agriculture Agricultural Research Service. (2012). USDA National Nutrient Database for Standard Reference, Release 25.

Source: National Institutes of Health Office of Dietary Supplements. (2012). *Dietary Supplement Fact Sheet.* Table 2. Selected Food Sources of Folate and Folic Acid. Retrieved from http://ods.od.nih.gov/factsheets/Folate-HealthProfessional/

can mask the symptoms of other vitamin B deficiencies such as a deficiency in vitamin B12. Vitamin B12 deficiencies can be harmful to the central nervous system and also can cause megaloblastic anemia, especially in older individuals.

Megan L. Norton and Lisa P. Ritchie

See Also: Megaloblastic anemia; Pregnancy and nutrition; Vitamins.

Further Reading

American Cancer Society. (2011). *Herbs, vitamins and minerals: Folic acid.* Retrieved from http://www.cancer.org/treatment/treatmentsandsideeffects/complementaryanda lternativemedicine/herbsvitaminsandminerals/folic-acid?sitearea=ETO

Centers for Disease Control and Prevention (CDC). (2013). *Folic acid: Birth defects COUNT.* Retrieved from http://www.cdc.gov/ncbddd/birthdefectscount/data.html

National Council on Folic Acid. (2013). Folic acid resources. *Folic Acid News.* Retrieved from http://www.folicacidinfo.org/index.php

National Institutes of Health, Office of Dietary Supplements. (2012, December 14). *Folate: Dietary supplement fact sheet.* Retrieved from http://ods.od.nih.gov/factsheets /Folate-HealthProfessional/

U.S. Department of Agriculture and U.S. Department of Health and Human Services. *Dietary guidelines for Americans, 2010* (7th ed.). (2014, December 4). Retrieved from http://www.health.gov/dietaryguidelines/dga2010/dietaryguidelines2010.pdf

Wolff, T. (2010). *Folic acid fact sheet.* Retrieved from http://womenshealth.gov /publications/our-publications/fact-sheet/folic-acid.html

Food Addiction

Food addiction refers to compulsive overeating and an obsessive relationship with food. Researchers who have studied food addiction think that people who say they are addicted to food might respond to certain foods in a fashion that physiologically and psychologically is similar to the response of people to addictive drugs, such as heroin and cocaine. Indeed, research suggests that people addicted to food meet the diagnostic criteria for substance dependence. Additionally, the behaviors associated with food addiction fit the criteria for other behavioral addictions, such as gambling. Although not yet recognized as a psychological disorder with an official diagnostic criteria, food addiction could contribute to binge-eating disorder, a recognized clinical diagnosis, although not everyone addicted to overeating develops binge-eating disorder (American Psychological Association, 2013).

Addiction refers to the compulsive use of a substance or performance of an activity even though the person experiencing the addiction knows it is causing or is likely to cause harm. Addiction also is characterized by a loss of control over the substance use or behavior. Addiction to both substances and behaviors involves activation of the brain's reward pathways. With addiction, the use of the substance or performance of the problem behavior also can change these reward pathways over time in ways that lead to tolerance (needing more of the substance/behavior to achieve a pleasurable feeling), craving (strong desires to use the substance/perform the behavior), and withdrawal symptoms (symptoms such as pain, irritability, restlessness, and difficulty sleeping) which develop when a person does not access the addictive substance or behavior.

People who describe themselves as addicted to food often experience significant distress regarding their lack of control over their food intake. This lack of control manifests in behaviors such as continuing to eat even though full and even though one wishes to not overeat. People addicted to food report emotional health problems such as anxiety, depression, and low self-esteem. They might feel sad or ashamed about eating or about their body weight, and report high levels of emotional overeating (overeating in response to negative emotions such as sadness, anger, or boredom). People with food addiction often say that they prefer to eat in private, avoiding social interactions because of eating behaviors and weight. People experiencing food addiction are more likely than others to develop obesity and obesity-related health disorders.

The Neurochemistry of Food Addiction

Scientists studying the brain's chemical response to foods have found a parallel between its response to food and to drugs. One of the most studied neurological pathways in research on food addiction is that of dopamine. Dopamine is a neurotransmitter—a chemical that sends messages from one nerve cell to another. Dopamine and its effects motivate people to eat as well as to engage in other "rewarding" behaviors, such as sex. Dopamine is known as the chemical that creates "wanting" and is essential for survival. Animals that lack dopamine, for example, starve to death because they have no motivation to eat.

Scientists have found that very obese people have lower levels of dopamine in the reward center of the brain as compared to people of normal weight. This is the same thing that occurs in cocaine addicts, alcoholics, and other addicts. This observation has led to the question, "Do people overeat because they are born with a dopamine system that doesn't respond, or do obese people have a low dopamine response because this area has been overstimulated by overeating?" To explore this question, a group of researchers fed rats calorie-dense foods that were high in sugar and fat, such as cookies and chocolate chips (Avena, Rada, & Hoebel, 2009). After a few months, the rats became obese and their reward center dopamine levels were less than those of rats fed a restricted diet. To see whether this change was the result of weight gain per se or the rats' diets, the researchers next fed the rats a restricted diet (of rat chow, not calorie-dense foods) having as many calories as that of the rats fed calorie-dense foods. This group also gained weight, but did not show a change in dopamine levels. In other words, the researchers found that the rats fed calorie-dense foods had a decrease in reward-center dopamine and the other rat group did not. This showed that weight gain alone did not cause a change in dopamine levels but the process of eating calorie-dense foods did (Avena, Rada, & Hoebel, 2009).

To test dopamine levels after weight gain in humans, one study examined 26 overweight and obese women (Stice, Yokum, Blum, & Bohon, 2010). The women who gained weight over a six-month period showed a lower dopamine response when they drank a milkshake than they had when the study began, six months earlier. The researchers suggested that a lower dopamine response might make one more likely to overeat in an attempt to restore normal dopamine levels, and yet, that same overeating can dampen the dopamine response further (Stice et al., 2011).

In a similar study, 30 teens who were at high risk for obesity (had two overweight or obese parents) were compared to 30 teens at low risk. All teens had a normal weight. The researchers found that the teens at high-risk for obesity had a greater dopamine response after drinking milkshakes than those that were at a low risk (Stice, Yokum, Blum, & Bohon, 2010). This study demonstrated that obese people could start out with an oversensitive dopamine system. This initial oversensitization could cause people to overeat, because eating is experienced as very leasurable. Over time, however, overeating could lead to a dampened response, which in turn leads to more overeating.

This research is important because it helps to establish the fact that food addiction has a physiological as well as a psychological basis, and that people who develop food addictions face strong cravings that drive them to overeat. This research helps both clinicians and those who feel addicted to food to better understand the problem of food addiction. It is hoped that this understanding also will lead to better strategies for prevention and treatment.

What Foods Are Most Addictive?

Many foods can activate reward pathways. The ingestion of chocolate, for example, causes one of the largest food-related rises in dopamine. In general, people with food addictions report being drawn to foods that are high in sugar and fat. Most of the foods people with food addiction crave are not found in nature, but instead are created in the kitchen or the laboratory. Most commonly craved are dessert foods such as cookies, cakes, donuts, and ice cream. These foods are calorie-dense, and it is easy to consume a lot of calories in a short span of time. The research described above suggests that, in vulnerable people, frequent consumption of these foods could alter reward pathways over time in ways that prompt further overeating.

Interesting research in rodents has found that addictive eating behavior, such as consuming a greater than normal amount of a given food, is more likely to occur when access to such foods is limited. Science writers have likened this observation to the experience of human beings "going on a diet," in other words, restricting access to certain foods (Liebman, 2012).

Treatment

After self-diagnosing or under clinical recommendation, some food addicts look for help in 12-step groups such as Food Addicts Anonymous, which have meetings in many regions or are available online. Others consult nutritionists, doctors, psychologists, counselors, or eating-disorder specialists. These professionals often help clients to better understand which situations trigger cravings and overeating, and to learn how to avoid them or respond to them with behaviors other than overeating. People addicted to food often need professional help to improve their ability to cope with unpleasant emotions and to develop better ways of managing stress.

Emily Ohrtman and Barbara A. Brehm

See Also: Eating disorders; Food cravings.

Further Reading

American Psychological Association (2013). *Diagnostic and Statistical Manual of Mental Disorders* (5th ed.). Arlington, VA: American Psychiatric Association.

Avena, N. M., Rada, P., & Hoebel, B. G. (2009). Sugar and fat bingeing have notable differences in addictive-like behavior. *Journal of Nutrition, 139* (3), 623–628. Retrieved from http://jn.nutrition.org/content/139/3. doi: 10.3945/jn.108.097584

Food Addicts in Recovery Anonymous. Retrieved from http://foodaddicts.org.

Liebman, B. (2012). Food & addiction: Can some foods hijack the brain? *Nutrition Action Healthletter 39* (4), 1–7.

Stice, E., Yokum, S., Blum, K., & Bohon, C. (2010). Weight gain is associated with reduced striatal response to palatable food. *Journal of Neuroscience, 30* (39), 13105-9. Retrieved December 4, 2014, from http://www.ncbi.nlm.nih.gov/pubmed/20881128. doi: 10.1523 /JNEUROSCI.2105-10.2010

Stice, E., Yokum, S., Burger, K. S., Epstein, L. H., & Small, D. M. (2011). Youth at risk for obesity show greater activation of striatal and somatosensory regions to food. *Journal of Neuroscience, 31* (12), 4360–4366. doi: 10.1523/JNEUROSCI.6604-10.2011

Food Additives

"Food additive" is a general term for substances added to food during the manufacturing process. There are three main types of additives: direct, indirect, and color. Direct additives are put in food products intentionally to keep them fresh and give them specific qualities, such as certain tastes or textures. Indirect food additives result from substances unintentionally entering food products during processing, packaging, and transport. Color additives are used to enhance natural color, maintain color despite storage conditions, or give foods a different color.

For centuries, humans have been adding salt, vinegar, and spices to food to reduce spoiling and enhance flavor. Today there are more than 3,000 substances included in the U.S. Food and Drug Administration's database of "Everything Added to Food in the United States" (U.S. Food and Drug Administration, 2013a), which can be accessed through the website (www.FDA.gov). Additives can be

Table 1. Types of Food Ingredients

Purpose	Additives	Examples of products that might contain these additives
Antioxidants: Preservatives used to prevent food discoloration and spoilage from the breakdown of fats from oxygen exposure.	Ascorbic acid, citric acid, calcium sorbate, butylated hydroxyanisole (BHA), butylated hydroxytoluene (BHT), vitamin E, propyl gallate	Cereal, chewing gum, snack foods, dried fruit
Antimicrobial agents: Preservatives used to prevent mold and fungus growth.	Sorbic acid, sodium benzoate, calcium propionate, salt	Cottage cheese, fruit juice, salad dressing
Artificial and alternative sweeteners: Used to sweeten foods with minimal calories.	Acesulfame K, aspartame, saccharin, sorbitol, stevia, sucralose, tagatose, xylitol	Diet soft drinks, reduced-sugar and sugar-free products
Bleaching agents: Used to whiten foods.	Ammonium chloride, bromates, peroxides	Flour, dairy products
Color: Used to make food look appealing or fun; used to associate a flavor with a specific color.	FD&C Blue Nos. 1 & 2; FD&C Yellow Nos. 5 & 6; annatto extract, beta carotene, grape skin extract, caramel color, saffron	Candy, cheese, vitamins, pickles, yogurt
Emulsifiers: Used to blend substances that frequently do not combine, such as oil and water.	Soy lecithin, monoglycerides and diglycerides, egg yolks, polysorbates	Baked goods, ice cream, mayonnaise, peanut butter
Flavoring and flavor enhancers: Used to give food specific tastes or to enhance flavors already present.	MSH, hydrolyzed soy protein, autolyzed yeast extract, salt, sugar, vanilla, monosodium glutamate (MSG)	Snack foods, soups, sauces, processed meats
Humectants: Used to retain moisture.	Glycerol, propylene glycol, sorbitol	Candy, dried coconut, marshmallows, rice cakes
Leavening agents: Used to make products rise and to achieve specific textures.	Baking soda, monocalcium phosphate, calcium carbonate	Bread, cake, cookies, crackers
Nutrient supplements: Used to enhance the nutrient content of foods. When nutrients are added to make up for those lost in processing, the product has been "enriched." When nutrients are added that were not there initially, the product is called "fortified."	Vitamins and minerals	Bread, cereal, milk, sports bars

Source: Types of Food Ingredients. In *Overview of Food Ingredients, Additives & Colors*, International Food Information Council (IFIC) and U.S. Food and Drug Administration, November 2004; revised April 2010. Retrieved from http://www.fda.gov/food/ingredientspackaginglabeling/foodadditivesingredients/ucm094211.htm

from natural or synthetic sources. Ascorbic acid (vitamin C), for example, can be extracted from citrus fruit, but it is more economical to make it in a laboratory. The table shows some of the more common food additives, why they are used, and examples of products in which they can be found.

Regulation

Food additive regulation varies greatly from one country to another. In the United States, the U.S. Food and Drug Administration (FDA) regulates food additives. When evaluating whether a substance should be approved for use as an additive, the FDA considers the chemical properties of the substance, the typical consumption amount, and the immediate and long-term health effects from consumption. If approved for use, the FDA creates standards for how much can be used and in what foods, and how it should be labeled. In general, the amount of additive allowed in a food product is 100 times less than the amount research animals have consumed with no observable effect. If evidence emerges that an additive in use might not be safe, then the FDA is responsible for conducting studies and, if necessary, preventing further use. On the production end, manufacturers must use additives only for their approved use, and must follow regulations known as Good Manufacturing Practices (GMP) that call for ingredients to be used only in the quantities necessary to achieve the desired effect.

The FDA does not regulate all substances added to food. If a substance is "generally recognized as safe" (GRAS), then it can be used by a manufacturer for its intended purpose without FDA regulation. To be considered GRAS, the substance must have a long history of safe usage in food, or have a body of scientific evidence confirming its safety (U.S. Food and Drug Administration, 2013b).

The safety of some food additives has caused some debate, including those additives regulated by the FDA as well as those considered GRAS. In 1958, the Delaney Clause of the Federal Food, Drug, and Cosmetic Act (named after New York congressman Jim Delaney) stated that no additive could be used that had been shown to cause cancer in humans or animals, even at doses much lower than typical human consumption levels. After numerous amendments, the Delaney Clause was repealed in 1996, and today the FDA considers an ingredient safe for consumption if there is "reasonable certainty in the minds of competent scientists that the substance is not harmful under its intended conditions of use" (U.S. Food and Drug Administration, 2013b).

Health Canada is the federal organization responsible for establishing safety, nutrition, packaging, advertising, and labeling standards for all foods sold in Canada. The Canadian Food Inspection Agency is responsible for enforcing these standards. Food additive approval includes a pre-market evaluation of the product's safety. Food additives must be effective for their intended purpose, and must not cause harm when used as intended. Proposals for new additives are reviewed by scientists from Health Canada. Canada does not have a list of GRAS substances, although the following substances are allowed to be added to foods without specific regulation: Salt, sugar, starch, vitamins, minerals, amino acids, spices, seasonings, agricultural chemicals, and food-packaging materials.

Lisa P. Ritchie

Research Issues

- What is the role of the government in regulating what people can and cannot eat?
    - If people want to eat it and businesses want to make it—despite possible risks—should the government allow it?
- How do regulatory agencies decide what is safe for consumption and what is not?
    - How are acceptable daily intake (ADI) amounts determined?
    - In the United States, what is required for a substance to be "generally recognized as safe" (GRAS)? Salt, sugar, and caffeine are GRAS—should they be? Why is refined stevia GRAS, but whole-leaf stevia is not?
    - Why do some countries approve ingredients that other countries do not?
- In 1958, the Delaney Clause was added to the Food, Drug, and Cosmetic Act. It stated that if any food additive was found to cause cancer in humans or animals, its use should not be allowed. In 1996, it was repealed as an archaic law incompatible with modern-day science. What do you think?
- How much and what type of research is needed to determine whether a food or food additive is safe?
    - Is a decade of research enough for a product that might be consumed daily for a lifetime?
    - Who is conducting the research? Some of the scientific studies proving the safety of artificial sweeteners were funded by the very companies who manufacture the sweeteners. Should this be allowed?
    - If a study determines a substance to be carcinogenic in animals, does that mean it will cause cancer in humans?

Center for Science in the Public Interest. (2012). *Chemical cuisine: Learn about food additives.* Retrieved from http://www.cspinet.org/reports/chemcuisine.htm

Weise, E. (2013, Aug. 8). Experts who decide on food additives conflicted. *USA Today.* Retrieved from http://www.usatoday.com/story/news/nation/2013/08/07/food-additives-conflict-of-interest/2625211/

See Also: Artificial sweeteners; Dietary supplements; U.S. Food and Drug Administration.

Further Reading

CNN. (2010, March 4). *FDA recalls food with flavor enhancer HVP.* CNNHealth. Retrieved from http://www.cnn.com/2010/HEALTH/03/04/flavor.enhancer.recall/indcx.html

CNN. (2010, June 22). *6 scary-sounding food additives—and what they really are.* Eatocracy. Retrieved from http://eatocracy.cnn.com/2010/06/22/9-scary-sounding-food-additives%E2%80%A6and-what-they-really-are/?iref=allsearch

Health Canada. (2013, May 31). *Food additives.* Retrieved from http://www.hc-sc.gc.ca/fn-an/securit/addit/index-eng.php

International Food Information Council (IFIC) and U.S. Food and Drug Administration. (2010, April*). Overview of food ingredients, additives & colors.* Retrieved from http://www.fda.gov/Food/IngredientsPackagingLabeling/FoodAdditivesIngredients /ucm094211.htm#why

U.S. Food and Drug Administration. (2013b, February 28). *Guidance for industry: Frequently asked questions about GRAS.* Retrieved from http://www.fda.gov/Food/ GuidanceRegulation/GuidanceDocumentsRegulatoryInformation/IngredientsAdditives GRASPackaging/ucm061846.htm

U.S. Food and Drug Administration. (2013a, March 13). *Everything added to food in the United States.* Retrieved from http://www.fda.gov/Food/IngredientsPackagingLabeling /FoodAdditivesIngredients/ucm115326.htm

Food Allergies and Intolerances

Food allergies involve activation of a type of immune response that, in some cases, can lead to life-threatening symptoms, a condition known as "anaphylaxis." People with severe food allergies, for example, can experience swelling of the throat and airways when they consume the offending food, making it difficult to breathe. Food intolerances are different from food allergies in that they do not involve the type of immune response that can lead to life-threatening symptoms. A food intolerance refers to a situation in which the ingestion of a certain food or food ingredient creates uncomfortable symptoms, often in the digestive tract, such as bloating or diarrhea. The most effective strategy for treating food allergies and intolerances is to identify and avoid the problematic foods. Digestive enzymes and other medical treatments might be available for some food intolerances. People who experience severe food allergies must carry medication, usually epinephrine, which is quickly injectable and can help counter the life-threatening symptoms of food allergies.

Food allergies affect about 4% of adults and about 5% of children in the United States; this number has increased significantly over the last decade (NIAID, 2012). Peanut allergies, for example, have tripled in the past 15 years (Slomski, 2012). It is unclear whether more diagnoses are being made as a result of increased knowledge or as a result of an actual increase in allergy frequency; it is also possible that some diagnoses are incorrect. Food intolerances affect a much greater number of people. Prevalence is difficult to estimate, because many people are never tested and instead simply avoid certain foods.

Food Allergies: Causes and Symptoms

A food allergy involves an adverse immune-system reaction to a food or component of food, usually a protein. There are several different ways in which the immune system can create an allergic response to food molecules. The most dangerous type of food allergy involves the production of an antibody known as

Food Allergy: Pregnancy, Breast-Feeding, and Introducing Your Baby to Solid Foods

Health care experts do yet not have enough conclusive evidence to tell pregnant women, nursing mothers, and mothers of infants how to prevent food allergies from developing in their children. It's essential to talk with a health care professional before changing your diet or your baby's diet. Health care experts, however, do know the following.

Pregnancy

- Pregnant women should eat a balanced diet.
- If allergic to a food, a pregnant woman should avoid consuming it.
- Pregnant women who have no food allergies—such as egg, tree nuts, peanut, fish, or cow's milk (all highly allergenic)—should not avoid them. There is no conclusive evidence that avoiding these foods will prevent food allergy from developing in an infant in the future.

Breast-Feeding

- Health care experts recommend that mothers feed their babies only breast milk for the first 4 months of life because of the health benefits of breast-feeding.
- Mothers who breast-feed do not need to avoid foods that are considered to be highly allergenic because there is no conclusive evidence that avoiding these foods will prevent food allergy from developing in their infants.

Introducing Solid Foods

- Health care experts in the United States currently suggest that you do not introduce solid food into your baby's diet until the baby is 4 to 6 months old.
- There is no conclusive evidence, however, to suggest delaying the introduction of solid foods after the baby 4 to 6 months old.
- There is no conclusive evidence to suggest delaying the introduction of the most common potentially allergenic foods (milk, egg, peanut) after the baby is 4 to 6 months old. Such delays will not prevent a child from developing an allergy in the future.

National Institute of Allergy and Infectious Diseases (NIAID). (2012, July 1). *Food allergy: An overview.* Retrieved from http://www.niaid.nih.gov/topics/foodallergy/documents/foodallergy.pdf

immunoglobulin (IgE). For reasons not yet understood, initial ingestion of the food allergen causes the body to mistakenly produce immunoglobulin antibodies to that particular food component. These antibodies then circulate in the bloodstream and attach to mast cells and basophils. Mast cells are located in all areas of the body, especially the respiratory system, the skin, and the gastrointestinal track. Basophils are found in the blood and in areas inflamed by an allergic reaction. When the food allergen is subsequently ingested, it binds to the immunoglobulin antibodies which then trigger the mast cells and basophils to release large amounts of chemicals called "histamine." Histamine triggers the inflammation and swelling associated with an allergic response.

In most cases, an immunoglobulin-mediated food allergy develops within an hour after eating the food. The consumer often notices common symptoms, such as hives, itching, skin rashes, swelling of the face or throat, wheezing, congestion, trouble breathing, abdominal pain, diarrhea, nausea, vomiting, dizziness, light-headedness, and fainting (Food and Drug Administration, 2013). A severe allergic reaction is called "anaphylaxis" and it produces life-threatening signs and symptoms such as swelling of the throat, shock, a drop in blood pressure, irregular or rapid pulse, and loss of consciousness. Anaphylaxis is potentially fatal.

Less-severe food allergies can be mediated by other types of immune responses. For example, immunoglobulin-mediated food allergies tend to develop more slowly with milder symptoms. Immunoglobulin-mediated responses might not be detected with standard diagnostic testing.

Food Allergies: Diagnosis and Treatment

To diagnose food allergies, health care providers might use a detailed history, an oral food challenge, an elimination diet, or skin or blood tests. The most reliable test for the diagnosis of a food allergy is to observe the symptoms that develop after a person has consumed a given food. This test is called an oral food challenge. Patients consume the potentially problematic food in increasing amounts, and alternating with placebo components, so that patients do not know when they are consuming the problem food. (It is possible to experience allergic reactions simply because one believes one has ingested a certain food, even when the food has not actually been ingested.) Because patients might develop a severe allergic response, many providers will not administer this test. In some cases, however, it is administered by experienced professionals in an environment that can provide immediate treatment should a severe reaction develop.

Elimination diets can take a variety of forms. The basic goal is to observe a person's response to a diet lacking—then later including—the potential food allergen. If allergic symptoms go away or do not appear when the food is absent, but appear when the food is added back into the diet, providers and patients can discover which foods are problematic. Elimination diets are not recommended for severe allergies, but can be helpful for milder food allergy symptoms.

Skin and blood tests measure levels of immunoglobulin antibodies, but can over-diagnose true allergies. This is because immunoglobulin antibodies could be present, but this does not indicate that a patient will develop a full-blown allergic response. Skin tests are rapid and usually are less expensive than a blood test. Two types of skin test commonly are used, the skin prick test and the intradermal test. The skin prick test is done by adding a drop of the alleged allergen onto the skin's surface which is either scratched or has a series of needle-pricks in it for the solution to enter. If the skin welts then the patient has a positive reaction and is allergic to the allergen. The intradermal test is done when the allergen did not test positive during the skin prick test, but is still thought to be the suspect. The intradermal test is a much more sensitive test. The allergen is injected right into the skin which is then observed for signs of irritation. The blood tests look for antibodies and generally are performed on patients who can't have skin tests.

The most reliable treatment for suspected food allergies is to avoid problematic foods. Some research has focused on training a person's immune system to tolerate an allergenic food by introducing very small amounts of allergens in a controlled environment over time (Slomski, 2012). Oral immunotherapy has the person eat a small portion of the food, and sublinguinal immunotherapy introduces microscopic amounts of the food (for example 1/100th of a peanut) under a person's tongue. Such therapies still are in the experimental phase, and must be administered in a controlled environment where medical treatment is available in case of a severe allergic reaction.

Anaphylaxis: A Medical Emergency

It is important for people with allergies to be prepared for unexpected exposure. They should wear a medical alert bracelet stating the possibility that they might have a severe allergic reaction; carry an auto-injector device that contains epinephrine; and seek medical help immediately if they experience allergic reactions.

Food allergies are particularly prevalent in children; therefore, food allergies are of particular concern in the school environment. Almost 20% of children with food allergies have had allergic reactions after accidentally ingesting food allergens at school. Up to 25% of anaphylaxis reactions in school occur in children who were not previously diagnosed with a food allergy (Centers for Disease Control and Prevention, 2013). It is vital that school personnel are ready to manage students with known food allergies and those who have not been diagnosed with any food allergy.

Common Allergens and Food Labeling

Eight foods account for 90% of all allergens in the United States: milk, eggs, peanuts, tree nuts (almonds, walnuts, pecans), soybeans, wheat, fish, and shellfish (crab, lobster, shrimp) (U.S. Food and Drug Administration, 2013). A major food allergen is defined as any one of the eight foods listed above or an ingredient that contains protein derived from the allergen food groups.

In 2004, the U.S. Congress passed the Food Allergen Labeling Consumer Protection Act (FALCPA), which went into effect in 2006 to protect those with food allergies. Under the FALCPA, food labels are required to clearly name the allergens in the list of ingredients, and state in a list beneath the ingredients whether a food contains one of the major eight food allergen (Food and Drug Administration, 2013).

Soon after the implementation of FALCPA, food labeling was revised to take into account possible allergen contamination of products because of cross-contact, when an allergen not normally present in a food product can accidentally be included in the product. Cross-contact can occur during harvesting, transportation, manufacturing, processing, or storage (Food and Drug Administration, 2013). To account for cross-contamination, labels now include statements such as "produced in a plant that processes wheat" or "may have come in contact with nut products." These advisory statements do not substitute for adhering to current and good manufacturing practices, and are required to be truthful and not misleading (Food and Drug Administration, 2013).

Food Intolerances

Food intolerance symptoms include intestinal gas, abdominal discomfort, diarrhea, hives, headaches, and irritability and usually come on gradually. These symptoms can result from an absence of an enzyme needed to fully digest a food, irritable bowel syndrome, food poisoning, sensitivity to food additives, reoccurring stress, and psychological factors (Li, 2013). Food intolerances include reactions to certain products that are added to foods to enhance the taste, add color, or protect against the growth of microbes. Food intolerances can be very uncomfortable but they are not immediately life threatening. Because symptoms of food intolerances often overlap with those of food allergies, people who experience such symptoms could benefit from allergy testing to rule out the possibility of a severe reaction. Two of the most common food intolerances include lactose intolerance and celiac disease.

Lactose is a sugar found in milk. Lactase is an enzyme in the lining of the gut that breaks down or digests lactose; when this enzyme is absent a person has lactose intolerance. The lactose stays in the digestive tract, producing a variety of digestive symptoms. Once it passes into the colon, it is broken down by bacteria, producing intestinal gas in this fermentation process.

Celiac disease is a food intolerance that elicits a unique physical response. Celiac disease, or gluten sensitive enteropathy, is an inherited condition that is triggered by foods containing gluten, and is present in about 1% of the population. People with celiac disease have an immune system that reacts negatively to the presence of gluten in the diet, but this response is not of the same nature as a typical allergic reaction, in that the immune system attacks the cells lining the small intestine, rather than stimulating anaphylaxis. Symptoms of celiac disease include abdominal pain, gas, bloating, diarrhea, constipation, malnutrition, fatigue, and weight loss. The damage to the inner lining of the small intestine reduces the ability of a person to absorb nutrients. If the symptoms are caught early enough and the person starts consuming a gluten-free diet, then the damaged tissues can heal. Diagnosis can include blood tests and a biopsy of the small intestine. Though food intolerances can provoke uncomfortable symptoms and bodily responses, they can usually be managed.

Mild forms of food intolerance often are referred to as "food sensitivities." People with food sensitivities find that certain foods "disagree" with them. They might feel that they have difficulty digesting the food, and they get a stomachache after eating it. People who have been on low-fat diets, for example, might find that eating a high-fat food such as quiche, french fries, or a fatty burger disagrees with them and feels heavy and uncomfortable in the stomach. Although food sensitivities are milder than food intolerances, food sensitivities can be problematic for some people.

Gabrielle Kassel Wolinsky

Research Issues

Researchers and clinicians are trying to understand why the prevalence of allergies is increasing so rapidly. Several theories have been proposed. It might be that people are more aware of the potential danger of severe allergic reactions, and are more likely to seek medical advice when they experience minor food-allergy symptoms; thus, more people are diagnosed. Similarly, clinicians might over-diagnose food allergies, thinking that it is better to avoid a severe allergic response even if this results in several incorrect diagnoses (telling people that they might have a food allergy, when they actually do not). Diagnostic skin and blood tests also can be somewhat unreliable.

The hygiene hypothesis speculates that the rise in the prevalence of allergies could be the result of an environment that contributes to a "confused" immune system. The hygiene hypothesis is based on the observation that allergies are more common in resource-rich countries and urban environments, and that people in poorer countries and rural environments have fewer allergies. The hypothesis suggests that the immune system functions best in an environment with a certain environmental bacterial mix, such as that found on a farm. Because people use antibacterial products, frequently take antibiotics for illness, and avoid contact with microbes, this "hygiene" might deprive the immune system of the stimulation it requires to correctly discriminate between dangerous and harmless proteins and other substances.

Some studies suggest that changes in infant feeding practices might increase allergy risk. The introduction of formula-feeding and the delayed introduction of potentially allergenic foods into an infant's diet both have been explored as possible explanations for the increase in allergy diagnoses.

Room for debate: The squishy science of food allergies. (2010, May 16). *New York Times*. The Opinion Pages. Retrieved from http://roomfordebate.blogs.nytimes.com/ 2010/05/16/the-squishy-science-of-food -allergies/?_r=0

See Also: Celiac disease; Digestion and the digestive system; Lactose intolerance; Microbiota and microbiome.

Further Reading

American Academy of Allergy, Asthma & Immunology. (2014). *Food intolerance defined.* Retrieved from http://www.aaaai.org/conditions-and-treatments/conditions-dictionary /food-Intolerance.aspx

Centers for Disease Control and Prevention. (2013). *Voluntary guidelines for managing food allergies in schools and early care and education programs.* Washington, DC: U.S. Department of Health and Human Services. Retrieved from http://www.cdc.gov /healthyyouth/foodallergies/pdf/13_243135_A_Food_Allergy_Web_508.pdf

Li, J. T. (2013, June 3). *Food intolerance vs. food allergy: What's the difference?* MayoClinic. Mayo Clinic Health and Food Allergy. Retrieved September 30, 2013, from http://www.mayoclinic.com/health/food-allergy/AN01109

National Institute of Allergy and Infectious Diseases (NIAID). (2012, July 1). *Food allergy: An overview.* Retrieved December 4, 2014, from http://www.niaid.nih.gov/topics /foodallergy/documents/foodallergy.pdf

Slomski, A. (2012). Treatment rather than avoidance may be within reach for children with food allergies. *Journal of the American Medical Association, 307* (4), 345–348. doi:10.1001/jama.2012.32

U.S. Food and Drug Administration. (2013, April 17). *Food allergies: What you need to know.* Retrieved December 4, 2014, from http://www.fda.gov/food/resourcesforyou /consumers/ucm079311.htm

Food Cravings

Food cravings can be defined as the overwhelming desire to consume a particular kind of food. People report that food cravings feel uncomfortable, in that the craving dominates a person's awareness until it either is satisfied or it passes. Research suggests that the brain reward circuitry response involved in food cravings is similar to that involved in drug cravings and addiction. Food cravings can range from mild to severe. Food cravings are not necessarily a problem if the craved food is obtainable and if eating it has no negative repercussions. If a person really wants a little cheese, for example, then he or she can eat a few small pieces of cheese and the craving is satisfied. Food cravings become problematic, however, for people who are trying to avoid overeating or who are restricting their food intake to lose weight. Many people report that food cravings can interfere with concentration and distract them from other activities. For some people, especially those with eating disorders, food craving can stimulate binge-eating behaviors that are experienced as distressing and uncontrollable. People tend to crave "forbidden" foods that are high in fat, sugar, and salt.

What Causes Food Cravings?

Researchers who have asked volunteers to record and analyze their food cravings think that a craving typically begins with thoughts about a particular food, often triggered by seeing the food or remembering something about eating the food. A person then might begin to focus on how good that food tastes or other positive associations about that food. Thinking about the food leads to an emotional "need" for it which then develops into an urge to obtain and eat that food. This explains why some people eat in response to viewing advertisements for food.

What determines which food is the object of a craving? There is little evidence to support the notion that people crave foods that supply a nutrient in which they have a deficiency. More likely, the food is associated with positive feelings in some way. Chocolate, for example, has chemicals that make some people feel good.

Similarly, carbohydrates help some people feel more relaxed. Cravings probably evolve from past experiences—both psychological and physiological—with the consumption of specific foods. For some people food cravings can trigger episodes of emotional overeating—a leading cause of obesity. Emotional overeating occurs when people eat to reduce emotional pain and relieve negative feelings.

Restrictive dieting can cause food cravings for several reasons. People are more likely to be drawn to foods categorized as "forbidden," because it seems to be human nature to want what one cannot have. Additionally, after following a bland diet for several days, people often begin to crave more flavorful foods, such as pizza. This is why nutrition professionals encourage people to see that all types of food can be included in a diet—if the food is consumed in reasonable portions and in the context of an otherwise well-balanced diet.

People also are more likely to experience food cravings when they are hungry. The hunger signal can evolve into a focus on a particular food. Restrictive diets also can make people feel stressed, grumpy, anxious, and depressed. These are the very emotions that can trigger the need for comfort foods—a need that can turn into cravings that increase the risk of emotional overeating.

Gender and Cultural Influences

Which foods are craved varies from culture to culture. Women in North America most commonly report craving chocolate, for example, and the most frequently craved food for women in Japan is sushi. In general, in North America women report experiencing more food cravings than men do. The causes for this difference can be complex. Women report experiencing more food cravings when they are premenstrual (a few days before the beginning of the menstrual cycle) and during the first few days of their periods than they experience at other times during the month. Researchers do not know whether hormonal changes cause different levels of hunger, or whether mood changes accompanying the menstrual cycle could be the motivating factor. In addition to the monthly hormone cycles, women are more likely than men to be restricting food intake and to feel hungry, factors that appear to stimulate food cravings. Food cravings also can increase during pregnancy. Although energy requirements do increase during pregnancy, scientists cannot explain why particular foods are craved.

Coping with Cravings

When eating a small portion of the craved food is not an option—because it tends to lead to overeating—exercise and mindfulness could be helpful. One interesting study suggests that exercise might help reduce cravings and consumption of craved foods, at least for chocolate (Oh & Taylor, 2011). Subjects were regular chocolate eaters who walked for 15 minutes or rested and were then given either a stressful task or an easier one. Throughout the tasks, chocolate was freely available. All volunteers had been deprived of chocolate for two days prior to the experiment, so cravings presumably were aroused. The subjects who exercised ate about half as much chocolate during the tasks as the subjects who did not.

Observations from alcohol addiction research might be applicable to food cravings. Researchers Ostafin and Marlatt encourage people in recovery and abstaining from alcohol to "surf the urge" (Ostafin & Marlatt, 2008). Many people fear that their feelings of craving will continue to increase—getting worse and more uncomfortable. According to Ostafin's and Marlatt's research, experiences of cravings actually rise and fall. The feeling of craving grows, then diminishes. When people become anxious about the craving, they feel much worse. The researchers advise people to allow themselves to mindfully observe and experience the craving, noticing the events, feelings, and thoughts that occur with the craving. Being "present" in the experience can make it less anxiety provoking. People who "surf the urge" usually observe that the craving gradually becomes less intense. Over time, the intensity of cravings tends to diminish as well (Ostafin & Marlatt, 2008).

One research study found that this theory did apply to a group of self-defined chocolate cravers (Moffitt, Brinkworth, Noakes, & Mohr, 2012). Ninety-four women and 16 men were randomly assigned to one of three groups: Wait-list control (for comparison purposes), cognitive restructuring, or cognitive defusion. The cognitive restructuring group was trained to become aware of unhelpful thoughts associated with food craving and change them to more helpful thoughts. If they found themselves thinking, "I want some chocolate," for example, they might reply to themselves, "I do not need chocolate. I can choose something more nutritious to eat." The cognitive defusion group similarly observed thoughts that were associated with food cravings, but instead of trying to change them, they simply acknowledged them and observed their thoughts and feelings. In response to the "I want some chocolate" thought, for example, they would think, "I notice I am having the thought that I would like to eat some chocolate."

All subjects carried bags of chocolate with them. At the end of the study the researchers compared how much chocolate was eaten by each group. The cognitive defusion group was more than three times as likely to abstain from eating chocolate as the cognitive restructuring group. Subjects reporting the most distress about cravings showed the most differences between groups (favoring the cognitive defusion training). In addition to eating less chocolate, the subjects in the cognitive defusion training group reported greater improvements in other eating behaviors and less distress regarding chocolate cravings.

Barbara A. Brehm

Research Issues

Very restrictive dieting in which certain foods or food groups—such as carbohydrates—are severely limited or prohibited is associated with a number of problems. One problem is the development of, or increase in the frequency and strength of, food cravings. Other problems include difficulty following the diet; rapid weight regain when the diet is stopped; and a decrease in resting metabolic rate if calorie intake is very low. Yet restrictive diets remain very popular. It is interesting to evaluate fad diets in the media, and to examine how restrictive they are, and whether they might lead to uncomfortable food cravings.

See Also: Chocolate; Cognitive restructuring; Food addiction.

Further Reading

Brehm, B. A. (2014). *Psychology of health and fitness*. Philadelphia: F.A. Davis.

Burrell, D. (n.d.) Stop the cravings! Academy of Nutrition and Dietetics. Retrieved from http://www.eatright.org/Public/content.aspx?id=6442469608#.URAx97tWr5E

Food "Cravings" and Diabetes. (2013). Joslin Diabetes Center. Retrieved from http://www.joslin.org/info/food_cravings_and_diabetes.html

Moffitt, R., Brinkworth, G., Noakes, M., & Mohr, P. (2012). A comparison of cognitive restructuring and cognitive defusion as strategies for resisting a craved food. *Psychological Health, 27* (Suppl. 2), 74–90.

Oh, H. & Taylor, A. H. (2011). Brisk walking reduces ad libitum snacking in regular chocolate eaters during a workplace simulation. *Appetite, 58* (1), 387–392.

Ostafin, B. D. & Marlatt, G. A. (2008). Surfing the urge: Experiential acceptance moderates the relation between automatic alcohol motivation and hazardous drinking. *Journal of Social and Clinical Psychology, 27* (4), 404–418.

Food Gardens

A food garden is an area where a variety of fruits, vegetables, and herbs are planted, cultivated, and harvested for the purpose of relatively small-scale consumption. A food garden often is planted on a section of land, but it can also consist of raised beds, where food is grown in soil placed in boxes or other containers. Food gardens should be distinguished from more expansive fields or farms, the purpose of which nearly always is to feed larger masses of people a somewhat more limited variety of crops. Involvement with farm-based food growth has declined in the United States and Canada over time. The number of citizens farming in these two countries has dropped from more than 30% of the workforce a century ago to less than 2% today (National Institute of Food and Agriculture, 2011; Statistics Canada, 2009). The popularity of small-scale, home-based food growth has been on the rise in recent years, however, with many people beginning a garden for the first time (Butterfield, 2009). At present, the practice is fairly common; an average of approximately 36 million households in the United States maintain gardens each year (Butterfield, 2009).

Victory Gardens

Over the past century, food gardens have been especially popular during periods of national turmoil, partly because of the food shortages sometimes affiliated with such tumultuous times. During World War II, for example, the United States faced a possible national food shortage, and many people began growing so-called victory gardens. These were vegetable gardens planted to assure adequate food

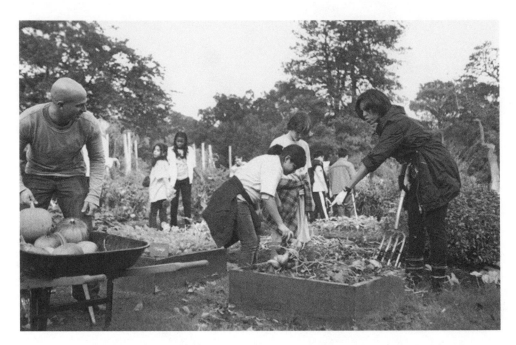

First Lady Michelle Obama, with Assistant White House Chef Sam Kass and students from Bancroft and Tubman Elementary Schools, works in the White House's organic kitchen garden on October 20, 2010. The first lady uses the garden to teach children the importance of nutrition and the value of eating locally grown food. (The White House)

availability for both civilians and the troops. In 1943, when the United States entered WWII, the U.S. president and first lady actively encouraged the installation of victory gardens across the United States. In addition to First Lady Eleanor Roosevelt's decision to install a victory garden at the White House, President Roosevelt himself issued a mid-war statement emphasizing the necessity of such gardens.

I hope every American who possibly can will grow a victory garden this year. We found out last year that even the small gardens helped. The total harvest from victory gardens was tremendous. It made the difference between scarcity and abundance. The Department of Agriculture surveys show that 42 percent of the fresh vegetables consumed in 1943 came from victory gardens. . . . Because of the greatly increased demands in 1944, we will need all the food we can grow. Food still remains a first essential to winning the war (Roosevelt, 1944).

Throughout the war, millions of various-sized victory gardens sprouted up in every corner of the nation, providing food for those who might have gone hungry and giving a sense of community to those who otherwise would have been left to cope with the coast-to-coast crisis alone.

Michelle Obama: Gardening and Health

After the war, White House food gardens of any substantial size were discontinued until 2008, when then-new First Lady Michelle Obama expanded Roosevelt's original blueprint and installed the first food garden at the White House in more than a half century (Burros, 2009). Mrs. Obama's garden was built for an entirely different reason than Mrs. Roosevelt's, however. Mrs. Obama's goal was to encourage healthy eating habits across a country in which growing rates of obesity were harming citizens' health. Coupling the revamped White House gardens with her overall campaign to help reverse the nation's growing obesity epidemic, Mrs. Obama particularly focused her outreach on a number of populations in which weight-related problems are especially high, including low-income and African-American communities. Her message: Homegrown foods are a relatively simple and cost-effective option, given the proper tools and education, for individuals seeking to revolutionize their family's—or their nation's—consumption patterns. In 2012, Mrs. Obama published a book, *American Grown: The Story of the White House Kitchen Garden and Gardens Across America,* discussing the White House gardens and promoting the idea that attaining healthier eating styles through home food gardening is an attainable and sustainable goal to pursue nationwide.

Motivations for Raising Food

Mrs. Obama's publicly touted experience with food gardening is both a hopeful gesture toward improving the health of vulnerable groups and a testament to the already changing landscape of food growth and consumption in North America. Of course, people have had food gardens for centuries, and those living in areas where farming is important and the soil is good have long planted and nurtured these gardens, whether living on a farm or in town. During the past several decades, however, food gardens have played new roles in the lives of many Americans. Although some gardeners still are concerned about food scarcity, most North American gardeners grow food to improve their health and quality of life. According to a Harris Poll conducted by the National Gardening Association, top reasons for gardening include to have better tasting food, to save money on food bills, to have better-quality food, and to grow food known to be safe (Butterfield, 2009). For some people gardening has become a much needed way to achieve the daily exercise necessary for long-term health; for others, gardening has come to provide a vital new means to control their food intake in ways that depart from the growing norm of mass-produced processed foods. Many people garden to obtain healthy organic foods without paying the high prices for comparable foods at grocery stores.

Community Gardens

Particularly in urban and suburban areas, aptly named "community gardens" have become increasingly popular and more widely supported in recent years. Such gardens involve large, staked-out areas of crop-hospitable land in which those who wish to grow food away from their own properties can buy or rent a plot of community land for the duration of a growing season. Community gardeners often begin gardening to gain access to fresh food and enjoy being outdoors. The promise of community, however, is what many later assert as their main reason for deciding to sustain the practice over the course of several growing seasons or years. The prospect of connection-by-garden is the prime motivator for many in the quickly expanding ranks of newly arrived immigrants to the United States, who frequently use community gardens to forge new connections while working to maintain cultural traditions (Twiss et al., 2003). Some schools also have begun to plant gardens not only to show students—whether from inner cities or the suburbs—how certain fruits and vegetables originate and grow, but also to encourage better, more tasty and nutritious eating habits.

Social Movements and Food Gardens

Common motivations often bind food gardeners together. The promotion of food gardens is a central focus of many social movements. Movements promoting sustainable agricultural practices value food gardens as a way of producing food that consumes fewer natural resources than traditional farming practices. Similarly, the locavore food movement, which encourages people to consume as much food as possible from locations relatively close to their homes, values home food gardens for similar reasons. The Slow Food movement was formed in opposition to the spread of fast food, and the eating style and agricultural practices associated with the production of fast food. The Slow Food movement believes food gardens further its mission, promoting the pleasure of good food and encouraging people to enjoy local food in season.

Erin K. McDaniel

Research Issues

Many schools have begun food-garden programs aimed at teaching youths to recognize, value, and eventually grow a wide variety of fruits and vegetables. Initial studies indicate that such focused instruction tends to increase students' knowledge of the foods on their dining tables and subsequently enhances their desire to consume healthier foods (Somerset, 2008). The eventual goal of these school-based campaigns is to transform the North American diet starting from the ground up—literally and figuratively—by giving young people the very basic tools they need to create, and sustain, more healthful eating patterns. Many people enjoy investigating gardening efforts in their local communities, interviewing gardeners and those involved in community gardening projects. In many schools, students have been the organizing force behind school gardens, initiating garden projects that serve as a laboratory for science and nutrition classes as well as a source of fresh produce.

See Also: The locavore movement; Organic food and farming; Slow Food movement; Sustainable agriculture.

Further Reading

Burros, M. (2009, March 19). Obamas to plant vegetable garden at White House. *New York Times*. Retrieved from http://www.nytimes.com/2009/03/20/dining/20garden.html?_r=3&partner=rss&emc=rss&

Butterfield, B. (2009). *The impact of home and community gardening in America*. National Gardening Association. Retrieved from http://www.gardenresearch.com/files/2009-Impact-of-Gardening-in-America-White-Paper.pdf

National Institute of Food and Agriculture. (2011). *About Us: Extension*. United States Department of Agriculture. Retrieved from http://www.csrees.usda.gov/qlinks/extension.html

Roosevelt, F. D. (1944, April 1). *Statement encouraging victory gardens*. Retrieved from http://www.presidency.ucsb.edu/ws/index.php?pid=16505

Somerset, S., & Markwell, K. (2008). Impact of a school-based food garden on attitudes and identification skills regarding vegetables and fruit: A 12-month intervention trial. *Public Health Nutrition, 12* (2), 214–221. Retrieved from http://journals.cambridge.org/download.php?file=%2FPHN%2FPHN12_02%2FS1368980008003327a.pdf&code=cede0b9d14c493000244640216120c97

Statistics Canada. (2009). *Canada's farm population: Agriculture-population linkage date for the 2006 Census*. Retrieved from http://www.statcan.gc.ca/ca-ra2006/agpop/article-eng.htm

Twiss, J., Dickinson, J., Duma, S., Kleinman, T., Paulson, H., & Rilveria, L. (2003). Community gardens: Lessons learned from California Healthy Cities and Communities. *American Journal of Public Health, 93* (9), 1435–1438. Retrieved from http://ajph.aphapublications.org/doi/pdf/10.2105/AJPH.93.9.1435

Food Security and Food Insecurity

"Food security" is the extent to which all individuals have access to adequate safe and nutritious food to maintain a healthful lifestyle. The Rome World Food Summit of 1996 defined the term as a right of all people in its Declaration on World Food Security. Attended by representatives from 185 countries, the summit's resulting Declaration and Plan of Action were adopted with aims to meet global nutritional needs. Specific dietary needs and food preferences, including culturally appropriate foods, must be available as part of a food secure environment. Food security also considers the appropriate use of food including level of basic nutrition knowledge and sufficient water and sanitation.

The primary obstacles to sustaining a food secure environment are poverty and the inability to maintain lasting peace. Strategies for fostering food security include implementation of policies that improve physical and economic access to food, as well as policies that support sustainable agriculture, fishery, and forestry practices. Further, preparation for natural disasters and other states of emergency ensure that resources are allocated and preserved in a manner that facilitates food security.

In the United States, different levels of food security have been described in detail by the U.S. Department of Agriculture (USDA), from very low to marginal to high food security. Characteristics of a household with very low food security include adults who have lost weight, are hungry but do not eat, or have not eaten for an entire day. These homes are marked by reduced and disrupted eating habits due to lack of resources. In 2011, the Economic Research Service determined that 85.1% of households in the United States were food secure, and 5.7% experienced very low food security at some point in the year (Coleman-Jensen, Nord, Andrews, & Carlson, 2012).

In Canada, Health Canada measures food security. Not all provinces administer the questionnaires each year. The most recent data for the country as a whole come from 2008. At that time, 92.3% of Canadians were food secure, and 2.7% were severely food insecure (Health Canada, n.d.). (It should be noted that the United States and Canada use different questionnaires, thus the data are not directly comparable.)

Patricia M. Cipicchio

Research Issues

Every country in the world has concerns about food security for at least part of its population. The World Health Organization (WHO) studies food security in all nations and examines the many variables associated with food security. The WHO urges countries to consider its citizens' food security in decision making on major policy issues. Trade regulations, for example, can affect how much local agricultural produce is available to a country's citizens versus how much is exported. Similarly, trade agreements might or might not ultimately provide better access to food for the country's population, for example, by influencing standard of living.

See Also: The poverty-obesity paradox; Supplemental Nutrition Assistance Program; Women, Infants, and Children, Special Supplemental Nutrition Program for.

Further Reading

Coleman-Jensen, A., Nord, M., Andrews, M., & Carlson, S. (2012). *Household food security in the United States 2011*. U.S. Department of Agriculture Economic Research Service. Retrieved from: http://www.ers.usda.gov/publications/err-economic-research -report/err141.aspx

Food security in the United States. (2012). U.S. Department of Agriculture Economic Research Service. Retrieved from http://www.ers.usda.gov/topics/food-nutrition -assistance/food-security-in-the-us/measurement.aspx

Health Canada. (n.d.). *Household food insecurity in Canada, 2007–2008*. Retrieved from: http://www.hc-sc.gc.ca/fn-an/surveill/nutrition/commun/insecurit/key-stats-cles-2007 -2008-eng.php

Trade, foreign policy, diplomacy and health. (n.d.). World Health Organization. Retrieved from: www.who.int/trade/glossary/story028/en/

Foodborne Illness and Food Safety

Foodborne illness, or "food poisoning," generally refers to sickness caused by consuming food that is contaminated by microorganisms, chemicals, and other substances hazardous to human health. People with foodborne illness often experience nausea, vomiting, diarrhea, and fever and the illness can take from minutes to weeks to develop. Because of its common symptoms and sometimes slow onset, many people do not recognize the actual cause of their sickness. Most cases of foodborne illnesses are mild and resolve without treatment, but some severe cases require hospitalization and sometimes cause deaths. According to the U.S. Department of Agriculture, preventable foodborne illnesses cause an estimated 48 million cases of sickness (one in six Americans) and 3,000 deaths each year in the United States, posing a serious challenge for public health (CDC, 2012).

Everyone is at risk of getting foodborne diseases. Many people, such as infants, young children, pregnant women, older adults and people with compromised immune systems, however, are at greater risk of experiencing more serious symptoms—and even death—once they become sick. According to USDA, foodborne sickness affects people so differently that some people can become seriously ill after ingesting only a few bacteria and others remain symptom-free even if they ingest thousands. Today, foodborne diseases can develop anywhere from the factory where the food is being produced and manufactured to the home kitchen where food is prepared and consumed. Some of the most common foodborne pathogens include the following.

Norovirus

Noroviruses are the most common cause of foodborne illness in the United States (CDC, 2013d). Noroviruses cause inflammation of the stomach and intestines, a condition known as gastroenteritis. Symptoms include diarrhea, vomiting, nausea, stomach pains and sometimes headaches. These symptoms usually go away within several days without treatment, but they easily can cause severe dehydration and infected people could require medical attention—especially infants, older adults, and people with other

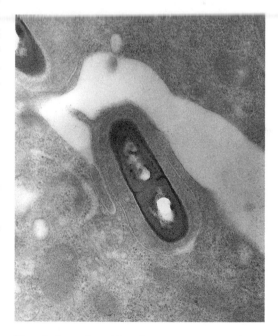

Listeria bacterium. Listeria monocytogenes is the microorganism responsible for listeriosis. The bacteria is found in soil, water, and animal feces. In the food supply, it is most commonly acquired from raw milk and soft cheeses. (Centers for Disease Control and Prevention)

illnesses. Noroviruses are highly contagious through food and feces, and cause illness more rapidly in closed and crowded environments such as hospitals, schools, nursing homes, and cruise ships. Norovirus illnesses can be acquired through eating food contaminated with norovirus, contact with the feces of infected persons, and or even touching the surface of a contaminated object.

Each year norovirus causes between 19 and 21 million cases of acute gastroenteritis and contributes to from 570 to 800 deaths (CDC, 2013d). Norovirus illness can happen any time of the year, but especially in winter. Any food that is served raw or handled after being cooked can contain norovirus, particularly leafy greens, fresh fruits, and shellfish. There is no specific treatment for people infected with norovirus, but drinking water and sports beverages (without alcohol or caffeine) can alleviate the dehydration. People can acquire norovirus repeatedly because there are many different types of viruses.

Salmonella

Salmonellosis is a common intestinal infection caused by the bacteria salmonella, and affects all age groups. It is estimated to cause approximately 1 million cases of foodborne illness and almost 400 deaths annually (CDC, 2012a). Symptoms include fever, vomiting, abdominal pain, and diarrhea, and generally resolve in around five to seven days. Long-term effects of salmonellosis include abnormal bowel movement for months and reactive arthritis, or joint pains, eye irritation, and painful urination. In severe cases—primarily in infants, older adults, and people with compromised immune systems—the infection can move from the gastrointestinal (GI) tract into the blood stream and to other organs of the body, and even cause death if not treated promptly with antibiotics.

Salmonella lives in the intestinal tract of humans, animals, and birds. Infection usually is caused by eating raw or undercooked meat, poultry, or eggs contaminated with the feces of animals harboring these bacteria. Antibiotics generally are not prescribed unless the infection has spread from the GI tract. Industrial use of antibiotics to promote weight gain in livestock has resulted in antibiotic resistance of some salmonella strains. The risk of contracting salmonellosis can increase when travelling abroad to countries with poor sanitation, when living in group housing, and even when owning a pet.

Escherichia Coli (E. Coli)

Escherichia coli (E. coli) is a group of usually harmless bacteria that live in human and animal intestines. A group of Shiga toxin-producing E. coli (STEC), however, can produce severe illness marked by bloody diarrhea, kidney failure, and sometimes even death. The most common E. coli bacteria in North America is STEC O157:H7. Symptoms of E. coli infection include stomach cramps, often bloody diarrhea, vomiting, and low fever, and usually go away within five to seven days. Severe cases can be life threatening. Approximately 5% to 10% of people infected with STEC develop hemolytic uremic syndrome (HUS), a potentially life-threatening form of kidney failure that develops about a week after infection (CDC, 2012b). The symptoms of HUS include less frequent urination, dark urine, and facial pallor. E. coli–infected persons usually get better in six to eight days.

Escherichia coli is spread via fecal matter and most commonly is caused by contaminated food, such as ground beef, unpasteurized milk, restaurant meals, contaminated water, and personal contact with animals and the feces of infected persons. In the case of E. coli O157:H7, no current treatment can cure the infection and relieve complications. Most people are advised to rest and increase hydration; antibiotics and anti-diarrheal agents should be avoided as they might increase the development of HUS (CDC, 2012b). People with severe cases should seek medical attention.

Clostridium Perfringens (C. Perfingens)

One of the most common causes of foodborne illness is C. perfringens, a bacterium found in the intestine of humans and animals. It is estimated to affect nearly one million Americans annually (CDC, 2014a). It causes food poisoning by producing spores that can survive in high temperatures and germinate—producing bacteria—during the cooling process. The most common food sources include beef, poultry gravies, and dried and precooked food, especially food that is cooked and kept warm for a long time before serving. As a result, outbreaks usually happen in large institutions like schools, cafeterias, and hospitals, and from catered food.

The bacteria produced by the spores produce a toxin that causes illness. Symptoms include diarrhea and abdominal pains, but no fever or vomiting, and usually last less than 24 hours; but severe cases can last up to two weeks. The infection is not contagious but older adults and infants are especially at risk. Infected persons should keep hydrated and seek medical assistance if dehydration occurs. Food associated with C. perfingens should be cooked thoroughly to recommended temperatures and be kept at a temperature that is either warmer than 140°F or cooler than 41°F (CDC, 2014a). Food should be served hot and perishable food should be refrigerated within two hours and heated before consumption.

Campylobacter

Campylobacteriosis, one of the most common causes of diarrheal illness in the United States, is caused by the bacterium campylobacter. It most commonly is acquired from raw and undercooked poultry, unpasteurized milk, and contaminated water. It is spread through fecal matter, but also can be acquired from the milk of infected cows. It is estimated to affect more than 1.3 million people in the United States each year, and approximately 76 people die annually from this illness (CDC, 2013b). Symptoms of campylobacteriosis include bloody diarrhea, cramping, abdominal pains, and fever. It usually resolves in one week without treatments, although some infected people might not experience any symptoms at all. Campylobacter can spread to the bloodstream and cause life-threatening symptoms for people with compromised immune systems. Preventive measures include cooking poultry meats to safe minimum temperature, separating raw meat, and avoiding unpasteurized milk.

Clostridium Botulinum (C. botulinum)

Foodborne botulism is a rare but serious disease caused by the ingestion of the neurotoxin C. botulinum, often found in improperly processed canned foods. Clostridium botulinum is one of the most toxic substances known, causing around 145 cases of botulism annually in the United States, of which 15% are foodborne (CDC, 2014d). Symptoms of botulism include double vision, drooping eyelids, slurred speech, difficulty swallowing, and muscle weakness. In rare cases, death can result from failure of the respiratory muscles, but people usually are treated in time with an antitoxin now medically available, and with respiratory support.

Clostridium botulinum neurotoxin is prevalent in soil and marine sediments, and its spores can be found on the surface of fruits, vegetables, and seafood. This neurotoxin can be killed in boiling water, but its spores continue to thrive under low-oxygen conditions, such as during the canning process. Clostridium botulinum cannot grow below the pH of 4.5, therefore most acidic food, such as most fruits, tomatoes, and pickles can be processed at home safely. Food with higher pH values, however, should be processed using a pressure cooker. Preventative measures include using approved processes for home canning, discarding spoiled canned food, and boiling home-processed canned food for more than 10 minutes before serving (USDA, 2011).

Listeria Monocytogenes

Listeriosis is a serious infection that results from ingesting food that contains the bacterium listeria monocytogenes, most often present in raw food, soft cheeses, processed meat, unpasteurized milk, and smoked seafood. Each year, listeriosis affects approximately 1,600 people in the United States—primarily older adults, pregnant women, newborns, and people with weakened immune systems—causing about 260 deaths per year (CDC, 2014b). Infection during pregnancy will result in fever, fatigue, and aches, and possibly lead to miscarriage, stillbirth, or life-threatening infections in newborns. Other people might experience fever, headache, loss of balance, and convulsions.

Shigella

Shigellosis, also known as "bacillary dysentery," is an infectious disease caused by acquiring the bacterium shigella, found in the stools of an infected person. It can be acquired by eating vegetables grown in infected sewage or soils, contact with infected persons, and consuming contaminated food. Shigella also can be found in water contaminated by sewage. Symptoms of shigellosis include diarrhea, fever, and stomach cramps and usually resolve in five or seven days. In healthy people, symptoms often are relatively mild, so the number of people who become infected each year is unknown; about about 14,000 cases are reported each year in the United States (CDC, 2013c).Young children might develop seizure and high fever in severe cases. Shigellosis can be prevented by good hygiene, especially after using the bathroom and changing soiled diapers. Shigellosis often occurs in high numbers in communities with poor sanitary conditions.

Staphylococcus Aureus

Staphylococcus aureus is a common bacterium found in the nose and on the skin of up to 25% of healthy people; its toxins are salt resistant and cannot be destroyed by heat (USDA, 2011). Staphylococcal food poisoning is a gastrointestinal disease that is acquired through contact with food workers with the bacterium and by eating contaminated food. Common sources of contamination are milk, cheese, sliced meat, puddings, some pastries, and sandwiches. Symptoms such as nausea, vomiting, stomach cramps, and diarrhea develop within one to six hours of consuming the contaminated food. Mild cases usually resolve in one to three days. Preventative measures include good hygiene; avoiding cooking when eye or nose infections are present; and refrigerating food properly.

Vibrio Vulnificus (V. Vulnificus)

Vibrio vulnificus is a bacterium that lives in warm seawater. Seafood contaminated with V. vulnificus can cause vomiting, diarrhea, and abdominal pains. For persons with chronic liver illness, it can infect bloodstream and cause fever and chills, blistering skin lesions, and septic shock (USDA, 2011). To prevent V. vulnificus infection, avoid eating raw oysters and other shellfish, cook shellfish thoroughly, avoid cross-contamination with raw seafood, and store leftovers properly in a refrigerator.

Hepatitis A

Hepatitis A is a highly contagious liver infection caused by the Hepatitis A virus. Symptoms might not occur until one month after exposure, and include jaundice, dark urine, fatigue, low-grade fever, and pale or clay-colored stools (CDC, 2014c). This infection most commonly is acquired through contaminated food or water, and through close contact with an infected person's blood, stool, or body fluids. Most mild cases can recover without treatment, and people with more severe cases are advised to rest and avoid alcohol or any substance that is toxic to the liver. Hepatitis A virus is found in infected people, fruits, vegetables, shellfish, and water. Preventative measures include vaccination, good hygiene, and avoidance of unclean water and food.

Bovine Spongiform Encephalopathy

Bovine Spongiform Encephalopathy (BSE), commonly known as "mad cow disease," is a progressive neurological disorder found in the nervous system of animals that are infected with prions, a modified form of normal protein. When animals eat tissues that are contaminated with abnormal prions, they can develop BSE. Abnormal prions are most likely to be found in the skull, brain, eyes, vertebral column, and spinal cord of cows at least 30 months of age; however, these body parts are not allowed in the human food supply (CDC, 2013a). Bovine Spongiform Encephalopathy has a very long incubation period—it can take months to years to develop symptoms after infection. Currently, BSE is fatal and incurable. There are some preventative measures that consumers can take, such as avoiding eating the body parts of cattle that are most likely to contain abnormal prions, and avoiding eating processed meat, especially meat from unknown sources.

Recommendations for Safe Food Practice

Consumers can take many measures to avoid contracting foodborne illnesses. First and foremost, personal hygiene is extremely important. It also is important for people handling food to clean their hands and the surfaces of work stations regularly. Secondly, food should be cooked or held at the correct temperature. Consumers should avoid leaving food in the "Danger Zone"—40° F to 140° F—in which foodborne bacteria grow very rapidly; food should be served hot and be refrigerated within two hours of serving (one hour during summer months) (USDA, 2011). Lastly, consumers should prevent cross-contamination by separating raw meat, poultry, and seafood during the purchasing, storage, preparation, and refrigerating processes.

Elise Bingyun Wang

See Also: Arsenic; Lead; Mercury.

Further Reading

Centers for Disease Control and Prevention (CDC). (2006, March 29). *Staphylococcal food poisoning*. Retrieved from http://www.cdc.gov/ncidod/dbmd/diseaseinfo/staphylococcus _food_g.htm

Centers for Disease Control and Prevention (CDC). (2012a, April 5). *Salmonella*. Retrieved from http://www.cdc.gov/salmonella/general/index.html

Centers for Disease Control and Prevention (CDC). (2012b, August 3). *E. coli (Escherichia coli)*. Retrieved from http://www.cdc.gov/ecoli/general/index.html

Centers for Disease Control and Prevention (CDC). (2012c, October 10). *CDC estimates of foodborne illness in the United States; CDC 2011 estimates: Findings*. Retrieved from http://www.cdc.gov/foodborneburden/2011-foodborne-estimates.html

Centers for Disease Control and Prevention (CDC). (2013a, February 21). *BSE (Bovine spongiform encephalopathy, or mad cow disease)*. Retrieved from http://www.cdc.gov /ncidod/dvrd/bse/

Centers for Disease Control and Prevention (CDC). (2013b, April 18). *Campylobacter*. Retrieved from http://www.cdc.gov/nczved/divisions/dfbmd/diseases/campylobacter/

Centers for Disease Control and Prevention (CDC). (2013c, May 14). *Shigellosis*. Retrieved from http://www.cdc.gov/nczved/divisions/dfbmd/diseases/shigellosis/

Centers for Disease Control and Prevention (CDC). (2013d, July 26). *Norovirus*. Retrieved from http://www.cdc.gov/norovirus/about/index.html

Centers for Disease Control and Prevention (CDC). (2014a, January 29). *Clostribium perfringens*. Retrieved from http://www.cdc.gov/foodsafety/clostridium-perfingens.html

Centers for Disease Control and Prevention (CDC). (2014b, March 12). *Listeria (Listeriosis)*. Retrieved from http://www.cdc.gov/listeria/

Centers for Disease Control and Prevention (CDC). (2014c, April 14). *Hepatitis A information for the public*. Retrieved from http://www.cdc.gov/Hepatitis/A/index.htm

Centers for Disease Control and Prevention (CDC). (2014d, April 25). *Botulism*. Retrieved from http://www.cdc.gov/nczved/divisions/dfbmd/diseases/botulism/

Foodsafety.gov. (2014, January 29). *Clostridium perfringens*. Retrieved from http://www.foodsafety.gov/poisoning/causes/bacteriaviruses/cperfringens/index.html

Foodsafety.gov. (2014, December 4). *Campylobacteriosis*. Retrieved from http://www.foodsafety.gov/poisoning/causes/bacteriaviruses/campylobacter/index.html

Insel, P., Ross, D., McMahon, K., & Bernstein, M. (2014). *Nutrition*. Burlington, MA: Jones & Bartlett Learning.

Mayo Clinic. (2014, April 2). *Norovirus infection*. Retrieved from http://www.mayoclinic.com/health/norovirus/DS00942

Mayo Clinic. (2014, April 5). *Salmonella infection*. Retrieved from http://www.mayoclinic.com/health/salmonella/DS00926

Mayo Clinic. (2014, August 1). *Diseases and conditions, E. coli; definition*. Retrieved from http://www.mayoclinic.com/health/e-coli/DS01007/DSECTION=treatments-and-drugs

United States Department of Agriculture (USDA). Food Safety and Inspection Service. (May 2011). *Foodborne illness: What consumers need to know*. Retrieved from http://www.fsis.usda.gov/wps/wcm/connect/602fab29-2afd-4037-a75d-593b4b7b57d2/Foodborne_Illness_What_Consumers_Need_to_Know.pdf?MOD=AJPERES

The French Paradox

"The French Paradox" refers to the observation that the French people have a lower incidence of heart disease than that of people in many other countries, despite their seemingly high-fat diets. This phenomenon challenges the widely accepted notion that high-fat diets increase the risk of heart disease. As researchers have tried to find explanations for this paradox, the concept has gained a substantial amount of media and scientific attention. The main explanation for this paradox is that one or many aspects of the French diet and lifestyle might help reduce the risk of heart disease. Several studies suggest that the lower incidence in heart disease can be at least partly attributed to a higher per capita consumption of red wine. Other dietary factors and eating behaviors also could help explain the French Paradox.

Serge Renaud, a French scientist, first coined the term "French Paradox" in the early 1990s. In 1991, Maury Safer featured this new term in the CBS television show "60 Minutes." Safer presented the idea that despite a diet that is high in saturated fat, the French have one-quarter the rate of coronary heart disease as compared to the rate in the United States. The show credited this concept to the French people's high consumption of red wine (Safer, 1991). This resulted in a significant increase in wine sales in the United States and epidemiological studies examining the association of wine and heart disease.

Hundreds of studies were published as scientists attempted to find explanations for the paradox. Some blamed the positive associations between wine consumption and a reduced risk of heart disease on a statistical error, and other researchers suggested that different dietary factors—such as a high fruit and vegetable intake—are the true explanation. Still, for many years, the hypothesis that moderate drinking of red wine is associated with a reduced rate of heart disease remained the most supported (Ellison, 2011). Since then, evidence has emerged that suggests red wine alone does not provide the significant health effects as was once thought. The high consumption of fruits and vegetables, in addition to fresh, local, quality ingredients and mindful eating is thought to be a more plausible explanation (Vendrame, 2013; Weil, 2013).

The French and Saturated Fat

When researchers first began to discuss the French paradox, saturated fats were thought to raise total and low-density lipoprotein (LDL) blood cholesterol levels. In a groundbreaking study examining 40 dietary factors spanning 40 countries, a significant positive correlation was identified between intake of saturated fat and cholesterol and death by cardiovascular disease (Ferrieres, 2004). In this same study, it was found that French citizens represented an outlier in the study, as they consumed far more high-fat foods but maintained low incidences of coronary heart disease.

The French diet is higher in saturated fats (such as butter and cheese) than that of people in nearly every other nation, including the United States. Each French citizen consumes an average of forty pounds of cheese per year (Safer, 1991). Due to the conventional knowledge of saturated fat intake and heart disease, researchers in the 1990s predicted that the French would have an exceptionally high rate of heart disease. Instead, the rate was found to be exceptionally low. At the time, this finding surprised researchers. More recent studies suggest that saturated fat per se is not as risky as was once thought (Malhotra, 2013).

The French and Red Wine

Many studies suggested that alcohol, itself, might be the component providing the protection against heart disease. In fact, one research group estimated that consumption of red wine reduces risk of cardiovascular disease mortality by about 30% to 50% (Vidavalur et al., 2006). Alcohol intake has been found to raise high-density lipoprotein (HDL) levels. Higher HDL levels are associated with reduced rates of blood clotting and reduced risk of heart disease.

Although light to moderate consumption of alcohol might reduce the risk of heart disease and other diseases, red wine consumption, as observed in the French, was thought to have a unique and stronger protective effect (Vidavalur et al., 2006). In fact, studies found that moderate wine consumption was associated with a decrease of 24% to 31% of all-cause mortality as compared with consumption of equivalent amounts (in terms of alcohol content) of beer or spirits (Ferrieres, 2004). This evidence suggested there is another component (or components) in red wine that makes moderate consumption that much more beneficial.

The hypothesized key ingredients in red wine linked to cardiovascular protection are polyphenols, particularly a polyphenol called "resveratrol." Resveratrol and other polyphenols are found in high concentrations in the skin and seeds of grapes and act to protect grapes from bacteria and fungi. Red wine is one of the largest sources of natural polyphenols in the diet. In red wine, polyphenols contribute to color, mouth feel, and, perhaps, the reduction of the risk of heart disease (Mochly-Rosen & Zalchari, 2010). Polyphenols might exert their effects through their antioxidant behavior. This behavior was thought to protect the heart in the following ways.

- Polyphenols might prevent blood clots—Polyphenols are known to decrease inflammation and increase the relaxation of blood vessels, which reduces obstruction to blood flow. A decrease in inflammation and an increase in artery relaxation reduce blood clot risk. Additionally, antioxidant polyphenols from red wine have been found to decrease the buildup of platelets, the blood compounds responsible for forming blood clots (Mochly-Rosen & Zalchari, 2010).
- Polyphenols might reduce oxidation of LDL cholesterol—Oxidized LDL initiates and encourages plaque accumulation in the artery lining. As LDL accumulates, the arteries begin to harden and narrow, a process called atherosclerosis. With this, the risk of heart disease increases. Thus, as resveratrol and other polyphenols reduce the oxidation, they also reduce risk of heart disease.

Over the years, there has been a strong and consistent amount of scientific data that indicates moderate alcohol consumption—especially of wine—has a beneficial impact on the heart. The U.S. Federal Dietary Guidelines indicate moderate consumption of red wine can be beneficial to health. In the United States, the Bureau of Alcohol, Tobacco, and Firearms and Explosives permits wine labels to include a statement regarding wine's health benefits (Insel, Ross, McMahon, & Bernstein, 2013). Unfortunately, there are both medical and societal risks of excessive or inappropriate use of alcohol. This makes the extensive use of wine for beneficial purposes—such as medical recommendations and treatments—difficult.

Although there is a strong association between moderate wine consumption and heart health, it is difficult to conclude that wine is the key factor reducing heart disease rates in France. Researchers have concluded that the amount of polyphenols in red wine probably is not enough to produce significant positive effects (Vendrame, 2013). In epidemiological studies, it is a well-known fact that association does not always indicate causation. In other words, although the increased intake of red wine by French people goes along with reduced risk of heart disease, this observation does not prove that red wine is the cause. Today, most researchers believe that although red wine might play a role in explaining the French Paradox, the paradox can be attributed to other factors of the French diet and lifestyle, as well.

The French Diet and Lifestyle

Current research suggests that the low heart-disease rates despite the high-fat diet among the French can be associated with moderate wine consumption in combination with mindful eating and more fruit and vegetable intake. The lesser rates of heart disease in the French population could derive from a thoughtful and wholesome approach to preparing and eating food (Pollan, 2004). Eating is considered a pleasurable experience enjoyed with family and friends. This allows the French to consume smaller portions as well as snack and skip meals less frequently. Also, due to France's higher value of and mindful approach to cooking and eating food, there is an emphasis on fresh, local, and high-quality ingredients (Weil, 2013).

As a whole, the French population consumes less sugar, processed flour, and trans fats (Weil, 2013). These processed foods have extremely damaging effects on the heart and increase the risk of heart disease. In fact, researchers are now finding these foods are the major drivers of heart disease. Instead of sugary and processed foods, the French consume a rich amount of unprocessed foods, particularly fruits and vegetables (Vendrame, 2013). Fruits and vegetables contain dietary fiber and many phytochemicals, which act in ways similar to the polyphenols found in wine to decrease risk and occurrence of heart disease.

Hannah O. Huggins

See Also: Alcohol; Cardiovascular disease and nutrition; Fatty acids; Polyphenols; Resveratrol.

Further Reading

Ellison, C. (2011). The French Paradox: 20 years later. *Journal of Wine Research, 22* (2), 105–108. Retrieved September 25, 2013, from the Academic Search Premier database.

Ferrieres, J. (2004). The French Paradox: Lessons for Other Countries. *Heart, 90* (1), 107–111.

Insel, P., Ross, D., McMahon, K., & Bernstein, M. (2013). *Nutrition.* Sudbury, MA: Jones and Bartlett Publishers.

Malhotra, A. (2013). Saturated fat is not the major issue. *British Medical Journal, 347,* f6340. doi: http://dx.doi.org/10.1136/bmj.f6340

Mochly-Rosen, D., & Zakhari, S. (2010). Focus on: The cardiovascular system—What did we learn from the French (paradox)? *Alcohol Research & Health, 33,* 76–86.

Pollan, M. (2004, October 17). Our National Eating Disorder. *New York Times.* Retrieved September 27, 2013, from http://www.nytimes.com/2004/10/17/magazine/17EATING .html?_r=0

Safer, M. (Director). (1991). The French paradox [Television show episode]. In *60 Minutes.* United States: CBS News.

Vendrame, S. (2013). The French paradox: Was it really the wine? *American Society for Nutrition.* Retrieved October 20, 2013, from http://www.nutrition.org/asn-blog/2013/01 /the-french-paradox-was-it-really-the-wine/

Vidavalur, R., Otani, H., Singal, P.K., & Maulik, N. (2006). Significance of wine and res- veratrol in cardiovascular disease: French paradox revisited. *Experimental and Clinical Cardiology, 11* (3), 217–225.

Weil, A. (2013). 8 Reasons the French are slim—Dr. Weil's daily tip. Dr. Weil's Tip of the Day. Retrieved October 30, 2013, from http://www.drweil.com/drw/u/TIP04979 /8-Reasons-the-French-are-Slim.html

Fructose

Fructose is a monosaccharide found in fruits and vegetables and is the sweetest of all natural sugars. Fructose commonly binds to glucose, forming the disaccharide sucrose. It is also found as a component of synthetic sweeteners such as high-fructose corn syrup, which is composed of water along with varying concentrations of fructose and glucose. Fructose also is called "levulose" and "fruit sugar." Fructose is absorbed by the small intestine and has mild effects on blood sugar levels as com-pared to other sweeteners. Unlike glucose—which can immediately enter the blood-stream from the small intestine and be metabolized throughout the body—fructose must be metabolized and converted to glucose by the liver before it can be used by the body. After fructose is processed by the liver the end product usually is glyco-gen, the body's form of long-term energy storage. When glycogen stores are full, fructose metabolism typically shifts toward generation of triglycerides and fatty ac-ids. In high amounts, serum triglycerides are associated with heart disease. In indi-viduals with fructose malabsorption, the small intestine does not absorb the sugar properly, leading to stomach pain and bloating, a condition that affects up to 40% of individuals in the Western Hemisphere (Hereditary Fructose Intolerance, 2011).

The average daily intake of fructose has increased during the past several de-cades with the introduction of high-fructose corn syrup into the food supply. This increase in consumption raises concerns about the long-term health effects of the sugar and its contribution to obesity. Conflicting reports on the topic, however, have made dietary recommendations regarding fructose tenuous. In animal mod-els, fructose has been shown to contribute to insulin resistance, hypertension and other vascular issues, fatty liver, metabolic abnormalities, and hyperuricemia, which precedes gout (Lee, Bruce, & Dong, 2009). Fructose also might contribute to certain cancers, particularly pancreatic and intestinal cancers (Port, Ruth, & Istfan, 2012). In normal human subjects, fructose has been shown to increase triglyceride levels after ingestion, but not after three hours, and it does not directly cause changes in body weight for people in energy balance (Dolan, Potter, & Burdock, 2010). In overweight and obese subjects, fructose could be linked to increased visceral fat and decreased insulin sensitivity. Although a definitive link between fructose and various dysfunctions has not yet been established in humans, the USDA considers consuming excess fructose—especially as a component of added sweeteners—to be undesirable.

Patricia M. Cipicchio

See Also: High-fructose corn syrup.

Further Reading

Dolan, L. C., Potter, S. M., & Burdock, G. A. (2010). Evidence-based review on the effect of normal dietary consumption of fructose on development of hyperlipidemia and obesity in healthy, normal weight individuals. *Critical Reviews in Food Science and Nutrition, 50*, 53–84.

HealthDay. (2013). *Is fructose making people fat?* MedlinePlus. Retrieved from: http://www.nlm.nih.gov/medlineplus/news/fullstory_132696.html

Hereditary fructose intolerance. (2011). *Genetics Home Reference*. National Library of Medicine. Retrieved from http://ghr.nlm.nih.gov/condition/hereditary-fructose-intolerance

Lee, O. Bruce, W. R., & Dong, Q. (2009). Fructose and carbonyl metabolites as endogenous toxins. *Chemico-Biological Interactions, 178* (1–3), 332–39.

Port, A. M., Ruth, M. R., & Istfan, N. W. (2012). Fructose consumption and cancer: Is there a connection? *Current Opinions in Endocrinology, Diabetes, and Obesity, 19* (5), 367–374. doi: 10.1097/MED.0b013e328357f0cb

Rizkalla, S. W. (2010). Health implications of fructose consumption: A review of recent data. *Nutrition and Metabolism, 7*. Retrieved from: http://www.medscape.com/viewarticle/733528

Functional Foods

Although no single, universally accepted definition exists, the term "functional foods" generally refers to foods containing one or more ingredients thought to provide physiological benefits beyond basic nutrition. Popular sources have used the terms "functional foods" and "nutraceuticals" interchangeably; however, functional foods are distinct from nutraceuticals—which are products isolated from foods and typically sold in liquid or capsule form.

Both whole and processed foods can be considered functional foods—the key ingredient can be naturally occurring or added during the manufacturing process. For example, both salmon and fortified eggs—when serving as sources of omega-3 fatty acids—would be categorized as functional foods, given the claim that adequate consumption of omega-3 fatty acids could reduce the risk of coronary heart disease. Functional food products are a multibillion-dollar industry, and food researchers and manufacturers are eager to develop food products that meet consumer demand.

History

The concept of functional foods originated in Japan in the 1980s, when the Ministry of Health and Welfare created the regulatory system known as Foods for Specified Health Use (FOSHU), in an effort to reduce rising health care costs (Hasler, 2002). Applicants seeking to have a product approved under FOSHU must demonstrate its safety and efficacy, presenting documentation of the basis for the health claim and the basis of the recommended intake of the functional ingredient. Functional foods gained popularity in the United States in the 1990s, but no comparable regulatory body has been established.

Health Claims and Marketing

Although functional foods are not legally defined in the United States, the Food and Drug Administration (FDA) does control the types of claims that can be made about functional foods. Manufacturers of these foods may include approved health claims in the advertising or packaging of their products, but cannot assert that the food treats disease or has an immediate effect—these claims are restricted to drugs. An oatmeal manufacturing company can claim that the fiber in its product "promotes heart health" or "reduces the risk of heart disease," but not that it treats existing cardiovascular issues. The FDA regulations also require that health claims for which there is limited or mixed scientific support include qualifying language to avoid misleading consumers.

Bioavailability and Physiological Relevance

A persistent concern with regard to functional foods is the bioavailability and concentration of the active ingredient. If the functional component is not readily available for absorption and utilization or if it is present in the food in very small amounts, then the product might not offer the desired health benefit (Academy of Nutrition and Dietetics, 2013). The example of omega-3 fatty acids provided above serves to illustrate this problem: Eggs produced by chickens fed flax seed contain mostly short-chain ALA, and salmon contains higher levels of the more bioavailable, long-chain fatty acids, eicosapentaenoic acid (EPA) and docosahexaenoic acid (DHA).

Some nutritionists are enthusiastic about the potential of functional foods in their modified form to improve the health of the general population without demanding drastic changes in diet, but others caution that products relying on added ingredients also tend to contain less of the compound of interest per serving, which can necessitate the consumption of unrealistic quantities of the food to obtain a sufficient amount of the functional component (Denny, 2013).

Laura C. Keenan

See Also: Dietary supplements; Phytochemicals.

Further Reading

Academy of Nutrition and Dietetics (2013). Position paper of the Academy of Nutrition and Dietetics: Functional foods. *Journal of the Academy of Nutrition and Dietetics, 113* (8), 1096–1103. Retrieved from http://www.eatright.org/About/Content.aspx?id=8354

British Nutrition Foundation (2009). *Functional foods.* Retrieved from http://www.nutrition.org.uk/nutritionscience/foodfacts/functional-foods

Denny, S. (2013). *Plates with purpose: What are functional foods?* Retrieved from http://www.eatright.org/Public/content.aspx?id=6442472528&terms=functional%20food

Hasler, C. M. (2002). Functional foods: Benefits, concerns and challenges—a position paper from the American Council on Science and Health. *Journal of Nutrition, 132* (12), 3772–3781. Retrieved from http://nutrition.highwire.org/content/132/12/3772.full

Health Canada. (2012). *What are functional foods and nutraceuticals?* Agriculture and Agri-Food Canada. Retrieved from http://www.agr.gc.ca/eng/industry-markets-and-trade/statistics-and-market-information/by-product-sector/functional-foods-and-natural-health-products/functional-foods-and-natural-health-products-canadian-industry/what-are-functional-foods-and-nutraceuticals-/?id=1171305207040

G

Gallbladder and Gallbladder Disease

The gallbladder is a small sac located underneath the liver. Its functions are to store and concentrate the bile produced from the liver, and release the bile as needed for digestion. Shaped like a pear, this organ holds about a quarter cup of bile. When the small intestine senses the presence of food—which enters the small intestine after leaving the stomach—the intestine releases a hormone called cholecystokinin (CCK). Cholecystokinin causes the gallbladder to contract, squeezing bile into the bile duct. The bile duct transports the bile to the upper portion of the small intestine. Bile is composed of bile salts, electrolytes, bilirubin, and cholesterol and other lipids, including the phospholipid lecithin, and usually is a yellowish color. As the bile mixes with the contents entering the small intestine, it enables fat globules to be broken down into smaller particles, a process called "emulsification," which aids in digestion and absorption.

Gallbladder disease refers to any condition related to the dysfunction of bile ducts or the gallbladder. Gallbladder diseases include those caused by gallstones, gallbladder inflammation, and gallbladder cancer (a rare disorder). The most common disorders by far are those caused by gallstones. Approximately 20 to 25 million people in the United States have gallstones—about 10% to 15% of the adult population (Stinton & Shaffer, 2012). Several factors increase risk for gallstone formation, including obesity and rapid weight loss. As rates of obesity increase worldwide, the prevalence of gallbladder disease has increased as well. Several effective treatments are available to treat gallbladder disease caused by gallstones.

Gallstones

Gallstones accumulate when substances in the bile harden into particles as small as a grain of salt or as large as a tennis ball. There are two main types of stones; the first type is made of the cholesterol that the liver produces. Gallstones form when the liver releases too much cholesterol and there are insufficient bile salts in the bile to break down the cholesterol. Another cause of gallstones is the gallbladder not emptying, thus allowing the bile to concentrate and form a sludge that can develop into stones (Stinton & Shaffer, 2012).

The second type of gallstone, known as "pigment stone," is made of bilirubin. Bilirubin is a substance formed from the remains of hemoglobin derived from the

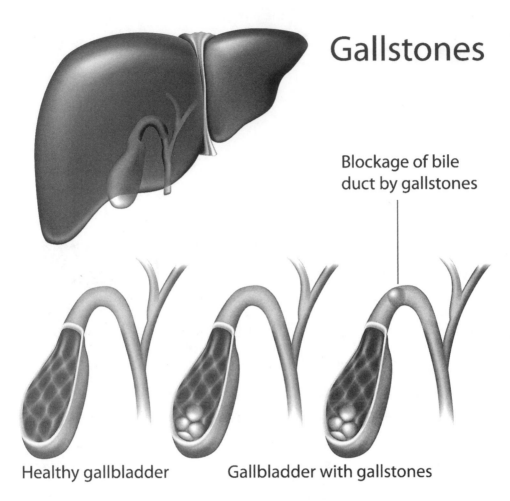

Gallstones

Blockage of bile
duct by gallstones

Healthy gallbladder   Gallbladder with gallstones

Comparison of healthy gallbladder and one with gallstones. A majority of gallstones are small
and pass through the bile duct without notice. However, if a gallstone lodges and blocks a
duct, severe pain results. Surgery may be necesssary for people with recurrent gallstones.
(Alila07/Dreamstime.com)

breakdown of red blood cells. In comparison to cholesterol stones, they are smaller
and darker. Pigment stones are classified as either brown or black. Black stones are
more common in patients who have cirrhosis, a liver disease, or sickle-cell anemia,
a blood disease. Brown stones have more cholesterol than calcium and can be
caused by infection. Asian patients more commonly have brown stones. Although
70% of gallbladder patients usually have cholesterol stones, it is possible for patients to have both cholesterol and pigment stones (Simon & Zieve, 2013). Of the
10% to 15% of Americans who will develop gallstones, 80% might never actually
suffer from discomfort or realize that they have stones (Stinton & Shaffer, 2012).
For those who do experience discomfort, pain arises when gallstones block bile

ducts, preventing the gallbladder from draining. Gallstones can affect the pancreas because the pancreas duct empties through the same opening as the bile duct (Choi & Silverman, 2013).

Symptoms of Gallbladder Disease

When a gallstone becomes lodged in any of the bile ducts, medically described as "choledocholithiasis," an individual could feel discomfort or pain. Pain duration might last from minutes to hours, and usually affects the upper abdomen. Other symptoms include nausea, vomiting, and sweating. Pain attack severity is described as feeling like that of a heart attack. Symptoms of fever, jaundice, chills, and severe abdominal pain can indicate that the gallbladder is inflamed, a condition that also is known as "cholecystitis"; that a stone is blocking pancreatic juices from leaving the pancreas; or that something in the gallbladder is infected (Choi & Silverman, 2013).

Diagnosis for gallbladder disease first starts with the patient describing symptoms of a gallstone attack. The presence of gallstones and gallbladder disease can be detected through x-ray or ultrasound (Choi & Silverman, 2013). A doctor then can recommend further ultrasound testing or CT scans, which can detect whether a bile duct is swollen and thus blocking the passage of bile. Endoscopic ultrasound can detect whether a gallstone is forming and if there are any changes in the pancreatic or biliary duct system. Endoscopic retrograde cholangiopancreatography (ERCP) also detects whether the gallbladder or bile ducts are blocked, and also can remove small blockages. ERCP diagnosis techniques are slightly invasive (Cedars-Sinai, 2013). They only involve a small incision in which the surgeon can then insert an endoscope to diagnose the patient. The endoscope can also be inserted through the mouth (Cedars-Sinai, 2014).

Treatment of Gallbladder Disease

Treatment for gallbladder disease should be pursued only if the individual experiences significant pain. This can be done either through surgery to remove the gallbladder or gallstones, or via drugs. The removal of the gallbladder is called "cholecystectomy" and is considered to be a low-risk operation. There are two forms of cholecystectomy. The most common form is larcoscopic cholecystectomy, which involves several small incisions made to enable a small video camera and surgical tools to view the abdomen and remove the gallbladder. In this surgery, the patient is put under general anesthesia and most patients can leave the hospital the same day or day after their surgery. The patient usually can expect to recover in the course of a week. Another form of cholecystectomy is an open cholecystectomy, in which a single, larger incision is used. The open cholecystectomy requires a longer recovery time. Although either form of cholecystectomy has low risks for patients, complications can include bile leak; bleeding; blood clots; heart problems; infection; damage to the bile duct, liver, or small intestine; pancreatitis; pneumonia; and even death (Mayo Clinic Staff, 2013). Gallbladder surgery is extremely successful, and because the gallbladder is a nonessential organ patients do very well after surgery. Some side effects of the surgery do include diarrhea and abdominal pain.

Other forms of gallbladder treatment include endoscopic retrograde cholangi-opancreatography (ERCP) (described above), which is only slightly invasive. Intracorporeal electrohydraulic lithotripsy (EHL) is another treatment for gallstones that breaks up stones that are too big to be removed through a bile duct. A doctor also can prescribe drugs that can dissolve gallstones over the course of half a year. This method is intended for patients who for whatever reason are not candidates for surgery. This is the least-effective method, as new stones can form once the patient goes off the medication.

Risk Factors for Gallbladder Disease

Not everyone suffers from the presence of gallstones and, of those who do, not all require gallbladder removal. Gallstones are most commonly found in adults age 40 and older. Women are at a greater risk for gallstones because estrogen can increase the levels of cholesterol in bile, which can minimize gallbladder movement and create gallstones. Women who take oral contraceptives also have an increased chance of developing gallstones. Other risk factors include diabetes; a family history of gallstones; a high level of serum triglycerides; inactivity; low levels of HDL cholesterol; pregnancy; and rapid weight loss (Weight-control Information Network, 2013). Obesity—especially extra fat in the torso—is a strong risk factor for gallstone formation. Researchers think this is because obesity is associated with a higher cholesterol output by the liver, leading to more cholesterol in the bile, and a higher risk of stone formation. Diets high in cholesterol, fat, and carbohydrates have been associated with increased risk for gallstones; and higher intakes of fiber, coffee, unsaturated fats, vitamin C, and calcium, and moderate consumption of alcohol have been associated with lower risk (Stinton & Shaffer, 2012).

Nutrition and Diet Following Gallbladder Surgery

Diarrhea is a common symptom following gallbladder surgery. After the gallbladder is removed, the bile simply drains into the small intestine from the liver, rather than being concentrated and stored, and delivered when stimulated by the presence of food in the small intestine. The diarrhea usually resolves on its own after a few months. Patients coping with this symptom should try consuming smaller, more frequent meals, and gradually consume more water-soluble fiber such as psyllium (Nelson, 2012). People whose diarrhea symptoms do not improve, or who continue to experience pain or weight loss should seek medical advice.

Christine S. Chang

Research Issues

Obesity, especially excess visceral adipose tissue, stimulates increased rates of cholesterol and triglyceride production by the liver. Conversely, fasting and very low-calorie diets reduce bile flow, and can contribute to gallstone formation as bile builds up in the gallbladder.

If both obesity and weight loss increase risk for gallbladder disease, what is a person dealing with obesity supposed to do? Rapid weight loss significantly increases risk for gallbladder disease, so much so that some bariatric surgeons prophylactically remove the gallbladder when they perform a weight-loss surgery—although this procedure is questioned by some. Slower forms of weight loss, however, have a much lower risk of gallstone formation (Johansson, Sundstrom, Marcus, Hemmingsson, & Neovius, 2013). People with obesity who are considering weight-loss surgery or weight-loss diets must take into account their obesity-associated health problems along with treatment risks, and choose their treatment options accordingly.

Johansson, K., Sundstrom, J., Marcus, C., Hemmingsson, E., & Neovius, M. (2013). Risk of symptomatic gallstones and cholecystectomy after a very-low-calorie diet or low-calorie diet in a commercial weight loss program: I-year matched cohort study. *International Journal of Obesity (London)* (2013, May 22), epub ahead of print. doi: 10.1038/ijo.2013.83

See Also: Digestion and the digestive system; Lecithin; The liver.

Further Reading

Cedars-Sinai. (2014). *Gallstones: Gallbladder disease.* http://www.cedars-sinai.edu/Patients/Health-Conditions/Gallstones-l-Gallbladder-Disease.aspx

Choi, Y., & Silverman, W. B. (2013). *Biliary tract disorders, gallbladder disorders, and gallstone pancreatitis.* American College of Gastroenterology. Retrieved from http://patients.gi.org/topics/biliary-tract-disorders-gallbladder-disorders-and-gallstone-pancreatitis/

Mayo Clinic Staff. (2013). *Cholecystectomy (gallbladder removal).* http://www.mayoclinic.com/health/cholecystectomy/MY00372/DSECTION=results

Nelson, J. K. (2012). *Can you recommend a diet after gallbladder removal?* MayoClinic.com. Retrieved from http://www.mayoclinic.com/health/gallbladder-removal-diet/AN02176/METHOD=print

Simon, H. & Zieve, D. (2013). *Gallstones and gallbladder disease.* University of Maryland Medical Center. Retrieved from http://umm.edu/health/medical/reports/articles/gallstones-and-gallbladder-disease

Stinton, L. M. & Shaffer, E. A. (2012). Epidemiology of gallbladder disease: Cholelithiasis and cancer. *Gut and Liver, 6* (2), 172–187. doi: 10.5009/gnl.2012.6.2.172 http://www.ncbi.nlm.nih.gov/pmc/articles/PMC3343155/

Weight-control Information Network. (2013). *Dieting and gallstones.* Retrieved from http://win.niddk.nih.gov/publications/PDFs/DietingandGallstones2002.pdf

Gamma Linolenic Acid

Gamma linolenic acid (GLA) is an omega-6 fatty acid found mainly in seed oils of borage, evening primrose, and black currant plants. These plant seed oils are sold as dietary supplement sources of gamma linolenic acid. Gamma linolenic acid also is found in human breast milk. The human body can make gamma linolenic acid from the essential fatty acid linoleic acid, which must be obtained from the diet. In humans, linoleic acid is obtained mostly from vegetable oils and egg yolks. Gamma linolenic acid is important for brain development, bone health, skin and hair growth, energy metabolism, and the health of the reproductive system. Gamma linolenic acid supplements are not needed by most people, because they can get more than sufficient linoleic acid from their diets and they are able to convert linoleic acid to sufficient quantities of gamma linolenic acid.

The human body uses gamma linolenic acid to manufacture prostaglandins, which are hormone-like substances that play important roles in many processes of the body. Prostaglandins help to control inflammation, make smooth muscles contract, and regulate body temperature. Although omega-6 fatty acids generally are thought to promote, rather than inhibit, inflammation, GLA might have anti-inflammatory effects, more commonly observed in the omega-3 fatty acids. Gamma linolenic acid has been promoted as a treatment for a variety of health problems, especially allergic skin conditions such as eczema, but evidence supporting a beneficial effect for eczema is fairly weak. A few small studies suggest that GLA might be somewhat helpful for the treatment of rheumatoid arthritis, hypertension, and diabetic neuropathy (Ehrlich, 2011)

Laboratory tests have shown that GLA can slow the growth of some types of human cancer cells in vitro, and GLA could enhance the effectiveness of some anticancer drugs (ACS, 2010). One interesting cell culture study found that gamma linolenic acid is able to stimulate apoptosis in leukemia K562 cells, and shows the capability of selectively inducing cell death in the cancer cells without causing damage to normal cells, which suggests that gamma linolenic acid someday might be an effective chemotherapeutic agent against cancer (Ge et al., 2009).

Fei Peng

See Also: Fatty acids; Linoleic acid.

Further Reading

American Cancer Society (ACS). (2010, May 13). *Gamma linolenic acid*. American Cancer Society. Retrieved from http://www.cancer.org/treatment/treatmentsandsideeffects /complementaryandalternativemedicine/pharmacologicalandbiologicaltreatment /gamma-linolenic-acid

Ehrlich, S. D. (2011, July 10). *Gamma-linolenic acid*. University of Maryland Medical Center. Retrieved from http://www.umm.edu/altmed/articles/gamma-linolenic-000305 .htm

Ge, H., Kong, X., Shi, L., Hou, L., Liu, Z., & Li, P. (2009). Gamma-linolenic acid induces apoptosis and lipid peroxidation in human chronic myelogenous leukemia k562 cells. *Cell Biology International, 33* (3), 402–410.

Garlic

Garlic, *Allium sativum*, is a bulb in the lily family. The bulb is segmented into smaller sections called "cloves." Around the world, garlic is used to flavor foods, and many people enjoy its pungent aroma and taste. A great number of cultures throughout time have also used garlic for medicinal purposes. Garlic has been shown to have multiple health benefits, including reducing the risk of cardiovascular disease, high blood pressure, and stomach and colon cancer. Garlic might help to prevent colds. Garlic has antifungal qualities when incorporated into a skin cream.

People in ancient Egypt used garlic medicinally, and buried pharaohs with garlic to give them health on their journey to the afterlife. Many cultures including the ancient Romans as well as modern European countries have used garlic poultices to prevent the infection of wounds. The well-known biologist Louis Pasteur was one of the first to demonstrate scientifically that garlic can kill bacteria. Garlic continues to be featured in folk remedies all over the world; many of these are gaining scientific support.

One of the active components of garlic is alliin. When garlic is crushed or cut, an enzyme is released that converts alliin to allicin and its derivatives. These contribute to garlic's strong odor and flavor. Although allicin is the most studied of garlic components, garlic contains many other compounds as well, including a number of trace minerals and essential fatty acids. For medicinal purposes, people use both raw and cooked garlic cloves as well as a variety of preparations, such as garlic powder and garlic oil formulas. Raw garlic exerts stronger physiological effects than garlic that has been cooked.

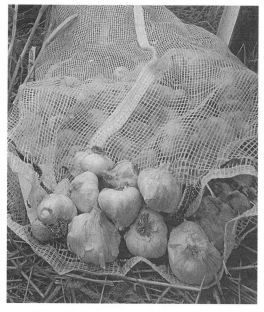

Garlic has been used as a health remedy around the world for thousands of years. It is a hardy plant that is relatively easy to grow. Garlic is usually grown by planting a single clove from a bulb of garlic. (U.S. Department of Agriculture)

Cardiovascular Effects: Blood Pressure and Artery Disease

When garlic is metabolized in the body hydrogen sulfide is released, which relaxes blood vessels. This relaxation of blood vessels results in a decrease in blood pressure, which is good for overall heart health. In addition to its effects on blood pressure, garlic also might reduce the risk of artery disease, which can cause heart attacks and strokes. Arterial plaque is most dangerous when it becomes inflamed and ruptures, releasing debris that can block arteries and interrupt blood flow. Garlic appears to exert anti-inflammatory effects in the body, increasing the release of immune-signaling molecules associated with decreased inflammation levels. Garlic preparations also are associated with decreased oxidation of low-density lipoprotein (LDL). Oxidized LDLs are believed to contribute to plaque deposition in the artery walls, thus accelerating the process of artery disease. Garlic also appears to boost the activity of the body's own powerful antioxidant systems, at least in laboratory animals.

Stomach and Colon Cancer

Garlic has been associated with a variety of anticancer effects in vitro, when human cancer cells in a glass dish are exposed to garlic. The application of this evidence in living people has not been as promising, however, probably because garlic does not come into direct contact with cancer cells, except in the digestive tract. In humans, several studies have found that people who consume more garlic have a lower risk of stomach and colon cancer.

Antimicrobial Effects

Garlic appears to have antimicrobial effects when it comes into contact with a variety of microbes, including bacteria, viruses, fungi, and protozoa. This does not mean that garlic can serve as a systemic antibiotic. The garlic must make direct contact with the microbe. This could explain why garlic preparations can serve as an effective treatment for fungal infections on the skin, or reduce oral bacterial concentrations when consumed raw. A few well-controlled studies have shown that consuming garlic can lead to decreased incidences and duration of common colds.

Safety and Side Effects

Garlic appears to very safe when consumed raw, cooked, or in supplement form. Side effects can develop, however, when large volumes of garlic—especially raw garlic—are used. Some people have experienced stomachaches, heartburn, nausea, diarrhea, and other symptoms of gastrointestinal distress after consuming garlic. Difficulty sleeping also has been observed in a minority of people. Garlic applied topically can cause skin irritation; raw garlic also can irritate the mouth and throat. Because garlic can have a blood-thinning effect, people taking anticoagulants probably should avoid ingesting large doses of garlic.

Elsa M. Hinds and Barbara A. Brehm

See Also: Allyl sulfides (organosulfurs).

Further Reading

Garlic (2012). Health Library. Retrieved from http://healthlibrary.epnet.com/GetContent .aspx?token=e0498803-7f62-4563-8d47-5fe33da65dd4&chunkiid=21729

Garlic (2011). MedlinePlus. Retrieved from http://www.nlm.nih.gov/medlineplus /druginfo/natural/300.html

Goldstein, M. C., & Goldstein, M. A. (2010). *Healthy foods: Fact versus fiction.* Santa Barbara, CA: Greenwood Press, pp. 133–138.

Tsai, C.-W., Chen, H.-W., Sheen, L.-Y., & Lii, C.-K. (2012) Garlic: Health benefits and actions. *BioMedicine, 2* (1), 17–29.

Gastroesophageal Reflux Disease

Gastroesophageal reflux disease (GERD) is a digestive disorder that affects people of all ages. The esophagus is a muscular tube that transfers ingested food and liquids from the mouth to the stomach. Gastroesophageal reflux (GER) occurs when the stomach's acid-containing digestive juices regurgitate from the stomach back up into the esophagus. It is also referred to as "acid reflux" or "acid regurgitation" because patients with gastroesophageal reflux report tasting food or acidic liquid in the back of their mouth. Patients often report burning feelings in the middle of their chests, directly behind the breastbone, a symptom known as "heartburn." The reflux of the acid can inflame the lining of the esophagus and can damage the muscles of the lower esophageal sphincter, causing it to not close properly. This allows for the contents of the stomach to travel back into the esophagus more easily, causing the more chronic gastroesophageal reflux disease (GERD). If GER is occurring twice a week or more, it could be a symptom gastroesophageal reflux disease. People who suspect that they might have GERD should seek medical attention. If left untreated GERD can cause serious health problems, including esophagitis, esophageal bleeding and ulcers, and strictures, and can increase the risk of developing esophageal cancer. Treatments for GERD include lifestyle change, especially dietary change; weight loss (if overweight); medications; and surgery.

Anatomy and Physiology of Gastroesophageal Reflex Disease

The esophagus, stomach, and esophagogastric junction (where the esophagus and stomach join) comprise the crucial anatomy of the gastrointestinal tract that is involved in gastroesophageal reflux disease. The cervical, thoracic, and abdominal sections make up the three parts of the esophagus with inner circular and outer longitudinal muscular layers maintaining the structure. The proximal esophagus accommodates the upper esophageal sphincter and is composed of striated and smooth muscle. The thoracic esophagus travels into the abdomen through the esophageal

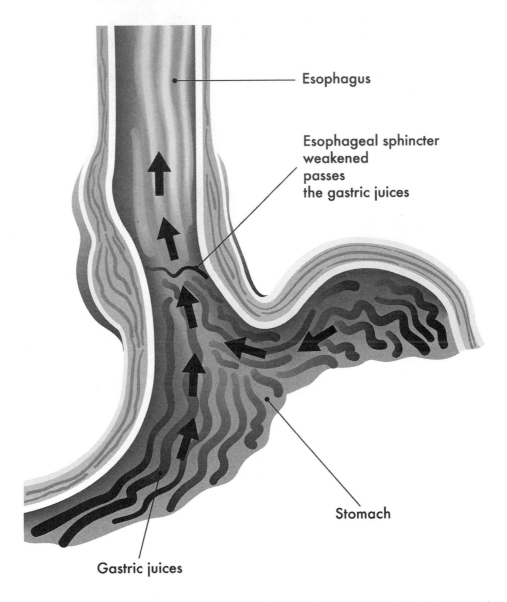

Acid reflux

Esophagus

Esophageal sphincter weakened passes the gastric juices

Stomach

Gastric juices

Gastroesophagel reflex refers to the movement of stomach contents up through the stomach and into the esophagus. The stomach has a specialized lining that prevents the acidic stomach contents from damaging the stomach. But the esophagus does not and is very vulnerable to damage caused by reflux. (Dreamstime.com)

Stomach Acid: A Good Thing or a Bad Thing?

"Heartburn" is a common name for "gastroesophageal reflux" (GER). When stomach contents are not digesting properly, fermentation begins, gas builds up, and the expanding stomach contents can press against the sphincter that separates the stomach from the esophagus. If this sphincter opens, the stomach contents, which are very acidic, can back up into the esophagus, causing pain, irritation, and even erosion of the esophageal lining.

Stomach acid actually is a good thing, thus the impulse to reach for antacids or proton pump inhibitors—drugs that reduce the stomach's production of hydrochloric acid and are marketed for GER—should be considered carefully. The highly acidic environment of the stomach disables many pathogens. Some research suggests that by reducing stomach acid, people are at increased risk for stomach cancer, initiated by the presence of bacteria in the stomach. Bacteria also increase risk of stomach ulcers.

Stomach acid increases the breakdown of food, facilitating separation of important nutrients so that they will be readily absorbed when they reach the small intestine. Stomach acid aids in the digestion of protein, for example. A highly acidic environment also helps calcium ions separate from food, thus making calcium more available in the small intestine. Studies suggest that people on long-term acid-reducing therapies decrease their absorption of calcium and thus increase their risk of osteoporosis.

Before reaching for products to reduce GER, it is important to try lifestyle measures first. Indigestion often is caused by eating too much too quickly, not chewing food enough, eating while feeling stressed, and consuming alcohol. Many people find that they have better digestion when they avoid high-fat meals, eat in a relaxing environment, chew their food thoroughly before swallowing, and consume smaller meals. Omitting alcohol can also aid digestion because alcohol can irritate the stomach. Meals should be consumed several hours before lying down so that gravity can assist stomach emptying. Some people also find relief with digestive enzymes such as papain and bromelain, which come from the fruits papaya and pineapple, respectively.

hiatus in the diaphragm, which creates a ring around the esophagus with right and left pillars. This allows for the esophagus to narrow when the diaphragm contracts. The phrenoesophageal ligament surrounds the esophagus at this level. The lower level of the phrenoesophageal membrane contains a fat pad on the anterior surface of the esophagus. The esophagogastric junction lies at the bottom of the esophagus in the abdomen, and contributes to the function of closure in the esophagus when intra-gastric and intra-abdominal pressures are at high levels.

The lower esophageal sphincter is a muscular valve between the esophagus and stomach that becomes strained or relaxed in individuals with gastroesophageal reflux disease. The lower esophageal sphincter is the most distal portion of the esophagus, ranging anywhere from 2 cm to 5 cm in length. The lower esophageal sphincter is responsible for keeping the top of the stomach closed and preventing the acidic contents of the stomach from traveling back up to the esophagus. Correct functioning of the lower esophageal sphincter is vital in preventing GERD.

Epidemiology

An estimated 7% to 10% of people in the United States experience GER symptoms on a daily basis, and 25% to 40% of Americans experience GERD symptoms at some point in their lives (Sawyer, 2013). Researchers believe that gastroesophageal reflux disease has become more common due to Western dietary habits, especially overeating, low intake of fruits and vegetables, and high alcohol intakes. It is as common in men as it is in women; however, white men are at a greater risk of Barrett esophagus and other adenocarcinomas than are other populations. GERD can occur in people of all ages, including infants. The prevalence of GERD is greater in people age 40 and older. Many individuals control symptoms with over-the-counter medications without consulting a medical professional, meaning that the actual number of people with GERD most likely is even greater.

Risk Factors

Several risk factors are associated with the development of GERD. Patients with asthma tend to have increased risk of developing GERD, as a relaxed lower esophageal sphincter causes asthma flare-ups. Asthma medications can worsen the acid regurgitation symptoms; however, it is not yet understood how or why. Reflux of the stomach's digestive acids also can worsen asthma symptoms by inflaming the lungs and airways. Irritated airways and lungs can trigger and cause more severe allergic reactions, because the irritation leaves people more sensitive to environmental conditions.

Abnormalities in the gastrointestinal system such as hiatal hernias also could be a casual factor. In hiatal hernias, part of the stomach is separated from the chest by the diaphragm. The upper part of the stomach pushes up into the chest and can slide through a gap (hernia) in the diaphragm. This opening is what can enable the stomach's digestive juices to travel back up through it, causing GERD. Other factors that could contribute to the development of gastroesophageal reflux disease are smoking, high alcohol intake levels, pregnancy, obesity, and certain medications such as calcium channel blockers, antihistamines, antidepressants, painkillers, and sedatives.

Signs and Symptoms

Common gastroesophageal reflux disease symptoms include regurgitation, heartburn, and dysphagia (difficult or painful swallowing). Excess and abnormal acid reflux can cause secondary esophageal symptoms such as bad breath, tooth cavities, sore throat, chest pain, wheezing, dry/chronic cough, asthma, nausea, vomiting, and otitis media (an infection of the middle ear). Long-term complications of GERD include esophagitis, strictures (a narrowing of the esophagus that causes difficulty swallowing), respiratory problems, and "Barrett's esophagus." Adults who have chronic forms of these complications can develop cancer of the esophagus. In the condition Barrett's esophagus, tissue of the intestinal lining replaces the tissue originally lining the esophagus in a process known as "intestinal metaplasia." People who develop Barrett's esophagus are more susceptible to esophageal adenocarcinoma, a rare and lethal type of cancer.

Diagnosis

A gastroenterologist is a physician who specializes in digestive diseases and can diagnosis GERD. A GERD-specific test does not exist for diagnosis but secondary symptoms can be measured with several other tests aiding in the diagnosis. The most common exams are the upper GI endoscopy, manometry, and 24-hour pH study. The endoscopy can aid in the confirmation of a reflux diagnosis by determining effects of the reflux by evaluating the anatomy of the esophagus. The manometry exam determines the pressure of the lower esophageal sphincter. The 24-hour pH test helps to confirm GERD in patients by determining if the pH levels of the esophagus are more acidic than normal. Upper GI imaging also might be ordered for a diagnosis with contrast into the stomach to determine if the contrast passes back up into the esophagus.

Treatment

Treatment for gastroesophageal reflux disease can include lifestyle changes, medication, and surgery. Lifestyle changes alone often are effective at reducing GERD symptoms, and usually are the first treatment approach. Lifestyle change strategies include losing weight, if a person is overweight; wearing loose-fitting clothing (tight clothing can constrict the GI tract and increase reflux); avoiding lying down 2 to 3 hours after meals (maintaining an upright position makes GER less likely); avoiding smoking; decreasing alcohol intake; and raising the top half of the bed 6 to 8 inches using stilts. Dietary changes that can reduce GERD-induced acid reflux and heartburn symptoms include avoiding foods and drinks that worsen symptoms such as carbonated beverages and spicy foods. Other dietary changes include decreasing meal portions and increasing meal frequency.

Most GERD medications are available over the counter; however if symptoms worsen or persist, patients should seek further medical attention from a professional. Antacids, such as Riopan and Alka-Seltzer, are the medical professional's first line of treatment to treat heartburn and other GERD symptoms. Zantac 75 and Axid AR are H2 blockers and decrease acid production. Proton pump inhibitors (PPIs), including omeprazole and lansoprazole, are more effective than H2 blockers at relieving symptoms and healing the esophageal lining. Prokinetics are used to empty the stomach faster; however they sometimes have psychological side effects including depression and anxiety. Antibiotics, such as erythromycin, have fewer side effects than prokinetics and also improve gastric emptying.

Surgery might be recommended when patients with GERD cannot manage their symptoms with lifestyle changes or medication. A fundoplication is performed as the standard medical treatment for GERD and leads to long-duration regurgitation control. The operation entails sewing the top of the stomach around the esophagus to the lower part of the esophagus, adding pressure that reduces regurgitation. Endoscopic techniques that sew and tighten the sphincter muscle are far less common and are less successful than the fundoplication.

Jessica M. Backus

See Also: Digestion and the digestive system; Esophagus; Stomach.

Further Reading

Gastroesophageal Reflux Disease. (2014). Medscape. Retrieved from http://www.nlm.nih .gov/medlineplus/gerd.html

Gastroesophageal Reflux (GER) and Gastroesophageal Reflux Disease (GERD) in Adults. (2013). NIH Publications. Retrieved from http://digestive.niddk.nih.gov/ddiseases /pubs/gerd/#GER

Sawyer, M. (2013). *Gastroesophageal reflux imaging*. Medscape. Retrieved from http:// emedicine.medscape.com/article/368861-overview

Silverthorn, D. U. (2012). *Human physiology* (5th ed.). Glenview: Person Education.

Genetically Modified Organisms

Genetically modified organisms (GMOs) are plants and animals whose genetic material has been altered using genetic engineering techniques. Although people have been genetically modifying food for centuries through cross-pollination, grafting, and other forms of crossbreeding, biotechnology experts have developed tools that allow them to alter an organism's genetic makeup with more precision, including inserting genes not naturally found in the target organism. The goal of genetic modification is to improve an organism, for example making a plant more resistant to disease or drought. Opponents of genetic modification worry that the long-term safety of these procedures is unknown in terms of impact on the consumer in the case of genetically modified food, and regarding the environment.

To create a food, such as a tomato, using a more traditional breeding technique, the DNA from one type of tomato is crossed with the DNA from another type via pollinization, with the hope of creating a plant with desired traits, such as increased sweetness, pest resistance, or more durability for the long journey to the supermarket. This process transfers both desired and undesired genes, however, therefore it can take many generations before the ideal traits are achieved, if at all. Biotechnology offers a more precise way to modify an organism's DNA. Popularly called "genetic modification" (GM), the terms genetic engineering (GE) and recombinant DNA (rDNA) biotechnology are more precise. Genetic modification, GE, and biotechnology often are used interchangeably. Recombinant DNA biotechnology enables scientists to take a specific piece of DNA from one plant or animal and combine it with a strand of DNA from another plant or animal. Instead of sharing thousands of genes (as with traditional breeding), genetic engineering

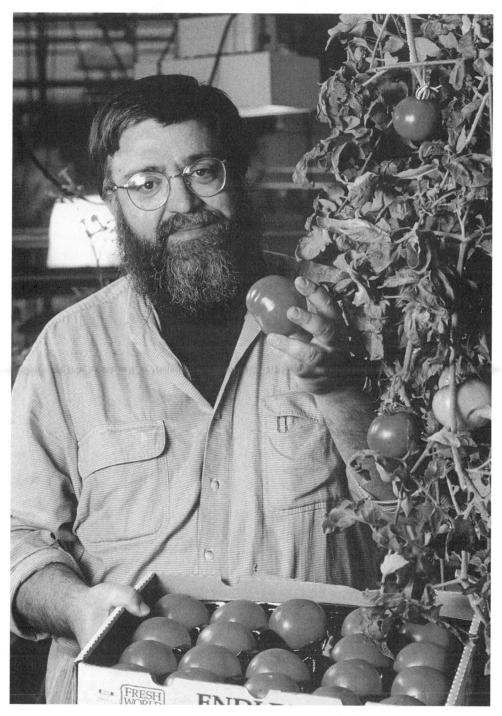

A plant physiologist displays a genetically modified tomato. Genetically modified foods do not require labeling in the United States, although many states are enacting legislation to require such labeling. Over 60 countries around the world, including those in the European Union, require labeling of genetically modified foods. (Agricultural Research Service/USDA)

permits a single gene to be exchanged. It also allows for combinations of DNA from organisms that never could be combined before.

Two methods are used to modify DNA through genetic engineering. One method uses a gene gun to shoot DNA-coated pellets into tissue of the receiving organism, some of which are incorporated into the cell nucleus. The second method uses the microbe *Agrobacterium tumefaciens*. Agrobacterium lives in the soil and infects the roots of plants. The agrobacterium infects by injecting an organism with a circular portion of its DNA called a "plasmid." Genetic engineers can replace the agrobacterium's plasmid with one they have created. The bacterium then transfers this DNA to the organism that the scientists are trying to modify.

"Cisgenesis" is the term used for gene transfer between two compatible organisms. The changes might have happened eventually through crossbreeding or evolution, but cisgenesis speeds up the process considerably. Cisgenesis also is referred to as "close transfer." "Transgenesis" refers to gene modification between organisms that are not sexually compatible, creating changes that most likely never would have occurred without genetic engineering. For example, DNA from the arctic flounder was injected into tomatoes to encourage frost-resistance. The experiment worked, although the tomatoes were not sold commercially. Transgenesis also is referred to as "wide transfer." Plants can also be "tweaked," meaning that genes within the plant are changed to create new expressions (Lemaux, 2008). "Genetically modified organism" (GMO) is the name given to a plant or animal that has been created through any type of genetic-engineering process.

The Flavr Savr tomato was the world's first commercially available "genetically modified" food and was introduced to consumers in supermarkets in 1994. It did not prove to be profitable, but it opened the door to a new era of food production. With its advent arose enormous questions of how, why, and when to use GMOs, and GM foods in particular.

Genetically Modified Foods

The United States is the largest producer of GM crops. More than 90% of all cotton and soybeans planted in the United States are genetically engineered, as well as 88% of corn (Allen, 2013). Other common GM crops include canola, alfalfa, and sugar beets. Most of these crops are engineered to tolerate herbicide or fight off pests. For example, Roundup Ready® soybeans are tolerant to RoundUp® herbicide (both products are produced by the same corporation, Monsanto). Other crops, such as Bt corn, contain DNA from a microorganism, *Bacillus thuringiensis* (Bt), which produces chemicals toxic to insects. *Bacillus thuringiensis* corn therefore produces its own insecticide against the European corn-borer insect.

The major GM crops are used to produce animal feed and food ingredients, such as corn starch, corn syrup, cottonseed oil, soybean oil, and canola oil. These ingredients are then used to make soups, salad dressings, cereals, chips, and other processed foods. Whole foods such as fruits and vegetables are less commonly made with genetic engineering, although that could change with increased consumer support. More than 70% of Hawaii's papayas are genetically engineered to resist the ringspot virus (Callis, 2013), and some varieties of disease-resistant squash, zucchini, and sweet corn also are on the market. In 1995, GM potatoes became available, but production ceased because the consumer market lacked interest. Several varieties of genetically engineered rice are in development, including "golden rice," which will include beta carotene, and rice that has been modified to contain the human enzymes lysostaphin and lysozyme, antibacterial agents that combat childhood diarrhea (Lemaux, 2008).

The most common use of genetic engineering among animals is for the creation of pharmaceuticals. In terms of foods, however, no meat, fish, or egg products created through GM are available for human consumption, although several have been or presently are being researched. In 1999, the University of Guelph in Ontario, Canada, developed a genetically engineered pig designed to create less pollution than conventional pigs. The project ended in 2012 because of lack of funding. Genetically modified rainbow trout and salmon also are being researched with the hopes of creating bigger, tastier fish in fish farms, thereby saving wild populations. Humans do consume milk that is the result of genetic engineering. Dairy cows are frequently given genetically engineered recombinant bovine growth hormone (rBGH) to increase milk production.

Regulation

Debate about GMOs frequently focuses on their regulation, which varies widely from country to country, and even from state to state within the United States because of new food labeling initiatives. In the United States, three federal agencies work in conjunction to regulate GMOs, the U.S. Food and Drug Administration (FDA), which is responsible for ensuring the safety of human and animal food; the U.S. Department of Agriculture (USDA), which is responsible for protecting agriculture from pests and disease; and the Environmental Protection Agency (EPA), which regulates food safety when connected with environmental concerns, such as pesticide use and crops that are genetically engineered to create their own pesticide, like Bt corn. Genetically modified foods must meet the same safety standards as traditional foods, as well as undergo tests for potential new toxins and allergens and any long-term risks from consumption. Nutrient levels between the GM crop and traditional crop also are compared.

Health Canada is the federal agency responsible for regulating GMOs grown and researched in Canada. Genetically modified foods have been sold in Canada since 1994, and all products must be approved before they can be marketed. More than 81 genetically modified foods have been approved, although not all are in commercial production.

The European Union (EU) has perhaps the most stringent GMO regulatory system. Few GM crops are grown in Europe, and those which are grown are predominately for research purposes. All GM crops require extensive testing, traceability, monitoring, and labeling, and many countries, such as Germany, have banned GM products altogether.

Arguments for and against GMOs

The genetic engineering of plants and animals is a complex issue with scientific, political, economic, and ideological implications. For every question answered, others are raised, and for every question raised, there are multiple answers. Some of the bigger issues are outlined in the table below, but the list is far from comprehensive in this ever-evolving debate.

Table 1. Genetically Modified Organisms

Issue	Arguments for GMOs	Arguments against GMOs
Risk to human health	• Substantial research shows that GM foods pose no health risks to humans. This position is supported by several large agencies, including the FDA, Health Canada, and the American Medical Association.	• Some research shows that there are risks to consuming GM foods. • Because this research is not positive regarding the corporations involved, it is hard to obtain funding and some researchers have lost their jobs because of their findings. • No studies can test the unknowns of new biotechnology. • GM foods only have existed for 20 years. Can research prove safe consumption for a lifetime when the products are so new?
Improved crop yield and pest resistance	• Plants genetically engineered to be disease resistant or herbicide resistant allow farmers to grow more per acre and use less pesticide, water, and fertilizer. Herbicide-resistant crops, for example, enable farmers to spray them with herbicide, which kills the weeds but not the crop.	• "Super weeds" have evolved that are herbicide resistant, causing more applications of herbicide rather than less. • The companies making the herbicide-resistant seeds also make the herbicide and are biased in their research and misleading in their marketing. • Increases in crop yields have not been significant.
Who benefits?	GM crops benefit everyone: • Farmers see increased profits • Food prices remain affordable • Developing countries are given resources to grow crops with improved nutritional value as well as crops more resistant to pests, disease, and extreme weather. • Technological innovation is nurtured by allowing corporations to patent their GM products.	• GM crops benefit the large corporations that develop them and patent their seeds. Farmers must buy patented seeds every year. Farmers have been sued by corporations for reusing patented seeds. • GM crops benefit large agribusinesses but not small farms or organic farms. • People in developing countries suffer from malnutrition because of lack of food. Food distribution must be improved, and not the food itself.

GMOs might spread to traditional plants and animals	• The risk of GMOs contaminating traditional plants and animals can be and has been managed effectively.	• There are numerous instances of GM crops contaminating GMO-free crops. Crops engineered to be weed-resistant, for example, cross-pollinate with the weeds, allowing the weeds to become resistant.
Regulation	• GM food is the safest food available because of the rigorous safety research required. • No food can ever be 100% safe.	• The FDA's regulation of GM foods is technically a voluntary consultation. • The GM food developers are the ones paying for the safety research. • Safety tests look for known risks; GMOs will have unknown risks.
Labeling	• Neither the United States nor Canada requires GM food to be labeled, although the FDA supports voluntary labeling of GM foods. • There is no reason to label because there is no real difference between GM foods and traditional foods. • Labels will cause uninformed consumers to think that GMO foods are unsafe.	• More than 60 countries require food made from genetically modified ingredients to be labeled. • If there is no risk to GM foods, why are companies afraid to label these products? • Consumers have a right to know what is in their food and make their own decisions about whether to buy it.
Additional Considerations	• Not all GMOs are the same and should be treated differently. • Not all GMOs are developed by large corporations. Many publically funded universities research and create GMOs. • Not all GMOs combine DNA from different species; some are combinations of similar species or even recombined DNA from the same species.	• All commercial varieties of GM crops are from the private sector, with the exception of papaya. • Tampering with the DNA of plants and animals changes evolution in a way that will have unexpected consequences. It could take a long time to know and understand the risks. Until more information is available, parties should proceed with caution—if at all.

Lisa P. Ritchie

Research Issues

Choose one of the arguments in Table 1 to investigate more thoroughly. Which side do you believe has the stronger argument?

See Also: Health Canada; Organic food and farming; Sustainable agriculture; U.S. Department of Agriculture; U.S. Food and Drug Administration.

Further Reading

Allen, K. (2013, June 16). *Is that corn genetically altered? Don't ask the FDA.* CNBC. Retrieved from http://www.cnbc.com/id/100814375

Callis, T. (2013, June 10). Papaya: A GMO success story. *Hawaii Tribune Herald.* Retrieved from http://hawaiitribune-herald.com/sections/news/local-news/papaya-gmo-success-story.html

Harmon, A. (2013, July 27). A race to save the orange by altering its DNA. *New York Times.* Retrieved from http://www.nytimes.com/2013/07/28/science/a-race-to-save-the-orange-by-altering-its-dna.html?pagewanted=all&_r=0

Lemaux, P. (2008, June). Genetically engineered plants and foods: A scientist's analysis of the issues (Part I). *Annual Review of Plant Biology, 59.* Retrieved from http://www.annualreviews.org/doi/full/10.1146/annurev.arplant.58.032806.103840

Sifferlin, A. (2012, Nov. 7). California fails to pass GM foods labeling initiative. *Time.* Retrieved from http://healthland.time.com/2012/11/07/california-fails-to-pass-gm-foods-labeling-initiative/

Tyson, P. (2001). *Should we grow GM crops?* PBS. Retrieved from http://www.pbs.org/wgbh/harvest/exist/

U.S. Food and Drug Administration. (2013, Apr 7). *Questions & answers on food from genetically engineered plants.* Retrieved from http://www.fda.gov/Food/FoodScienceResearch/Biotechnology/ucm346030.htm

Ginger

Ginger is the rhizome, or underground stem, of the *Zingiber officinale* plant and is used as a spice and medicinal herb. Originally from Southeast Asia, the plant has been used since ancient times in India and China as a remedy for gastrointestinal distress, especially nausea. Ginger can be consumed in a variety of forms including fresh, dried, powdered, candied, pickled, and ground. The main bioactive ingredients in ginger are called gingerol compounds, more than 31 of which have been

---

Is Ginger Always a Healthful Food?

Ginger is sold in many forms. It is interesting to compare the labels of these products to evaluate ginger content, as well as note the presence of other ingredients. Ginger slices coated with sugar, for example, often are marketed as a healthy snack. This product, however, can contain a great deal of sugar, sometimes more than 30 g of sugar in 6 small slices of ginger, providing more than 125 kcals. This is equivalent to the amount of sugar in a 12-oz serving of some soft drinks.

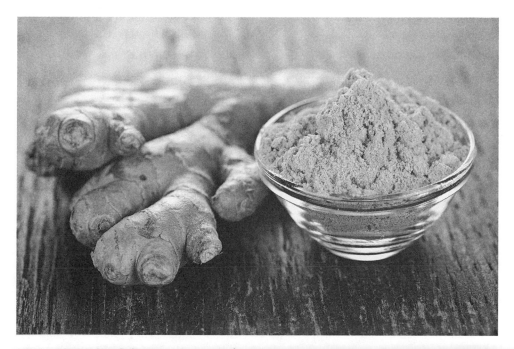

Fresh and powdered ginger root are popular spices in many countries. Ginger root comes from the ginger plant, a perennial, herbaceous plant that grows in tropical climates. (Elena Elisseeva/Dreamstime.com)

isolated. The most-studied is [6]-gingerol, which is found in the rhizome's oleoresin, or oily resin (University of Maryland Medical Center, 2011). The concentration of gingerols and other bioactive substances vary widely based on the preparation, including in mass-produced supplement products where contents are not heavily standardized.

Ginger has been used for thousands of years in traditional medicine. Many scientific studies also have explored the efficacy of ginger for a variety of symptoms and disorders. Ginger is best known as an antinausea agent because of its ability to break up and get rid of intestinal gas. It has been suggested that its interaction with serotonin receptors has a role in its soothing qualities in the digestive tract (Bode, 2011). People experiencing nausea and vomiting induced by motion sickness and possibly from chemotherapy might benefit from ginger consumption. Ginger also helps relieve inflammation. A few studies have found that ginger supplements (250 mg, 4 times per day, for three days) can reduce pain associated with menstrual periods (National Institutes of Health, 2012). Similarly, some benefit has been found for knee pain associated with osteoarthritis. Although a small number of studies suggest that ginger can reduce muscle pain following exercise, other studies have not found a benefit. In animal models, ginger has been observed to suppress several forms of cancer by inducing cell death and serving as an antioxidant, although a lack of clinical trials in humans leaves its practical utility questionable at present.

The U.S. Food and Drug Administration (FDA) recognizes ginger as being safe overall, although generally it is suggested that adults ingest less than 4 g daily. Because ginger could affect blood sugar and blood pressure regulation, people taking medications for diabetes or hypertension should consult their health care providers before using ginger. Ginger also can have a blood-thinning effect, so people taking anticoagulant medications should consult their providers before taking ginger supplements. Ginger might be somewhat effective for the treatment of morning sickness (nausea and vomiting) associated with pregnancy. Pregnant women should check with their providers before taking ginger supplements, however, and should not take more than 1 g of ginger per day.

Patricia M. Cipicchio

See Also: Dietary supplements; Inflammation.

Further Reading

Bode, A. M., & Dong, Z. (2011). Chapter 7: The amazing and mighty ginger. In *Herbal Medicine: Biomolecular and Clinical Aspects*, I. F. F. Benzie & S. Wachtel-Galor (Eds.). Boca Raton, FL: CRC Press.

Goldstein, M. C., & Goldstein, M. A. (2010). *Healthy foods: Fact versus fiction*. Santa Barbara, CA: Greenwood Press.

National Institutes of Health. (2012). *Ginger*. MedlinePlus. Retrieved from: http://www.nlm.nih.gov/medlineplus/druginfo/natural/961.html

University of Maryland Medical Center. (2011). *Ginger*. Retrieved from: http://www.umm.edu/altmed/articles/ginger-000246.htm

Ginkgo Biloba

The Ginkgo biloba or "maidenhair" tree is native to China. Its leaves are used in alternative medicine, especially with the intent of improving memory and concentration. The tree is one of the oldest living species on the planet, and some individual trees are estimated to be more than 1,500 years old. The Gingko's leaves and nuts have been a part of traditional Chinese herbal medicine as far back as the Yuan dynasty (1280–1368 BCE) and have been used to treat a variety of maladies from pulmonary disorders to alcohol abuse (Birks & Grimley, 2009). The Ginkgo biloba tree is a resilient organism, immune to many diseases and pests, and can thrive in heavy pollution. Although few other living species survived, six Ginkgo trees are known to have lived through the 1945 atomic bomb in Hiroshima, Japan.

Contemporary medicine has seen the development of a widely used standardized Ginkgo leaf extract. The active components of this extract are its flavonoids and terpenoids, a pair of organic acid groups unique to plants. The flavonoid compounds have been shown to exert antioxidant effects. The terpenoids act to dilate blood vessels and reduce platelet stickiness, thus improving blood flow. Gingko biloba preparations are available as supplements, are widely prescribed in many European countries, and have been the subject of an array of pre-clinical and clinical trials. Most studied has been the effectiveness of Gingko biloba supplements for the treatment of Alzheimer's disease and other forms of dementia. Although the Cochrane Database of Systematic Reviews has yet to affirm Ginkgo biloba as a clinically significant treatment for dementia or cognitive impairment, multiple trials have shown some improvement in cognitive symptoms in those with Alzheimer's and other dementias (Birks & Grimley, 2009). It is possible that the supplement could help a subgroup of dementia patients that is yet to be clearly identified.

The Natural Medicines Comprehensive Database (Gingko, 2014) rates supplements on their possible efficacy, based on the available scientific evidence. According to this group, Gingko biloba supplements are rated as "possibly effective" for Alzheimer's disease and other forms of dementia. Evidence suggests possible efficacy for improving cognitive ability in both young and old people. Ginkgo could improve circulation and relieve the pain associated with Raynaud's syndrome, a disorder characterized by severely reduced blood flow in the hands and feet. The supplement also might improve circulation and relieve the pain of peripheral vascular disease, such as intermittent claudication in the deep veins of the legs. Some studies suggest Ginkgo supplements have helped some with people with vertigo and dizziness. Ginkgo also might be effective in reducing symptoms associated with premenstrual syndrome (PMS).

The Gingko biloba leaf preparations generally are safe for most people, although reported side effects include upset stomach, headache, and skin rashes. Gingko supplements also might increase risk of bruising and bleeding, and should not be taken for several days before surgery. The roasted seed of the tree might be unsafe, and the fresh seeds are poisonous. Consumption of the fresh seed can lead to seizures and even death. Gingko biloba supplements appear to interact with a large number of prescription medications, so people on any kind of medication should check with their health care providers before taking gingko supplements (Ginkgo, 2014).

Patricia M. Cipicchio

See Also: Alzheimer's disease and nutrition; Antioxidants; Dietary supplements.

Further Reading

Birks, J. & Grimley, E. J. (2009). Ginkgo biloba for cognitive impairment and dementia. *Cochrane Database of Systematic Reviews,* 1, CD003120. Retrieved from http://www.ncbi.nlm.nih.gov/pubmed/19160216. doi: 10.1002/14651858.CD003120.pub3

Ehrlich, S. D. (2010). *Ginkgo biloba.* University of Maryland Medical Center. Retrieved from http://www.umm.edu/altmed/articles/ginkgo-biloba-000247.htm

Ginkgo. (2014, July 7). MedlinePlus. Natural Medicines Comprehensive Database. Retrieved from http://www.nlm.nih.gov/medlineplus/druginfo/natural/333.html

Vitamins and Supplements Lifestyle Guide: Ginkgo Biloba. (2012). WebMD. Retrieved from http://www.webmd.com/vitamins-and-supplements/lifestyle-guide-11/supplement-guide-ginkgo-biloba

Ginseng

Ginseng is a plant species used for a variety of pharmacological and clinical applications. It only grows in Eastern Asia and North America and its roots have been prized in China, Korea, and Japan for more than 2,000 years in traditional folk medicine. The ginseng root's gnarled appearance often is characterized by its human-like form. It is important to note that there are different kinds of ginseng which have different uses and effects. The most well-known ginseng plant is Panax ginseng, a name derived from the Greek word "panacea," which refers to a universal remedy. When the root is heated through sun drying or steaming, it becomes what is known as "Red ginseng," which typically is the form available for commercial distribution. Ginseng recently has gained wider acceptance in Western culture as one of the top 10 herbal dietary supplements in the United States, but is not as commonly used in food products because of its earthy, bitter taste (Chung, Lee, Rhee, & Lee, 2011). American ginseng, or *Panax quinquefolius*, is in the same genus but has different medicinal effects than Panax ginseng.

The primary bioactive components of ginseng are a diverse group of compounds called ginsenosides. These substances might play a preventative role for certain types of cancer, as well as inhibit tumor growth and reduce metastasis (the breaking off and spreading of tumors) (Wee, Park, & Chung, 2011). Additionally, treatment of diabetic animal models and humans with ginseng, especially *Panax quinquefolius*, suggest that the plant could reduce blood glucose and prevent development of type 2 diabetes.

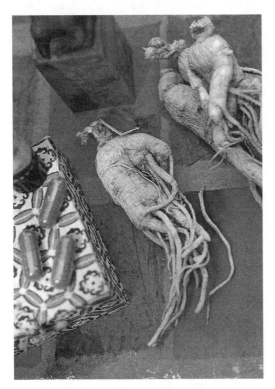

Ginseng root is used in Chinese and other herbal medicine traditions. The English word "ginseng" is derived from the Chinese words for "person" and "plant root," since the roots often resemble the human form. (Antaratma Images/Dreamstime.com)

Memory and neurodegeneration also could be affected positively by ginseng by reducing programmed cell death and facilitating the formation and retrieval of memories (Wee, Park, & Chung, 2011).

In addition to reducing blood sugar, The Natural Medicines Comprehensive Database, as reported in Medline, rates American ginseng as "possibly effective" for the prevention of cold and flu symptoms. The database also rates Panax ginseng to be "possibly effective" for improvement of thinking and memory and treating erectile dysfunction (NIH, 2012). Panax ginseng supplements typically are formulated to contain 4% to 7% ginsenosides, and are sold in 200 mg tablets. Therapeutic doses range from 200 mg to more than 2,000 mg per day. Some people also use raw ginseng, 1 g to 2 g daily during the treatment period. Ginseng is usually taken for only a 2- to 3-week period. Side effects are rare, although occasional cases of restlessness, sleeplessness, and hypertension have been reported. No toxicity level has been set, although users should exercise caution.

Patricia M. Cipicchio

See Also: Blood sugar regulation; Cancer and nutrition; Dietary supplements.

Further Reading

Chung, H. S., Lee, Y. C., Rhee, Y. K., & Lee, S. Y. (2011). Consumer acceptance of ginseng food products. *Journal of Food Science, 76* (9), 16–22.

National Institutes of Health (NIH). (2012). *Ginseng, Panax*. Retrieved from http://www.nlm.nih.gov/medlineplus/druginfo/natural/1000.html

Wee, J. W., Park, K. M., & Chung, A. (2011). Chapter 8: Biological activities of ginseng and its application to human health. In *Herbal Medicine: Biomolecular and Clinical Aspects*. Boca Raton, FL: CRC Press.

Global Hunger and Malnutrition

Currently, the world produces enough food to feed 10 billion people (Gimenez, 2012), yet from 2011 to 2013, more than 842 million people—roughly 12% of the world's population—were estimated to be suffering from chronic hunger (FAO, 2013). Of the one in eight people experiencing hunger and its associated health implications—which include fat accumulation in the central region of the body, insulin resistance in adults, hypertension, poor mental development in children, and behavioral abnormalities—approximately 827 million live in developing regions of the world such as parts of Africa, Asia, Latin America, and Oceania (FAO, 2013).

In the context of malnutrition, hunger is defined as the discomfort or weakness caused by a chronic lack of food. Malnutrition, literally "bad nutrition," often is characterized by an inadequate food intake, resulting in nutrient deficiencies. Malnutrition also can occur with adequate energy (calorie) intake but insufficient amounts of specific nutrients. Malnutrition generally is characterized by protein-energy deficiency or by vitamin-mineral deficiency. Protein-energy malnutrition (PEM) tends to be pervasive in resource-poor regions and essentially is the lack of energy and protein necessary for proper growth and development and for the maintenance of health. Commonly, PEM results in two similar but distinct diseases—marasmus and kwashiorkor—and their overlapping condition, marasmic-kwashiorkor. Marasmus refers to the chronic lack of energy needed to maintain body weight, and kwashiorkor is typified by the abnormal accumulation of fluid underneath the skin (edema), irritability, a distended abdomen, and an enlarged liver (FAO, 1997).

The second type of malnutrition—micronutrient deficiency—manifests in a variety of forms. The most prevalent form of malnutrition, iron deficiency, affects billions of people around the world and inhibits cognitive development. Vitamin A deficiency affects 140 million preschool children in 118 countries; increases the risk of dying from measles, malaria, and diarrhea; and is a leading cause of child blindness in developing countries. Iodine deficiency impacts 780 million people and results in mental developmental problems in newborns when women consume inadequate amounts during pregnancy. Zinc deficiency leads to weakened immunity in young children and contributes to about 800,000 child deaths per year (WFP, 2014).

Factors Influencing Global Hunger and Malnutrition

Chronic hunger and malnutrition can be caused by a wide variety of factors that limit people's access to food. These factors can grouped into four broad categories—availability, access, utilization, and stability.

Food availability describes the overall quantity of food for a given population supplied by domestic production and imports. Food production is dependent on a variety of factors including weather patterns, pest control, land management, and livestock management. Food importation is influenced by infrastructure, economic, political, and other factors.

As demonstrated by the fact that, in the early 1990s, 80% of all malnourished children lived in countries with food surpluses, access is a vital component to food security (FAO, 2002). Factors influencing access to food typically are divided into two categories—economic and physical. Economic access relies on disposable income, food prices, and sufficient social support. Physical access is determined by the availability of land resources; labor; inheritance; yields from agriculture, aquaculture, fisheries, and forests; and the ability of existing infrastructure such as roads, railways, communication, food storage facilities, and ports to facilitate market activity.

Poverty is a leading contributor to undernourishment and malnutrition. Market fluctuations due to policy changes, globalized trade, political conflict, and infrastructure management all potentially can impact a household or community's income and purchasing power, the local and regional allocation of food, and consequently the health of an entire area. Even if physical and economic accesses are controlled, full access to food still might not be achieved due to the tendency for some to prioritize the purchasing of some goods and services over food. Furthermore, the intra-household distribution of food might not allow individual household members adequate access to food to meet their physiological requirements (IFPRI, 2012).

Often seen as the interface between food availability and human health, food utilization encompasses both anthropometric indicators of undernourishment and malnutrition, such as height for age scores, height for weight scores, weight for age scores, and other measurements. It also includes and is affected by the sanitary conditions and preparation of the food (FAO, 2013). Although increased availability and access to food could help to correct global, regional, and household conditions, it does not necessarily follow that food utilization on an individual level will adequately address symptoms of hunger and malnutrition. Hunger and malnutrition could be exacerbated by diseases, for example, such as malaria, AIDS, and tuberculosis, which prevent individuals and caregivers from obtaining, preparing, and consuming adequate food. Food utilization also is influenced by the handling, preparation, and storage of food. Prior to ingestion and dependent on access to clean water, the hygiene and nutritional quality of food must be adequately maintained to ensure good health and nutrition absorption.

Stability is the measure of the transitory and permanent vulnerability of a food system. Instability can result from changes in water supply (due to the uncertainty of drought); the ability of foreign exchange reserves to pay for food imports; local supply and production of food; and overall food prices. Volatility of food prices and supply can be strongly influenced by national and global institutions such as the U.S Department of Agriculture, the World Bank, the International Monetary Fund, and the World Trade Organization. Increasingly, however, unpredictable droughts, hurricanes, and flooding due to climate change could lead to substantial decreases in income and food production for smallholders, pastoralists, and poor consumers, especially in parts of the world such as Africa, Latin America, and the Caribbean, which have experienced the greatest variability in food supply since 1990 (FAO, 2013).

The Green Revolution

Serious efforts to address world hunger and malnutrition took place from the 1940s through the 1960s with "The Green Revolution." The Green Revolution is said to have begun in 1940 when an American scientist, Norman Borlaug, conducted research on disease-resistant high-yield varieties (HYV) of wheat in Mexico. The term was officially coined by a U.S. Agency for International Development administrator, and the Green Revolution picked up momentum through the 1950s due to its success in Mexico. Combining Borlaug's wheat with mechanized agricultural technologies, Mexico began producing more wheat than domestically needed, and by the 1960s was a leading exporter of the crop (IFPRI, 2002). During the mid-1960s, with widespread hunger and malnutrition still prevalent in Asia and back-to-back droughts in India, for example, Green Revolution technologies had room to expand. The Rockefeller and Ford Foundations established an international agricultural research system to help adapt scientific advances in developing countries and began developing varieties of wheat and rice that would mature quicker, resist major pests and diseases, and retain desirable cooking and consumption traits (IFPRI, 2002).

By about 1990, 70% of wheat and rice in developing countries was converted to high-yield varieties (HYV), and by 1995 cereal production in Asia had doubled (IFPRI, 2002). Latin America also experienced significant gains, but Sub-Saharan Africa was only moderately impacted by the Green Revolution due to high transport costs, limited investment in irrigation, and market policies that made new technologies too expensive. A significant decline in global hunger and malnutrition, however, still is attributed to the agricultural growth of the Green Revolution (IFPRI, 2002). In many cases, raised incomes and reduced food prices that resulted from this rapid development have contributed to better nutrition. People have been able to consume added calories and a more diverse diet, as illustrated by increases in per capita consumption of vegetable oils, fruits, vegetables, and livestock products in Asia (IFPRI, 2002).

The Future

According to the Food and Agriculture Organization of the World Health Organization, 50% of the increase in crop yields in the recent years has come from irrigation and fertilizer and the other 50% has come from new seed varieties (FAO, 2010). Despite this yield increase and its ability to reduce poverty and hunger rates in developing countries, however, opponents of the Green Revolution argue that significant environmental and anthropological ramifications gradually have surfaced. When overused or used inappropriately, the high external inputs—namely fossil-fuel-based pesticides, fertilizers, and mechanization technologies—needed to ensure the production of HYVs in turn disrupt soil fertility, pollute waterways, kill beneficial wildlife, and poison agricultural workers (IFPRI, 2002).

The monocultures of wheat, soybean, corn, and rice cultivated by this process often require highly irrigated and high-potential rain-fed areas, resulting in an unquenchable reliance on groundwater, and economic and agricultural stagnation in areas with low rainfall. Moreover, this dependence on high-yield monocultures limits diet diversity, particularly the diets of poorer residents, by replacing a variety of nutrient-dense food crops from local food systems. The importance of biodiversity and the potential of wild crop varieties largely have been overlooked. The FAO estimates that throughout the 20th century, as much as 75% of crop diversity was lost. The FAO also has predicted that by 2055, 22% of the wild relatives of peanuts, beans, and potatoes will disappear due to climate change (FAO, 2010).

In response to issues regarding environmental quality and biodiversity, and subsequently human health and nutrition, methods of sustainable intensification have become more prevalent. Focused on increasing production, reducing food waste, moderating demand for resource-intensive foods, and improving the resiliency and efficiency of governance systems, many experts believe sustainable intensification is an alternative framework through which to achieve food security (Garnett et al., 2013). It advocates for practices such as cover cropping (planting extra crops before or after the regular growing season to improve the soil), contour farming, organic farming, rain harvesting, zero-tillage farming, sheet mulching, and agroforestry. These practices produce higher yields from the same area of land and lessen environmental impacts such as soil salinization, desertification, and soil erosion (Godfray et al., 2010). Unlike industrialized agriculture strategies furthered by the Green Revolution—strategies that reduce biodiversity, limit ecosystem services, and contaminate natural resources—sustainable intensification offers a way in which to rethink food production. Whether it is through site-specific, hands-on land-management strategies; integrated pest management systems; or integrated livestock-waste management systems and their simultaneous interface with animal welfare, institutional priorities, economic systems, and social capital, sustainable intensification provides an alternative approach to the problem of world hunger and malnutrition.

Tyler L. Barron

See Also: Climate change and global food supply; Food security and food insecurity; Sustainable agriculture.

Further Reading

Food and Agriculture Organization of the United Nations (FAO). (1997). *Human nutrition in the developing world*. Retrieved from http://www.fao.org/docrep/w0073e/w0073e00.htm

Food and Agriculture Organization of the United Nations (FAO). (2002). *Crops and drops: Making the best use of water for agriculture*. Retrieved from ftp://ftp.fao.org/docrep/fao/005/y3918e/y3918e00.pdf

Food and Agriculture Organization of the United Nations (FAO). (2010, October). *Crop biodiversity: Use it or lose it*. Retrieved from http://www.fao.org/news/story/en/item/46803/icode/

Food and Agriculture Organization of the United Nations (FAO). (2013). *The state of food insecurity in the world: The multiple dimensions of food security*. Retrieved from http://www.fao.org/docrep/018/i3434e/i3434e.pdf

Garnett, T., Appleby, M.C., Balmford, A., Bateman, I.J., Benton, T.G., Bloomer, P., Burlingame, B., Dawkins, M., Dolan, L., Fraser, D., Herrero, M., Hoffmann, I., Smith, P., Thornton, P. K., Toulmin, S. J., Vermeulen, C., & Godfray, H. C. J. (2013, July). Sustainable Intensification in Agriculture: Premises and Policies. *Science, 5* (341), 33–34. doi: 10.1126/science.1234485

Gimenez, E. (2012, May 2). We already grow enough food for 10 billion people—and still can't end hunger. *The Huffington Post*. Retrieved from http://www.huffingtonpost.com/eric-holt-gimenez/world-hunger_b_1463429.html

Godfray, H. C. J., Beddington, J. R., Crute, I. R., Haddad, L., Lawrence, D., Muir, J. F., Pretty, J., Robinson, S., Thomas, S. M., & Toulmin, C. (2010). Food security: The challenge of feeding 9 billion people. *Science, 327*, 812–818. Retrieved from http://www.sciencemag.org/content/327/5967/812.full

International Food Policy Research Institute (IFPRI). (2002, December). *Green revolution, curse of blessing?* Retrieved from http://www.ifpri.org/sites/default/files/pubs/pubs/ib /ib11.pdf

International Food Policy Research Institute (IFPRI). (2012, March). *The food security system: A new conceptual framework.* Retrieved from http://www.ifpri.org/sites/default /files/publications/ifpridp01166.pdf

World Food Programme (WFP). (2014, December 5). *Hunger FAQS.* Retrieved from http:// www.wfp.org/hunger/faqs

Glucosamine

Glucosamine is a natural compound present in human cartilage. Glucosamine is an amino monosaccharide, which is a sugar and protein composite. Glucosamine levels decline with age, causing researchers to question whether glucosamine supplements might help slow this decline, and perhaps even prevent the development of osteoarthritis (a condition marked by a loss of the cartilage that covers bones in the joints). Glucosamine sulfate often is taken with chondroitin—another component of cartilage—to relieve arthritis pain. Studies suggest it might not actually slow the process of osteoarthritis (which tends to worsen over time), but might be helpful for reducing pain, especially in people with moderate to severe knee pain caused by osteoarthritis.

Glucosamine injections initially were used in veterinary medicine in the 1970s as a treatment for larger animals that had joint pain, and treatments seemed to be successful. In the early 1990s, the Italian company Rottapharm combined glucosamine with sulfate to create the first supplemental form for humans. Several studies suggested that glucosamine supplements were helpful for many people with osteoarthritis (Towheed et al., 2009). The supplement came to the attention of the National Center for Complementary and Alternative Medicine—one of the centers that is part of the National Institutes of Health—which funded a well-controlled study of 1,583 people with osteoarthritis of the knee. This double-blind study was called the "Glucosamine Arthritis Intervention Trial" (GAIT). Researchers divided subjects into several groups and compared the effectiveness of glucosamine alone, chrondroitin alone, or the combination of both to a usual care group and a placebo group (Clegg et al., 2006). The researchers did not find much difference in pain levels among the groups, except for subjects in the glucosamine plus chondroitin group that had moderate to severe knee pain. Follow-up results did not show much difference between this group and the placebo group for arthritis progress; however, the placebo group had unusually slow progression, which could have muddied results (Clegg et al., 2006).

Glucosamine and chondroitin sulfate supplements did appear to be helpful for some subjects, with minimal side effects; therefore many experts suggest that patients suffering from arthritis pain should try using these supplements. Because dietary supplements in the United States are regulated as foods rather than drugs, it is important to be sure the supplements come from a reliable source. Supplements used in research studies came from the Rotta Research Laboratorium in Europe. Glucosamine is sold in a variety of forms; the most effective form is glucosamine and chondroitin sulfate.

Barbara A. Brehm, Amber Faith Walton, and Jessica M. Backus

See Also: Arthritis and nutrition; Dietary supplements.

Further Reading

Clegg, D. O., Reda, D. J., Harris, C. L., et al. (2006). Glucosamine, chondroitin sulfate, and the two in combination for painful knee osteoarthritis. *New England Journal of Medicine, 354,* 795–808. doi: 10.1056/NEJMoa052771

National Standard Research Collaboration. (2014). *Glucosamine.* Retrieved from http://www.mayoclinic.org/drugs-supplements/glucosamine/background/hrb-20059572

Towheed, T., Maxwell, L., Anastassiades, T. P., et al. (2009). Glucosamine for asteoarthritis. *Cochrane summaries.* Retrieved from http://summaries.cochrane.org/CD002946/glucosamine-for-osteoarthritis

University of Maryland Medical Center. (2011). *Glucosamine.* Retrieved from http://www.umm.edu/altmed/articles/glucosamine-000306.htm

U.S. National Library of Medicine, National Institutes of Health. (2011). *Glucosamine sulfate.* Retrieved from http://www.nlm.nih.gov/medlineplus/druginfo/natural/807.html

Glucose

Glucose is the most common simple carbohydrate compound (monosaccharide) in both plants and animals. In people, it is the primary source of energy for cellular metabolism. The term "blood sugar" refers to the glucose that is carried in the bloodstream. Blood glucose level is very important because cells in all body organs depend upon a reliable supply of glucose to carry out cellular functions. Glucose is the building block from which many other carbohydrates are made, including glycogen (the starch animals store in skeletal muscles and the liver) and many plant starches and fibers.

Extensive progress in understanding the structure of glucose occurred in the late 1800s in the laboratory of Hermann Emil Fischer in Germany. According to the scientist's autobiography, as a young man, Fischer was not very successful in his family's lumber business, wishing instead to study science. Fischer wrote that his father had declared that Fischer was not smart enough to succeed in business, so he had better be a student (Nobel Foundation, 1966). Fischer was an excellent student, received his doctorate in chemistry, and became a professor and researcher. He studied the chemical structure of a number of important molecules. Some of Fischer's most important work involved elucidating the structure of several monosaccharides—including glucose—and synthesizing glucose and other molecules from glycerol (a component of fatty acids). Fischer received the Nobel Prize in Chemistry for his work in 1902.

Plants produce glucose with the process of photosynthesis, using energy from the sun to combine water and carbon dioxide. Plants also combine units of glucose to make a variety of starches and fibers; can convert glucose into other monosaccharides; and can combine monosaccharide units to form disaccharides (two monosaccharide units joined together). All disaccharides contain at least one unit of glucose. People obtain glucose from food containing carbohydrates, or the body converts other nutrients, such as amino acids (from proteins) and glycerol (from fats) into glucose. Glucose also is found in the diet as an ingredient in processed foods, where it is called "dextrose."

Barbara A. Brehm

See Also: Blood sugar regulation; Carbohydrates; Digestion and the digestive system; Hyperglycemia; Hypoglycemia.

Further Reading

Brain, M. (2014, December 5) *How food works.* How Stuff Works. Retrieved from http://science.howstuffworks.com/innovation/edible-innovations/food2.htm

Nobel Foundation. (1966). The Nobel Prize in Chemistry 1902: Emil Fischer. In *Nobel lectures, chemistry 1901–1921.* Amsterdam: Elsevier Publishing Company. Retrieved from http://www.nobelprize.org/nobel_prizes/chemistry/laureates/1902/fischer-bio.html

Glutamine

Glutamine is the most abundant amino acid in the human body and is produced primarily in muscle tissue, the lungs, and the brain. Because it is synthesized by the body by combining the molecules ammonia and glutamate, it is not considered essential. In high-stress circumstances, however, such as after extreme workouts or trauma, the body must consume outside sources of glutamine. Dietary sources of glutamine include meat, milk, ricotta and cottage cheese, raw spinach, parsley, and cabbage.

Glutamine serves to remove the waste product ammonia from the body and is heavily utilized by cells in the immune system, particularly by white blood cells known as "lymphocytes" and "macrophages." There also is high demand for glutamine in the gastrointestinal tract, where it can help to protect the lining of intestines. Glutamine levels in muscle and blood plasma are reduced after surgery and radiation treatment as well as injury and burns. Although moderate exercise can promote increased glutamine synthesis, heavy endurance exercise and excessive training depletes glutamine and slows synthesis over time (Agostini, 2010). Low glutamine can compromise the functioning of the immune system and gut, leaving individuals vulnerable to more significant health issues.

Glutamine supplementation has proven beneficial in recovering from illness and surgery, leading to a reduced death rate in those with critical illness and trauma. Reduced levels of infection and shorter hospital stays also were found in a group that received glutamine following bone-marrow transplants. Patients considering glutamine supplementation should work with their health care providers, because excess amino acids can be harmful for people with reduced kidney function. In strenuous exercise, glutamine has been employed to boost the characteristically depressed immune system and to promote muscle growth and muscle glycogen stores (Gleeson, 2008). Although the supplement is well tolerated over time, clinical evidence is not sufficient to prove its efficacy in these areas. Protein supplements often include glutamic acid, an amino acid very similar in structure to glutamine. The body easily converts one form to another depending upon need.

Patricia M. Cipicchio

See Also: Amino acids.

Further Reading

Agostini, F. & Biolo, G. (2010). Effect of physical activity on glutamine metabolism. *Current Opinion in Clinical Nutrition and Metabolic Care, 13* (1), 58–64.

Gleeson, M. (2008). Dosing and efficacy of glutamine supplementation in human exercise and sport training. *Journal of Nutrition, 138* (10), 2045S–2049S.

Therapeutic Research Faculty. (2009) *Glutamine*. Natural Medicines Comprehensive Database WebMD. Retrieved from http://www.webmd.com/vitamins-supplements/ingredientmono-878-GLUTAMINE.aspx?activeIngredientId=878&activeIngredientName=GLUTAMINE

University of Maryland Medical Center. (2011). *Glutamine*. Retrieved from http://www.umm.edu/altmed/articles/glutamine-000307.htm

Glutathione

Glutathione is one of the body's most powerful antioxidants, low levels of which are associated with chronic illness and aging. Synthesized exclusively by the body and found in greatest concentrations in the liver, glutathione is a nonessential nutrient composed of the amino acids cysteine, glycine, and glutamine. Unlike most antioxidants, the molecule is located within nearly every cell, allowing it to directly scavenge free radicals and toxins. Glutathione not only neutralizes harmful reactive oxygen species directly, but it primarily is responsible for restoring the antioxidant potential of other useful antioxidants like vitamins C and E. Additionally, optimal levels of glutathione are important for supporting the activation of transcription factors that help control the expression of genes in cells.

Many factors can contribute to decreased glutathione levels, including poor diet, stress, and medications. Glutathione metabolism is regulated by several genes—some of which commonly are impaired in the general population. Many individuals are missing genes that regulate enzymes critical for making and recycling glutathione, for example, and this genetic profile (lacking the effective genes) might be associated with increased risk for certain diseases, such as several types of cancer (Yeh et al., 2010). Low levels of glutathione leave individuals less able to detoxify cells (Hyman, 2010). Research shows chronic diseases such as heart disease, cancer, autoimmune disease, diabetes, and arthritis nearly always are accompanied by glutathione deficiency. High-intensity exercise has been shown to immediately decrease plasma glutathione by increasing reactive oxygen species, therefore creating greater demand for the molecule's antioxidant properties (Elokda & Nielsen, 2007). Over time, however, exercise appears to increase plasma glutathione levels by increasing the ability of skeletal muscle to push glutathione into circulation, which increases its availability for the body (Kretzschmar & Muller, 1993).

Glutathione is present in most foods, especially protein foods. Supplementation has not proven beneficial, because the body breaks down the protein during digestion. Supplementation also has been associated with reduced endogenous production of glutathione. Instead, consumption of N-acetyl cysteine and alpha lipoic acid as well as folate, vitamin B6, and vitamin B12 could help boost glutathione levels (Hyman, 2010). High-quality whey protein also can provide the raw materials needed for glutathione production. (People allergic to milk products should avoid consumption of whey protein supplements.) The herb "milk thistle" helps to prevent depletion of the molecule in the liver (Das & Vasudevan, 2006).

Patricia M. Cipicchio

See Also: Antioxidants.

Further Reading

Das, S. K., & Vasudevan, D. M. (2006). Protective effects of silymarin, a milk thistle (Silybium marianum) derivative on ethanol-induced oxidative stress in liver. *Indian Journal of Biochemistry and Biophysics, 43* (5), 306–311.

Elokda, A. S., & Nielsen, D. H. (2007). Effects of exercise training on glutathione antioxidant system. *European Journal of Preventative Cardiology, 145*, 630–37.

Glutathione. (2012). Health Library. Retrieved from http://healthlibrary.epnet.com/GetContent.aspx?token=e0498803-7f62-4563-8d47-5fe33da65dd4&chunkiid=108306#ref32

Hyman, M. (2010). Glutathione: The mother of all antioxidants. *Huffington Post.* Retrieved from http://www.huffingtonpost.com/dr-mark-hyman/glutathione-the-mother-of_b_530494.html

Kretzschmar, M., & Muller, D. (1993). Aging, training and exercise. A review of effects of plasma glutathione and lipid peroxides. *Sports Medicine, 15* (3), 196–209.

Palkhivala, A. (2001). *Glutathione.* MedicineNet. Retrieved from http://www.medicinenet.com/script/main/art.asp?articlekey=50746

Yeh, C.-C., Lai, C.-Y., Hsieh, L.-L., Tang, R., Wu, F. Y., & Sung, F. C. (2010). Protein carbonyl levels, glutathione S-transferase polymorphisms and risk of colorectal cancer. *Carcinogenesis, 31* (2), 228–233. doi: 10.1093/carcin/bgp286

Gluten-Free Diets and Foods

Gluten is a protein found in certain grains, including wheat, rye, and barley. Gluten-free diets refer to diets that contain minimal amounts of gluten (or none); gluten-free foods refer to foods that contain minimal or no gluten. Many gluten-free foods are naturally gluten-free, for example all vegetables, fruits, meats, and dairy products that have no added ingredients. Some food products—such as breads and baked goods that typically are made from wheat flour—can be made with wheat substitutes containing no gluten. Gluten-free foods often are consumed by people who must or who choose to avoid gluten, but who still wish to eat such products—which are very popular and common in the diet of most North Americans.

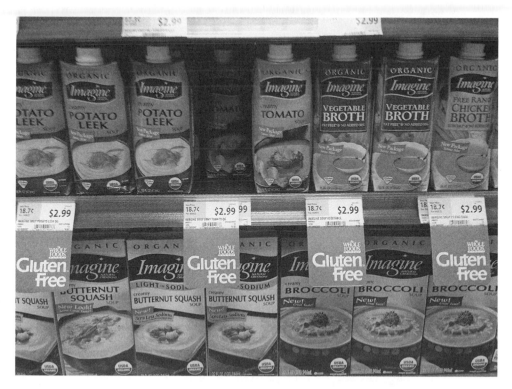

Gluten-free products on a grocery store shelf. In the United States, products labeled "gluten-free" have to contain less than 20 parts per million of gluten. (AP Photo)

People avoid gluten for a variety of reasons. In about 1% of the population, gluten elicits an autoimmune response, in which immune cells mistakenly attack the lining of small intestine. People with this autoimmune response and the accompanying damage to the small intestine are diagnosed with celiac disease, which is an inherited disorder. The only treatment for celiac disease is a lifelong gluten-free diet and avoidance of all gluten-containing foods, beverages, and medications, as no cure currently exists.

Some people avoid gluten because they are allergic to wheat. A wheat allergy is a type of food allergy. Allergic responses are characterized by a range of symptoms, from hives, rashes, and swelling to difficulty breathing and loss of consciousness. In severe cases, food allergies can be fatal. Wheat allergies are thought to affect about 0.1% of people in North America (Gaesser & Angadi, 2012).

Some people without celiac disease or wheat allergies could experience distressing symptoms, such as intestinal gas, bloating, pain, and constipation, as well as non-GI symptoms such as fatigue and headaches, when they consume gluten-containing foods, a condition known as non-celiac gluten sensitivity (NCGS). To receive a diagnosis of NCGS people must test negatively for celiac disease; experience the functional negative symptoms associated with celiac disease, such as bloating and pain after ingestion of gluten-containing foods; and show symptom improvement with a gluten-free diet. Recent research suggests that many people currently diagnosed or who have self-diagnosed themselves with NCGS actually could be sensitive to food components other than gluten, such as certain types of small carbohydrate groups common in grains (Biesiekierski et al., 2013; Catassi et al., 2013). These components have been called "FODMAPs," an acronym that stands for fermentable oligo- , di- , and mono-saccharides and polyols. FODMAPs are poorly absorbed in the GI tract of people with functional bowel disorders, such as irritable bowel syndrome. When the FODMAPs reach the large intestine, the microbes living there metabolize these molecules, releasing gas in the process. The gas increases feelings of bloating, pressure, and pain, and can interfere with normal colon motility. The elimination of gluten-containing foods concomitantly reduces intake of these FODMAP components, leading to an amelioration of NCGS symptoms.

People who suspect that they might have a gluten sensitivity of some sort should seek medical advice and be tested for celiac disease, rather than self-diagnosing this condition. Celiac disease is a serious illness that can compromise long-term health if untreated.

Gluten-free diets and foods have become popular even among people with no adverse GI reactions to gluten. One survey performed by a market-research company found that 30% of respondents expressed a desire to cut back on gluten consumption (Hamblin, 2013). This might be attributable to popular media that have sensationally painted gluten as a food ingredient responsible for everything from autoimmune diseases to brain disorders such as autism, anxiety, depression, and Alzheimer's disease. Although a few research studies have linked gluten consumption to neurological disorders in animals and a small number of humans, especially people with celiac disease, the research is very preliminary at this point (Hamblin, 2013).

Even though gluten-free diets have been promoted as successful weight-loss strategies, evidence supporting this claim is lacking. Temporary weight loss often occurs when people eliminate foods from their diet. Several studies suggest that gluten and other components of gluten-containing whole grains could have important health benefits for people without celiac disease, wheat allergies, or NCGS, including better colon microbiome composition (beneficial bacteria in the gut) and protection from colon cancer. A diet high in cereal fibers appears to contribute to healthful blood pressure regulation, blood sugar regulation, and blood fat levels (Gaesser & Angadi, 2012). These observations suggest that eliminating wheat, barley, and rye from the diet of people without celiac disease, wheat allergies, or NCGS could have negative impacts on pubic health.

Food products must meet certain standards to make a gluten-free label claim. In the United States such claims are regulated by the Food and Drug Administration (FDA). According to FDA regulations, a product may claim to be gluten-free if it has less than 20 ppm of gluten (FDA, 2014). Consumers should note that gluten-free products such as baked goods are not automatically healthful foods, but actually can contain significant amounts of added sugars, salt, and fats.

Barbara A. Brehm

See Also: Celiac disease; Fiber; Food allergies and intolerances; Intestinal gas; Irritable bowel syndrome; Microbiota and microbiome.

Further Reading

Biesiekierski, J. R., Peters, S. L., Newnham, E. D., Rosella O., Muir, J. G., & Gibson P. R. (2013). No effects of gluten in patients with self-reported non-celiac gluten sensitivity after dietary reduction of fermentable, poorly absorbed, short-chain carbohydrates. *Gastroenterology, 145* (2), 320–8.e1-3. doi: 10.1053/j.gastro.2013.04.051

Catassi, C., Bai, J. C., Bonaz, B., et al. (2013). Non-celiac gluten sensitivity: The new frontier of gluten related disorders. *Nutrients, 5* (10), 3839–53. doi: 10.3390/nu5103839

Food and Drug Administration (FDA). (2014, June 5). *Gluten and food labeling: FDA's regulation of "gluten-free" claims.* Retrieved from http://www.fda.gov/Food/ResourcesForYou/Consumers/ucm367654.htm

Celiac Foundation. (2014, December 5). *Gluten sensitivity.* Retrieved from http://celiac.org/celiac-disease/non-celiac-gluten-sensitivity/

Gaesser, G. A., & Angadi, S. S. (2012). Gluten-free diet: Imprudent dietary advice for the general population? *Journal of the Academy of Nutrition and Dietetics, 112* (9), 1330–1333. doi: 10.1016/j.jand.2012.06.009

Hamblin, J. (2013, December 20). This is your brain on gluten. *The Atlantic.* Retrieved from http://www.theatlantic.com/health/archive/2013/12/this-is-your-brain-on-gluten/282550/5/

Strom, S. (2014, Feb 17). A big bet on gluten-free. *New York Times*. Retrieved from http://www.nytimes.com/2014/02/18/business/food-industry-wagers-big-on-gluten-free.html?_r=0

Glycemic Index and Glycemic Load

The glycemic index (GI) of a food is a measure of the food's impact on blood glucose level following its ingestion. Specifically, glycemic index is a measure of how quickly glucose appears and how high its level rises in the blood after a given portion of carbohydrate from that food is consumed, relative to the blood glucose response of a standard food such as pure glucose or white bread. Foods such as sugar, white bread, and instant white rice have a high glycemic index. The sugars and starches in those foods are digested and absorbed very quickly. Foods such as whole-grain breads, oatmeal, and berries have a lower glycemic index, which means it takes the body longer to digest and absorb the sugars and starches in these foods. Knowing a food's glycemic index is helpful for people who want to raise their blood sugar quickly, as would be the case for someone with hypoglycemia (low blood sugar). People who are trying to avoid high blood sugar, such as people with diabetes, also can benefit from knowing the GI of foods so they can avoid foods that might raise their blood sugar level too high.

In terms of chronic health issues, such as heart disease, the glycemic index of a particular food is not as important as a variable called glycemic load (GL), which represents the glycemic index multiplied by the grams of carbohydrate in the actual serving of food, divided by 100. Although GI is measured for a standard amount of carbohydrate, GL reflects the typical serving size of foods and better represents what people actually eat. For example, cooked beets have a relatively high glycemic index (64) but a fairly small amount of carbohydrate per serving, and thus a low GL (4). Macaroni has lower glycemic index (45) but quite a bit of carbohydrate per serving, and thus a high GL (22). Studies suggest that people consuming a relatively high-glycemic-load diet throughout their lives tend to have higher rates of chronic disease, especially heart disease (CQC, 2013). A high glycemic load is correlated with higher blood glucose levels after meals, which appear to be related to greater risk of disease progression, perhaps through higher levels of insulin and obesity.

Calculating Glycemic Index and Glycemic Load

Glycemic Index is calculated by measuring blood sugar changes in people after they consume standard amounts of specific foods. For example, to calculate the GI of apples, the subjects first might consume 50 grams of carbohydrate from pure glucose, the standard to which apples will be compared. Scientists monitor the subjects' blood glucose levels over time, noting how quickly and how high blood glucose levels rise, and how long it takes for blood sugar to return to normal. These measures are plotted on a graph, and the area under the curve is calculated. On a separate occasion, the same participants would consume a portion of apples containing 50 g of carbohydrate under test conditions identical to the glucose trial. To calculate GI, the area under the apple curve is divided by the area under the glucose curve for each subject, and the results are averaged. The GI for apples is about 40. This means that the area under the curve for apples is about 40% of the area under the curve for pure glucose.

A number of different organizations have calculated the GI for various foods. The GI of a variety of foods can be found at www.glycemicindex.com, a GI database overseen by the University of Sydney, Australia. The GI of a given food can vary somewhat among databases, as some use different reference foods (for example, white bread rather than glucose) or a different variety of food being tested, such as different varieties of apples. This means that GI is simply a relative value rather than a precise number. In general, a GI of 55 or less is considered low; 56 to 69 is medium; and 70 or more is high.

To calculate the GL of an apple, multiply the GI, in this case 40, by the grams of carbohydrate present in a typical serving, 15 g, and then divide that number by 100 (to standardize values to a 100 g serving). This gives a GL of about 6.

$$\frac{40 \times 15 \text{ g}}{100 \text{ g}}$$

In general, a GL of 10 and under is considered low; 11 to 19, is medium; and 20 or greater is high. Some calculations of GL use 1,000 kJ (a measure of energy content equivalent to about 139 kilocalories) in the denominator to standardize for a food's energy value rather than its weight (CQC, 2013).

Factors That Influence Glycemic Index and Glycemic Load

Several factors influence a food's glycemic index and glycemic load. Of course, the food must contain carbohydrates, such as sugars or starches. Foods such as oils and meats that do not contain carbohydrate do not release glucose into the bloodstream; thus these foods do not have a GI.

The nature of the carbohydrates contained in a food influences that food's GI. The digestive system breaks down carbohydrates in foods and transports the resulting monosaccharides (basic carbohydrate structures), such as glucose and fructose, into the bloodstream. The liver converts fructose to glucose and releases some of the glucose back into the bloodstream. The speed of the digestion and absorption of a food depends upon the amount of simple carbohydrates (sugars) versus complex carbohydrates (starches) in the food, and the structure of the molecules. Some starch formations, for example, are broken down more quickly than others.

Additionally, the other structures in a given food influence the speed of digestion and absorption. Dietary fiber (especially water-soluble fiber) and fats slow down the digestion and absorption of carbohydrates. Interestingly, pasta has a fairly low GI, even though it has very high levels of carbohydrate. This is because the carbohydrate is bound up with a protein called gluten, found in wheat and some other grains, that makes the carbohydrate less accessible to digestive enzymes.

The composition of other foods consumed at the same time as the carbohydrate food impact digestion and absorption. A baked potato, for example, has a fairly high GI. If it is consumed with high-fat toppings such as chili, cheese, and sour cream, however, then the potato and its toppings stay in the stomach longer, and the digestion and absorption of carbohydrates from the potato occurs more slowly. (Carbohydrate digestion and absorption occur primarily in the small intestine; thus when food stays in the stomach longer, carbohydrate absorption slows.)

Applications

Epidemiological studies of dietary and lifestyle factors associated with chronic diseases and premature mortality are increasingly including glycemic load as a risk factor, as risk of all-cause mortality increases with GL (e.g., Baer, Glynn, Hu, et al., 2011). An international panel of experts suggests that reducing GL can be especially helpful for improving blood sugar regulation in people with type 2 diabetes, and for reducing risk of cardiovascular disease (CQC, 2013). This same group also suggests that low GL diets might reduce risk by decreasing insulin response, improving blood lipid levels, and reducing levels of systemic inflammation, although more research is needed to explain and quantify these relationships (CQC, 2013). Knowledge of a food's GI or GL alone is insufficient to guide dietary choices. Research on GL, however, generally reinforces other advice on healthful eating that urges people to consume healthful proteins and fats; choose whole grains rather than refined grains; consume a wide variety of carbohydrate foods, including fruits, nonstarchy vegetables, and legumes; and limit foods with added sugars and refined grains, especially soft drinks and dessert goods such as cookies and cakes.

Barbara A. Brehm

Research Issues

Knowing a food's glycemic index (GI) or glycemic load (GL) can be helpful for anyone trying to exert control over blood sugar levels, including athletes. Athletes sometimes speak of low- and high-glycemic-index foods as "slow" and "fast" carbohydrates. Fast carbohydrates (high GI) foods are helpful for coping with exertional hypoglycemia (low blood sugar that results from high levels of exercise) and replenishing depleted carbohydrate (glycogen) stores as quickly as possible. Athletes looking for ways to refuel during physical activity, for example, will find that high glycemic foods have a quicker impact on blood sugar. The same is true for athletes who exercise more than once per day; fast carbohydrates help restore glycogen and blood sugar levels between workouts or competitions. Fruit juices, sports beverages, and other high-sugar foods low in fat and fiber allow carbohydrate to enter the bloodstream quickly. Conversely, consuming high GI foods too soon before exercise can lead to a high insulin response, and then a drop in blood sugar levels that leave an athlete tired at the beginning of a workout or contest. Hundreds of food products—including sports drinks, bars, goos, and gels—have been designed for athletes seeking optimal glycogen and blood sugar levels.

See Also: Blood sugar regulation; Carbohydrates; Diabetes, type 1; Diabetes, type 2; Digestion and the digestive system; Fiber; Glucose; Insulin.

Further Reading

Atkinson, F. S., Foster-Powell, K., & Brand-Miller, J. C. (2008). International tables of glycemic index and glycemic load values: 2008. *Diabetes Care, 31* (12), 2281–2283.

Baer, H. J., Glynn, R. J., Hu, F. B., et al. (2011). Risk factors for mortality in the Nurses' Health Study: A competing risks analysis. *American Journal of Epidemiology, 173* (3), 319–329.

Carbohydrate Quality Consortium (CQC). (2013). *Glycemic index, glycemic load and glycemic response: Scientific consensus statement.* Retrieved from http://www.glycemicindex.com/blog/2013/July/GI%20Summit%20Consensus%20Statement.pdf

Higdon, J. (2010). *Glycemic index and glycemic load.* Linus Pauling Institute, Oregon State University. Retrieved from: http://lpi.oregonstate.edu/infocenter/foods/grains/gigl.html

University of Sydney. (2012a). *GI database.* Retrieved from www.glycemicindex.com

University of Sydney. (2012b). *Frequently asked questions.* Retrieved from http://www.glycemicindex.com/faqsList.php

Grains

Grasses that are cultivated for food have seeds which are called "grains." True grains belong to the Poaceae botanical family. Nutritionists generally include several other plants, such as amaranth, buckwheat, and quinoa in the "grain" family, as they are prepared and consumed in similar ways. Grains provide a significant portion of the daily energy intake in most countries around the world. The whole grain consists of three parts: the bran is the outermost layer that protects the grains from the environment, the endosperm is what provides food for the seedling, and the germ is the plant embryo. What makes whole grains whole is they have not been milled—a process that removes some or all of the bran and germ along with the nutrients and fiber found in those components. Grains can be consumed as whole or milled grains or when made into other products. Public health campaigns are encouraging consumers to replace some of the milled or refined grain products in their diets with whole grains and whole grain products, to improve diet quality.

Grains commonly cultivated and consumed include the following (Whole Grains Council, 2014; CDC, 2012).

- Amaranth: This grain usually is popped and eaten like popcorn and is especially high in fiber and protein. Like quinoa and buckwheat it is not a true grain.
- Barley: Barley often is used in soups and stews and is a great source of fiber.
- Buckwheat: This pseudo-grain is one the most heart-healthy choices because it is high in helpful phytochemicals and magnesium.

- Corn: Many people think of corn as a vegetable but it actually is a grain. Corn is high in fiber and beneficial phytochemicals.
- Millet: This grain often is served like rice and is high in magnesium, manganese, and phosphorous.
- Oats: Oats are one of the most popular grains, consumed whole, rolled, or in a variety of products. The soluble fiber in oats helps to lower blood cholesterol levels.
- Popcorn: Popcorn is a familiar grain to moviegoers. Once this whole grain is popped and drenched in fats and salts, its health benefits are reduced. Popping in healthful oils and adding small amounts of salt along with other herbs and spices can create a more healthful snack.
- Quinoa: This pseudo-grain offers more protein than any other grain, and the protein is complete, meaning that it has all nine essential amino acids.
- Rice: Brown rice (a whole grain) contains greater amounts of vitamins, minerals, and fiber than does white rice, which is polished to remove the outer covering.
- Rye: Rye usually is used in breads and is an excellent source of manganese.
- Teff: Teff is the smallest grain in the world.
- Triticale: The triticale grain is a hybrid of wheat and rye.
- Wheat: Many varieties of wheat are found in the food supply, including durum, bulgur, faro, spelt, and kamut. Wheat products include breads, pasta, and couscous, along with baked goods made from wheat flours.
- Wild Rice: Wild rice actually is not a type of rice, but is a grain that has a strong nutty flavor and is an excellent source of fiber and protein.

Nutritional Content

Whole grains contain many vitamins as well as dietary fiber. Whole grains offer a high concentration of B vitamins such as riboflavin, thiamin, and niacin, as well as minerals such as calcium, magnesium, and potassium. Whole grains also have significant amounts of fiber and protein. High antioxidant activity is associated with many of the phytochemicals found in whole grains. Common grain phytochemicals include lignans, phenolic compounds, tocotrienols (forms of vitamin E), tannins, enzyme inhibitors, and phytic acid.

Refined grains are grains that have been milled, a process that removes the bran and germ. Removing these components extends the shelf life of the grain product and creates a finer flour texture. Despite not being as healthful, refined grains and their products are popular in many countries. Refined grains include white flour and white rice. Grain flours are used to make white bread, cereals, crackers, pastries, and desserts.

Enriched and fortified grain products have added nutrients. Enriched means that nutrients typically removed during the milling process, such as B vitamins, are added back to the product. Fortified means extra nutrients, such as iron, that were not present in the original grain are added to the product. These added nutrients are listed on the labels of food products.

Grains and Health

Grains supply consumers with a rich source of complex carbohydrates. Although carbohydrates serve as an important fuel substrate for energy production, obesity can result if too many calories—including calories from carbohydrates—are consumed. Grain products such as donuts and dessert foods also can be high in added fats and sugars. Therefore, the health effects of grain consumption hinge on how grains are consumed.

Studies support the idea that a moderate consumption of whole grains prepared in healthful ways contributes to good health for people in energy balance, that is, people not consuming excess calories. Epidemiological studies suggest that the consumption of whole grains, rather than refined grains and grain products, is associated with a decreased risk of cardiovascular disease (CVD) (Jonnalagadda et al., 2011). Researchers believe the benefits of whole grains for cardiovascular health probably are attributable to the higher intake of cereal fiber. Other components in whole grains like antioxidants, lectins, and phytic acid also might reduce risk for CVD (Slavin, 2004).

Some studies indicate that consumption of whole grains is associated with reduced rates of gastrointestinal cancer and possibly other cancers. Whole grains contain selenium, vitamin E, and phytochemical antioxidants that might help slow carcinogenic processes in cells. Many phytochemicals found in grains, including digestive enzyme inhibitors, saponins, phytic acid, and phenolics could act as cancer inhibitors, as they might have the ability to prevent the formation of carcinogens as well as being able to block the interaction of carcinogens with cells (Slavin, 2004).

Rates of type 2 diabetes have been increasing dramatically in the United States and many other countries. This disease often can be controlled through lifestyle changes that produce weight loss, for those who are overweight, and prevent high blood glucose levels. Reducing consumption of carbohydrate foods often is part of type 2 diabetes treatment. Along with reducing carbohydrate intake, replacing the intake of refined grains with whole grains is recommended to increase fiber intake and diet quality. Researchers think that people consume fewer calories per day when their diets contain more fiber. It is possible that increasing dietary fiber content might help people eat less and could prevent weight gain.

Labeling of Whole Grain Products

The term "100% whole grain" means something different according to which agency is defining it. According to the U.S. Department of Agriculture Food and Nutrition Service, a food is considered whole grain when it meets one of three requirements: (1) it has 8 g of whole grain per serving; (2) it is 51% whole grain by weight; or (3) it has a whole grain as the first ingredient (Whole Grains Council, 2014).

Grains and Gluten

People with celiac disease, gluten intolerance, non-celiac gluten sensitivity, and wheat allergies must avoid foods that contain a protein called gluten. Gluten is found in all varieties of wheat and wheat products, barley, and rye. Other grains, including the pseudo-grains amaranth, buckwheat, and quinoa, do not contain gluten. Consumers should be aware, however, that these gluten-free grains can become contaminated with wheat and other gluten-containing grains during processing. Food labels can help consumers find out which products should be gluten free.

Improving Grain Choices

The *Dietary Guidelines for Americans* recommends that adults should consume at least half of their grains as whole grains. The purpose of this recommendation is to reduce the consumption of grain products of lower nutrient density, possibly reducing the consumption of dessert foods with added fats and sugars, and increase people's intake of cereal fiber. The consumption of whole grains is much lower than what is recommended; Americans on average have less than one serving of whole grains per day and 40% of adults don't have whole grains in their diet at all (Whole Grains Council, 2014).

How to Increase the Consumption of Whole Grains

One way to increase the consumption of whole grains is to simply substitute a refined-grain product with a whole-grain product, such as replacing white bread with whole-grain bread, or using brown rice instead of white rice, or whole-wheat pasta instead of white pasta. Whole-grain breakfast cereals are a good way to add more whole grains to the diet. Another easy way to increase whole grains in the diet is to eat popcorn, which itself is a whole grain; if it is air popped with very little salt and butter it is a healthful snack.

Caroline A. Kushner

Research Issues

Can grains be harmful to a person's health? Sensational book titles such as *Wheat Belly* and *Grain Brain* suggest that this can be the case. What is the evidence? Many people do consume too many calories, too many carbohydrates, and too much junk food, all of which elevate blood sugar. High blood sugar, in turn, damages arteries, thus increasing risk of heart disease, stroke, and dementia. High blood sugar and excess calories lead to too much adipose tissue, and the increased risk of developing the cardiometabolic syndrome and type 2 diabetes. When people eliminate grains from their diets, diet quality often improves if they replace grains with fruits and vegetables, and reduce intake of refined grain products with added fats and sugars. It is likely, however, that most people in energy balance can benefit from consuming small portions of whole grains.

See Also: Carbohydrates; Celiac disease; *Dietary Guidelines for Americans*; Enrichment and fortification; Fiber; Phytochemicals.

Further Reading

Centers for Disease Control and Prevention. (2012). *Nutrition for everyone: Basics: Carbohydrates*. Retrieved from http://www.cdc.gov/nutrition/everyone/basics/carbs.html

Jonnalagadda, S. S., Harnack, L., Liu, R. H., McKeown, N., Seal, C., Liu, S., & Fahey, G. C. (2011). Putting the whole grain puzzle together: Health benefits associated with whole grains—summary of American Society for Nutrition 2010 Satellite Symposium. *Journal of Nutrition, 141* (5), 1011S–1022S.

Mayo Clinic Staff. (2014, July 19). *Whole grains: Hearty options for a healthy diet.* MayoClinic.com. Retrieved from http://www.mayoclinic.com/health/whole-grains /NU00204

Slavin, J. (2004). Whole grains and human health. *Nutrition Research Reviews, 17* (1), 99–110.

United States Department of Agriculture (USDA). *Tips to help you eat whole grains.* ChooseMyPlate.gov. Retrieved from http://www.choosemyplate.gov/food-groups /grains-tips.html

Whole Grains Council. (2014, December 5). *Whole grains A to Z.* Retrieved from http:// wholegrainscouncil.org/whole-grains-101/whole-grains-a-to-z

H

Health Canada

Health Canada is Canada's federal department responsible for public health. Its mission statement highlights objectives to support scientific research and evaluation, as well as to ensure the quality of medical products and health care. Health Canada regulates and approves a wide range of products including food, consumer goods, medical devices, biologics, natural health products, pharmaceuticals, pesticides, and toxic substances. Health Canada promotes public health through a variety of educational programs.

Health care in Canada largely was privately funded and delivered before World War II. In 1957, the first specific set of health care services provided under universal coverage were outlined by the federal government in the Hospital Insurance and Diagnostic Act. These legislations eventually were consolidated to establish a system that was more accessible and comprehensive. Currently, Health Canada sets and administers principles and guidelines for the national health care system through the Canada Health Act.

Food safety and nutritional adequacy are key responsibilities for the promotion of public health. Health Canada establishes policies and standards for food safety and nutritional value as mandated by the Food and Drug Act. Surveillance of nutrition and food data informs many aspects of food safety, nutrition-related health outcomes, and nutrient intakes. Novel foods such as food additives, genetically modified foods, and biotechnology-derived foods are reviewed for approval by Health Canada. Before public distribution, companies producing novel foods are required to submit detailed scientific data for assessment. The organization is also responsible for providing safety warnings on food products currently in production. Potential food-related hazards are addressed in the Recalls and Safety Alerts Database, a regularly updated, comprehensive list of advisories and recalls.

As an authoritative voice in nutrition education, Health Canada focuses on the role of healthy eating in human development and disease prevention. Various public health programs and education initiatives are created through the Office of Nutrition Policy and Promotion and the Food Directorate. Topics addressed by the agency include prenatal nutrition and infant feeding as well as achieving healthy weight and activity levels in the general population.

Eating Well with Canada's Food Guide outlines information on nutrition and healthy eating. The guide is useful for learning basic nutrition facts, calculating individual energy requirements, and understanding recommended daily nutrient intakes. Serving suggestions are provided for four food groups—vegetables and fruits, grain products, milk and alternatives, and meat and alternatives. Whole grains such as barley, quinoa, wheat, oats, and wild rice are recommended. To ensure the intake of a variety of micronutrients, Canadians are encouraged to eat at least one green vegetable and one orange vegetable per day. The food guide also suggests increased consumption of meat alternatives such as beans, lentils, and tofu in addition to two servings of low-mercury fish each week. Additional tools for nutrition support are found in the shopping tips, meal ideas, and recommendations for maintaining healthy habits. Interactive guides teach the importance of reading nutrition labels and understanding nutrition claims.

Ana Maria Moise

Further Reading

Health Canada. (2011). *Eating well with Canada's food guide*. Retrieved from http://www.hc-sc.gc.ca/fn-an/food-guide-aliment/index-eng.php

Health Canada. (2014). *About Health Canada*. Retrieved from http://www.hc-sc.gc.ca/ahc-asc/index-eng.php

Herbs and Herbal Medicine

An herb is a plant or plant part that is used for its flavoring, scent, and/or medicinal qualities. Botanists use the word "herb" to refer to seed-producing plants that do not develop woody branches (as do shrubs and trees), but which die after the growing season. The term also is used to mean any plant that provides desired components for food or medicine—which is the use that is discussed here.

Plants have provided the foundation of most human diets throughout the ages, and people in all cultures have developed ways to use plants for foods, medicines, and other purposes. Examples of popular herbs used in North America for health benefits include echinacea and ginkgo biloba. Garlic and ginger are examples of herbs that are used in the diet both to flavor food and as components of dietary supplements for health benefits. Soy products, such as edamame, provide nutrients and energy, along with flavors and health benefits.

Although herbs contain a range of chemicals that contribute flavor and health benefits when consumed, plant components also can be toxic and have been used intentionally as poisons in many cultures throughout time. Some plant compounds used for healing have both health benefits and risks. Kava, for example, can reduce feelings of tension and stress but has also been associated with liver damage. Current pharmacopeias—books with official lists of medical drugs' uses and compositions—contain many medical formulas taken directly from ancient herbalists. Herbs traditionally used in cooking are regulated as food. In the United States, food and drug regulations define and regulate herbal products as dietary supplements.

History of Herbal Medicine

The healing effect of herbs for numerous human diseases has been observed since before recorded history. One of the oldest known medical documents is the Edwin Smith Papyrus, and it documents the recommended use of herbal medicine over magic in Egypt in 1500 BCE. Other surviving papyrus documents from the period list more than 700 substances that mostly consist of plant derivatives. Information regarding herbal remedies spread from the ancient Near East along trade routes and disseminated into the medical practices of the ancient Greek world.

The ancient Greeks and Romans linked many of their gods and goddesses to specific herbs. Greek mythology, for example, documents the goddess Demeter being closely associated with barley water mixed with fresh mint through her asking for a glass of that concoction after the her nine-day search for abducted daughter Persephone (D'Andrea, 1982). Another example associates the myrtle plant with Venus, whereby it commonly became depicted as a symbol of marriage and indication of being a bride. Greek mythology hints at the power of herbal medicine as a life-saving remedy. Classical Greek medicine attributed the healing properties of herbs to their god Apollo and his son Asclepius, the herbalist of the gods.

The medical school of Alexandria, founded in 260 BCE, established an international reputation in its day as a top medical school. Medical treatises which included herbal remedies were translated and shared throughout the ancient world. Dioscorides, a surgeon in the Roman army, wrote a five-volume series on how to make drugs—primarily from herbs—and titled *De Materia Medica*. It became the prominent medical handbook of its century and spread throughout the Roman Empire.

Historical scholars claim Hippocrates (ca. 460 BCE–ca. 370 BCE) as the founder of Western modern medicine. Hippocrates was one of the first practitioners to abandon supernatural beliefs in the occult and turn his focus toward observation and scientific method, a major step that revolutionized the practice of medicine. Many of his remedies included pure herbs without alteration. Historical scholars also recognize Theophrastus (ca. 372 BCE–ca. 287 BCE) as the first scientific botanist. Theophrastus made a systematic analysis of herbs. His book, *Enquiry into Plants*, had a profound effect on herbal medicine during the medieval period and antiquity. Theophrastus outlined plant parts used, scientific and superstitious practices, and included expert advice from druggists and herbalists regarding the cultivation and use of herbs.

Through legend and education, the apparent healing effects of herbal medicine were passed down through generations. The three main influences on medieval medical botany in Europe were Greco-Roman school medicine; Christianity's interpretations of orthodoxy; and pagan folk beliefs, which incorporated the use of magic. After the fall of the Roman Empire, Christian monks preserved the knowledge of herbal medicine within their illuminated manuscripts.

Abd-Allah Ibn Al-Batir—a Muslim scientist and botanist of the 13th century—compiled a pharmacopeia titled *Simple Drugs and Food*, which became the most frequently translated book of the Middle Ages (Jorda, 2008). This publication had far-reaching effects promoting herbal medicine beyond the Arab world into North Africa.

The use of herbs for both health maintenance and healing purposes has been central to many Asian medical traditions for thousands of years, including in Indian Ayurvedic medicine, traditional Chinese medicine, Tibetan medicine, and Japanese herbal medicine (known as "Kampo") (NCCAM, 2013).

Plants: Food and Phytochemicals

Plants can provide nutrients including carbohydrates, protein, fats, minerals, and vitamins. Plants also supply dietary fiber and and many other compounds, known as "phytochemicals." Phytochemicals include both primary and secondary metabolites. "Metabolites" are the intermediates and products produced during an organism's metabolism. Primary metabolites are substances that the plant requires to survive and are directly involved in the plant's normal growth, development, and reproduction. They include carbohydrates, fats, and proteins. Although not essential for survival, secondary metabolites are recognized as having beneficial effects upon an organism's health. Secondary metabolites include plant pigments that protect plants from too much sunlight, for example. When people consume these pigments, the pigments appear to exert helpful antioxidant activity in the human body. People also are able to utilize many of the secondary metabolites found in herbs for medicine and flavoring. Both primary and secondary metabolites are believed to have medicinal qualities, but the exact effects of many of these substances on the human body are largely unknown.

Ubiquity of Herbs and Herbal Remedies

Herbs continue to play a major role in the complementary and alternative treatment of ailments around the world. Traditional Chinese medicine, for example, still is popular today. It combines acupuncture and massage with prescriptions of herbal remedies. Naturopathy is another holistic approach to medicine focusing on noninvasive treatment and natural cures using herbs and herbal extracts. Homeopathy was established in 1876 with the premise of "like cures like." Homeopathic remedies are made from plants, minerals, and animal products. Allopathic medicine, also known as "modern biomedicine," treats chronic aliments by alleviating symptoms with drugs that often are extracted and refined from herbal sources. Aromatherapy uses extracts of essential oils from plants and herbs to alter a person's cognitive state, such as mood, in an effort to promote better health.

Regulation of Herbs

Primary metabolites as components of plants consumed as food have been part of the human diet throughout history. These foods and components therefore usually are unregulated as a result of their history of being harmless. Derivatives of these primary metabolites, however, can be artificially modified to create new forms never before seen in the diet. The Dietary Supplement Health and Education Act (DSHEA) of 1994 currently classifies herbs as dietary supplements which are not subject to drug requirements of proof of efficacy and safety tests. Because herbs are deemed "natural" they often are assumed to be safe, but this is not always the case. Consumers should research herbal products—especially dietary supplements—before consuming any.

Jinan M. Martiuk

See Also: Dietary supplements; Phytochemicals.

Further Reading

Bent, S. (2008). Herbal medicine in the United States: Review of efficacy, safety, and regulation. *Journal of General Internal Medicine, 23* (6), 854–859. Retrieved from http://www.ncbi.nlm.nih.gov/pmc/articles/PMC2517879/. doi: 10.1007/s11606-008-0632-y

D'Andrea, J. (1982). *Ancient herbs.* Malibu, HI: The J. Paul Getty Museum.

Daniel, M. (2013). *Medical plants: Chemistry and properties.* Plymouth: Science Publishers.

Jorda, E. G. (2008). Sacred herbs. *Clinical & Translational Oncology, 10* (11), 685–687. Retrieved from http://link.springer.com/article/10.1007%2Fs12094-008-0274-x#page-1

National Center for Complementary and Alternative Medicine (NCCAM). (2013). *Traditional Chinese medicine: An introduction.* Retrieved from http://nccam.nih.gov/health/whatiscam/chinesemed.htm

Stannard, J. (1999). *Herbs and herbalism in the Middle Ages and Renaissance.* Brookfield, VT: Ashgate Publishing Limited.

TCM healing modalities. (2014) Traditional Chinese Medicine World Foundation. Retrieved from http://www.tcmworld.org/what-is-tcm/tcm-healing-modalities/

Heterocyclic Amines and Polycyclic Aromatic Hydrocarbons

Heterocyclic amines (HCAs) are chemicals that include an amine (nitrogen) group and a heterocyclic ring. A heterocyclic ring is a ring of carbons that includes an atom of an element that is not carbon, such as nitrogen, oxygen, or sulfur. Not all HCAs are harmful, but researchers and consumers have become concerned about a group of carcinogenic HCAs that are produced from cooking muscle meats such as beef, pork, fish, and poultry at high temperatures, particularly during grilling and frying. Polycyclic aromatic hydrocarbons (PAHs) are a type of chemical produced during the incomplete burning of organic substances such as meat, tobacco, and coal, and are composed of aromatic rings fused together. An aromatic ring is a closed chain of six carbons, each bonded to a hydrogen, as in a benzene ring. Heterocyclic amines and polycyclic aromatic hydrocarbons are capable of causing genetic mutations that can initiate the development of cancer. Although high exposure to HCAs and PAHs can cause cancer in animals, the link between humans and

HCA and PAH consumption still is unclear. Epidemiological studies have found an association between consumption of well-done meats and grilled meats, especially grilled processed meats such as hot dogs, and some types of cancer. Apart from avoiding consumption of grilled meats, using certain cooking techniques can reduce the risk of HCA and PAH formation. These include microwaving the meat or marinating meat before cooking it.

Heterocyclic amines are formed when amino acids, sugars, and creatine react at high temperatures. Formation is greater in well-done or medium-well-done grilled or barbequed chicken and steak. This is especially true for meats cooked at temperatures greater than 300°F. Polycyclic aromatic hydrocarbons in food usually are produced during the grilling of meats. Fats and other juices from the meat drip onto the coals beneath the meat being cooked, and produce PAHs. Flames and the smoke produced from the drippings carry the PAHs back up to the meat, where they adhere to the meat's surface. When enzymes in the body break them down, HCAs and PAHs become capable of damaging DNA. Both of these carcinogens usually are concentrated in the burnt or charred areas of the meat. When chicken is grilled or barbequed, the skin has more than eight times the amount of HCAs as the meat contains.

Research has found a link between the consumption of HCAs and certain forms of cancer. When HCAs are introduced to the diet of mice, the mice develop tumors in organs such as the colon, breast, and prostate (Sugimura, Wakabayashi, Nakagama, & Nagao, 2004). Although the amount of HCAs consumed by humans is less than the doses given to laboratory mice, human epidemiological studies have shown a positive correlation between preference for high-temperature cooked meat and an increased risk of cancer, including cancers of the prostate, pancreas, breast, colon, and rectum (American Association of Cancer Research, 2009; National Cancer Institute, 2010). In one study, 62,581 participants—including 208 people diagnosed with pancreatic cancer—were interviewed about their meat intake. Researchers found that the participants with a preference for well-done steak were about 60% more likely to develop pancreatic cancer than those participants who ate rare or medium rare steak, or did not consume steak (American Association of Cancer Research, 2009).

Research on the association between PAHs and cancer originated with studies of workers with occupational exposure to these chemicals. Workers in coal carbonization and gasification in 1936, for example, were found to have higher rates of lung cancer mortality (CDC, 2011). Animal studies have confirmed the carcinogenicity of PAHs, which appear to particularly increase risk of skin cancer, along with cancers in the pulmonary, gastrointestinal, renal systems (CDC, 2011).

There are several ways to prepare meat to lower consumption of HCAs and PAHs. Instead of grilling or barbequing, cooking meats on low heat using techniques such as steaming or stir-frying minimizes the formation of HCAs and PAHs. Microwaving the meat before grilling or pan-frying produces well-done meat without the prolonged exposure to high temperatures. Marinating meat before grilling also reduces production of HCAs and PAHs. Grilling vegetables does not produce carcinogenic chemicals, therefore consuming dishes such as a shish kebab composed mostly or entirely of vegetables is less harmful than eating a large charbroiled steak.

Janet Ku

See Also: Cancer and nutrition; Nitrates and nitrites, dietary.

Further Reading

American Association of Cancer Research. (2009). *Pancreatic cancer risk: Associations with meat-derived carcinogen intake.* Presented at the April 18–22, 2009, American Association of Cancer Research (AACR) Meeting, Denver, CO. First author: Kristin Anderson, PhD, associate professor and cancer epidemiologist with the University of Minnesota's School of Public Health and Masonic Cancer Center. Retrieved from http://www.cancer.org/cancer/news/news/eating-charred-well-done-meat-may-increase-pancreatic-cancer-risk

Centers for Disease Control and Prevention (CDC). (2011). Polycyclic aromatic hydrocarbons (PAHs). *Toxic substances portal.* Agency for Toxic Substances and Disease Registry. Retrieved from http://www.atsdr.cdc.gov/substances/toxsubstance.asp?toxid =25

John, E. M., Storn, M. C., Sinha, R., & Koo, J. (2011). Meat consumption, cooking practices, meat mutagens, and risk of prostate cancer. *Nutrition and Cancer, 63* (4), 525–37. doi:10.1080/01635581.2011.539311

Larsson, S.C., & Orsini, N. (2013). Red meat and processed meat consumption and all-cause mortality: A meta-analysis. *American Journal of Epidemiology.* Retrieved from http://www.ncbi.nlm.nih.gov/pubmed/24148709

National Cancer Institute. (2010, October 15). *Chemicals in meat cooked at high temperatures and cancer risk.* Retrieved from http://www.cancer.gov/cancertopics/factsheet /Risk/cooked-meats#r1

Sugimura, T., Wakabayashi, K., Nakagama, H., & Nagao, M. (2004). Heterocyclic amines: Mutagens/carcinogens produced during cooking of meat and fish. *Cancer Science, 95* (4), 290–09. Retrieved from http://www.ncbi.nlm.nih.gov/pubmed/15072585

High-Fructose Corn Syrup

High-fructose corn syrup (HFCS) is a common sweetener used in many food products. It is called "high fructose" because the syrup contains more fructose than regular corn syrup. Food engineers developed high-fructose corn syrup during the 1960s to serve as a sugar alternative. The abundance of corn has made HFCS cheaper than regular table sugar. High-fructose corn syrup became a popular ingredient in food products in the 1970s. Recently, consumers have questioned the safety of HFCS and other sugars in the diet, as studies show that too much sugar poses many health risks, including risk for obesity and type 2 diabetes.

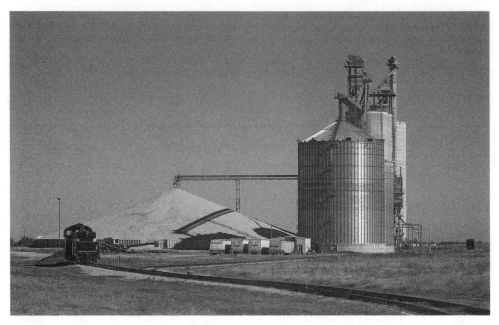

Grain elevator with surplus corn pile in Nebraska. (Jeff Wilson/Shutterstock)

History

The process of converting starches to sugars was first developed in Japan in the 1800s using arrowroot (Cavette, 2009). The process became more popular in 1811, when Russian chemist Gottlieb Kirchhoff added sulfuric acid to starch and obtained starch-derived sweeteners. The method was brought to the United States in 1831 when chemist, physician, and inventor, Samuel Gutherie, explored the possibilities of creating sugar from potato starch (Warner, 2011). Americans soon adapted the new method to create cornstarch, and later began to derive glucose from corn. In 1866, a plant in Buffalo, New York, produced the first corn sweeteners. An enzyme-conversion method was discovered to yield high-fructose corn syrup in 1967.

The Market

Because of American agricultural subsidies, corn is both abundant and cheap, making high-fructose corn syrup one of the most common commercial sweeteners. Many American food manufacturers turned to corn syrup after 1977 when new tariffs and sugar quotas made importing sugar significantly more expensive (Goldstein, 2012). By 1996, 28 corn-refining plants existed in the United States, and about 25 billion pounds of corn were converted into corn syrups and other corn sweeteners (Cavette, 2009). Corn-based products provide more than 50% of nutritive sweeteners in the United States.

Processing

High-fructose corn syrup is mostly composed of fructose and glucose, but it also contains water and a small amount of other sugars. The two types of HFCS most commonly produced commercially are HFCS-42 and HFCS-55. The former consists of 42% fructose and 53% glucose; the latter consists of 55% fructose and 42% glucose. The percentage of fructose in the solution is positively correlated with the sweetness of the solution, as fructose is naturally sweeter than glucose. HFCS-42's sweetness is comparable to that of sucrose, whereas HFS-55 is sweeter than sucrose.

Not only is HFCS sweet, but it also can be used as a flavor and texture enhancer. High-fructose corn syrup also is used as a preservative, and it can help maintain levels of moisture in packaged foods. Although sugar derived from cane or beets undergoes a less complex process, corn syrup is more cost effective because of the availability of the corn crop. Therefore, the overall lower production cost yields greater profits for food producers.

Food manufacturers use high-fructose corn syrup in a variety of processed foods. HFCS appears most obviously in sweet foods, but it also is an ingredient in many savory products, which could account for the large quantities of HFCS that Americans today unknowingly consume. Corn syrup is used as a sweetener in foods like soft drinks, candy, baked goods, jams, sports drinks, pancakes, breads, fruit drinks, and flavored yogurt. HFCS is used as a flavor enhancer in products such as salad dressings, frozen pizza, macaroni and cheese, tonic water, and ketchup. High-fructose corn syrup also is used for added texture and prolonged shelf life.

Fructose Metabolism

Fructose, like glucose, is a six-carbon sugar. Although fructose is naturally occurring in foods such as fruit and honey, dietary fructose is not necessary for humans. Fructose metabolism occurs primarily in the liver, and favors the metabolic pathway leading to lipogenesis (formation of triglycerides). Several studies have found that a high-fructose intake increases circulating lipid levels; this happens with other sweeteners as well.

Health Risks

Although high-fructose corn syrup appears in a large number of food products that people consume, it is an ingredient that many people try to avoid. Because obesity rates increased during the same time period, researchers wondered if HFCS might be responsible. Several studies have found that excessive consumption of high-fructose corn syrup, like excessive consumption of other sugars, could pose many health risks, especially weight gain and the health problems associated with obesity. Rodent studies suggest that high-fructose corn syrup might cause greater weight gain than table sugar, and increase the risk of cardiometabolic syndrome. In humans, a high consumption of HFCS has been associated with increased risk for the development of hypertension, kidney damage, type 2 diabetes, and cardiometabolic syndrome. But over time, researchers have found that the health risks associated with HFCS appear to be similar to those for other added nutritive sweeteners, including sugar (White, Foreyt, Melanson, & Angelopoulos, 2010). This is not surprising as cane sugar, beet sugar, and HFCS all are approximately 50% fructose.

Preliminary evidence suggests that fructose could fuel the growth of cancer cells (Boros et al., 2010). One research team observed pancreatic cells in vitro and found that pancreatic cancer cells given fructose grew faster than normal. The study revealed that—even though it is known that cancer cells use glucose to proliferate—they can just as readily use fructose, unlike other cells. More research is needed before these results can be applied in vivo. Fructose comes not only from HFCS and sucrose, but from fruits and vegetables as well. Public health experts recommend that all people limit their intake of food products with added sugars to prevent obesity and obesity-related health risks.

Environmental Impacts

The United States produces more corn than any other country. Corn is the biggest cash crop in the United States, occupying approximately 84 million acres of land (EPA, 2013). Many factors have led to corn being America's number one crop, including the introduction of high-fructose corn syrup. Monoculture corn production has a number of environmental impacts. Corn requires more synthetic fertilizers and pesticides than any other crop (Hartman, 2008). The fertilizers and pesticides are made from fossil fuels, and their hazardous chemical components are incorporated into runoff and subsequently contaminate the soil and bodies of water. Many consumers also are concerned about the prevalence of genetically modified corn in the United States and many other countries.

Megan J. Park and Gabriella J. Zutrau

See Also: Fructose; Obesity, causes; Sugar-sweetened beverages.

Further Reading

Boros, L. G., Heaney, A. P., Huang, D., Liu, H., McArthur, D., & Nissen, N. (2010). Fructose linked to pancreatic cancer tumor growth—UCLA Study. *Pancreatic Cancer Action.* Retrieved December 2, 2013, from https://pancreaticcanceraction.org/news/fructose -linked-to-pancreatic-cancer-tumour-growth-ucla-study-2/

Cavette, C. (2009). *Corn syrup. How products are made.* Retrieved October 12, 2013, from http://www.madehow.com/Volume-4/Corn-Syrup.html

Goldstein, M. C. (2012). High fructose corn syrup. In S. Zoumbaris (Ed.), *Encyclopedia of Wellness: From Açaí berry to yo-yo dieting* (pp. 448–457). Santa Barbara, CA: ABC-CLIO.

Hartman, E. (2008, March 9). High-fructose corn syrup: Not so sweet for the planet. *Washington Post*. Retrieved March 30, 2014, from http://www.washingtonpost.com /wp-dyn/content/article/2008/03/06/AR2008030603294.html

United States Environmental Protection Agency (EPA). (2013, April 11). Major Crops Grown in the United States. U.S. Environmental Protection Agency. Retrieved March 30, 2014, from http://www.epa.gov/agriculture/ag101/cropmajor.html

Warner, D. J. (2011, September). *Sweet stuff: An American history of sweeteners from sugar to sucralose*. Washington, DC: Rowman & Littlefield.

White, J. S., Foreyt, J. P., Melanson, K. J., & Angelopoulos, T. J. (2010). High-fructose corn syrup: Controversies and common sense. *American Journal of Lifestyle Medicine, 4* (6), 515–520. Retrieved from http://www.medscape.com/viewarticle/735543_3

Honey

Honey is made from the nectar of flowering plants, which honeybees break down into simple sugars and store in honeycombs. The shape of the honeycomb and the beating the bees' wings then cause much of the remaining moisture to evaporate, forming honey. Beekeepers remove frames of honeycomb from their hives and extract the honey. The honey then is strained, sometimes by using heat to speed the process, and bottled. Honey has different flavors, colors, aromas, sugar ratios, and antioxidant chemical content depending upon the flowers from which the bees collected the nectar. In North America there are more than 300 types of honey available, such as alfalfa, clover, and orange blossom. Humans have enjoyed honey's delicious flavor and sweetness throughout history. Honey also has been used for medicinal purposes in many cultures.

The honey produced by bees provides a source of energy for all of the bees in the hive. Nectar itself would ferment, and therefore does not serve as a suitable food source for use during the winter. To make honey, bees swallow the nectar as they collect it, storing it in an organ called the honey stomach. Enzymes in this organ act upon the nectar, converting the nectar's sucrose into glucose and fructose. The bees then regurgitate the product back at the hive, where other bees also ingest it, break it down further, and then regurgitate it. The honey then is stored in the honeycomb. After the water has evaporated, the honey maintains its nutritional qualities for extended periods of time.

Honey is predominantly composed of fructose and glucose. The fructose content gives honey a lower glycemic index than that of other popular sweeteners. Because it is concentrated, honey has more calories per tablespoon than granulated, powdered, or brown sugar. Honey also contains phenolics, peptides, organic acids, enzymes, and Maillard-reaction products which, combined, give honey its antioxidant capacity. Additionally, honey is a prebiotic; it contains a type of fiber that is not digested in the human digestive tract but instead feeds the beneficial bacteria that live in the intestines. A study in laboratory mice found that feeding the mice a food mix with honey led to a more beneficial mix of intestinal bacteria as compared to feeding them a food mix containing sugar (Ezz El-Arab et al., 2006).

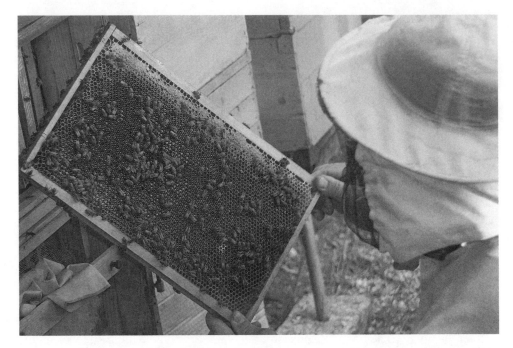

A beekeeper examines a framed beehive panel. Many commercial beekeepers transport their bees to various locations around the country, freeing the insects in orchards so they can pollinate the crops. However, Colony Collapse Disorder poses a threat to the livelihood of migratory beekeepers, commercial growers, and U.S. consumers. (iStockPhoto.com)

The American Academy of Pediatrics recommends withholding honey from children younger than one year old, because spores from the Clostridium botulinum bacteria occasionally migrate from the soil into beehives. People older than one year have stronger immune systems and can cope effectively with the minute traces of the bacteria which occasionally occur in honey products, but infants could develop botulism infection.

All honey contains hydrogen peroxide, produced by bee enzymes in the honey-making process, and also has antimicrobial and antibacterial properties. Honey has been used on wounds to prevent infection, although that practice has become less common over time. Manuka honey, made from the pollen of the manuka bush in New Zealand, has been found to have antimicrobial, antibacterial, and antifungal properties, and has been made into a product called Medihoney, which was approved by the FDA in 2007.

Honey is a humectant, meaning it attracts and retains moisture. For this reason it often is used in moisturizers and to soothe and coat sore throats and suppress coughing. A couple of well-controlled studies have shown that honey might provide an effective treatment for cold symptoms. One study found that, as compared to a sweet placebo, honey increased sleep time and reduced nighttime coughing in

300 children 1 to 5 years old who had upper respiratory tract infections (Cohen et al., 2012).

Helene M. Parker

See Also: Glycemic index and glycemic load; Microbiota and microbiome.

Further Reading

Cohen, H. A., Rozen, J., Kristal, H., et al. (2012). Effect of honey on nocturnal cough and sleep quality: A double-blind, randomized, placebo-controlled study. *Pediatrics, 130*, 1–7. doi: 10.1542/peds.2011-3075

Edgar, J. (2011). *Medicinal uses of honey*. Web MD. Retrieved from http://www.webmd.com/diet/features/medicinal-uses-of-honey

Ezz El-Arab, A. M., Girgis, S. M., Hegazy, E. M., & Abd El-Khalek, A. B. (2006). Effect of dietary honey on intestinal microflora and toxicity of mycotoxins in mice. *BMC Complementary and Alternative Medicine 6*, 6. doi:10.1186/1472-6882-6-6

Gheldof, N., Wang, X., & Engeseth, N. (2002). Identification and quantification of antioxidant components of honeys from various floral sources. *Journal of Agricultural and Food Chemistry, 50* (21), 5870–5877. Retrieved from http://pubs.acs.org/doi/abs/10.1021/jf0256135.

National Honey Board. (January 2013). *How honey is made*. Retrieved from honey.com

Hunger, Biology of

Hunger is defined as the internal, physiological drive to find and consume food. Individuals often interchange the words "hunger" and "appetite." There is a key difference between these terms, however, and they are easily distinguishable. Hunger often is experienced as a negative, physical sensation when prolonged, and appetite is a psychological desire for food and often is a positive sensation. Hunger often begins with the sensation of an empty stomach or hunger pangs. The regulation of hunger also is controlled by an area in the brain called the lateral hypothalamus. Additionally, two important hormones—leptin and ghrelin—signal the brain when there is a lack of nutrients or when fullness is reached. There are believed to be more than 50 different chemicals, however, that play an integral part in regulating hunger and eating behavior (Insel, Ross, McMahon, & Bernstein, 2014).

Although hunger has a negative connotation and is thought of as something that must be "fixed" or "eliminated," hunger is an essential physical drive that ensures animals, including humans, obtain the food necessary for survival. This drive is helpful in many situations, but researchers are studying how hunger is related to overeating. It is important to know about the various regulations and the physiology of hunger because of the high rates of obesity worldwide. Understanding hunger and its physiological regulation could greatly improve the understanding and treatment of obesity.

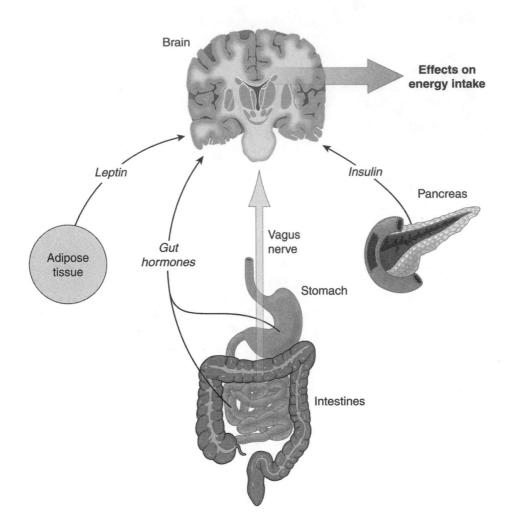

Many factors affect the sensation of hunger. These include leptin levels, gut hormones, and the hormone insulin. (Legger/Dreamstime.com)

Biology of Hunger

The basic purpose of eating is to satisfy the body's need for nutrients and energy. Hunger typically is characterized by the aching and empty feeling that the stomach experiences. It is the body's first demand for essential nutrients. As the feeling persists and goes unsatisfied, the sensations grow into an uncomfortable pang, which most people call a "hunger pang." It can be distinguished as a growling stomach or a contracting pain in the abdominal area. This easily is relieved by ingesting food.

The hypothalamus plays a very important role in coordinating the chemicals that regulate hunger. The hypothalamus is located in the forebrain region, just above the brainstem and below the thalamus. There are three sections of the hypothalamus that are involved in the regulation of hunger; the lateral, the ventromedial, and the paraventricular. Damage to the ventromedial section of the hypothalamus produces a condition known as hyperphagia, which causes animals to overeat and gain enormous amounts of weight. Damage to the lateral hypothalamus produces aphagia and adipsia, which is the total lack of drive to eat or drink, respectively.

The hypothalamus regulates hunger through the release and monitoring of certain hormones. These specialized hormones circulate within the body and act as initiators or terminators of hunger. The lateral hypothalamus stimulates hunger. It produces the hormone orexin when blood sugar levels are too low. The ventromedial hypothalamus is responsible for controlling the amount of food consumed. When this area of the hypothalamus is stimulated, it reduces the feeling of hunger.

There are two mechanisms that influence the regulation of hunger—the short-term and long-term mechanisms. The short-term mechanism reflects daily energy balance, in which food intake is balanced with energy expenditure. The second mechanism, the long-term regulation, is the storage mechanism. Excess energy (calories) is stored so that it will be available for later use or use when emergency energy is needed spontaneously. This stored energy is in the form of fat within the adipose tissues and cells. The short-term mechanism generally is assumed to be closely related to monitoring blood glucose levels and when that level becomes too low, hunger is induced. The long-term mechanism involves monitoring the body's fat level and induces hunger when fat stores become too low.

Hunger Hormones

Neuropeptide Y is a major neurotransmitter that acts in the brain and in the autonomic nervous system. In the autonomic nervous system it is mainly produced by neurons of the sympathetic nervous system. Neuropeptide Y is produced in various locations in the brain, including the hypothalamus. In laboratory animals, elevating the activity of neuropeptide Y results in the increase of food intake.

Peptide YY is a short protein that is released by the cells in the ileum (the lower portion of the small intestine) and the colon. In humans, it appears to reduce hunger after a meal. Peptide YY works by decreasing hunger and increasing water and electrolyte absorption in the colon. Peptide YY works by slowing gastric emptying; it increases the effectiveness of the digestion process and nutrient absorption after a meal. Peptide YY signals the brain to sense that it is not hungry.

Leptin is a hormone produced by fat cells that appears to be involved with the long-term regulation of hunger. Increasing leptin levels appear to decrease the production of neuropeptide Y, thus decreasing hunger. Experiments on mice have revealed that leptin hormone levels are greater when more fat is present; however, other contributing factors—such as sleeping and eating patterns—also affect leptin levels. Additionally, it is possible for the body to become leptin-resistant. A person who is leptin-resistant does not experience the normal increase in satiety and then stop eating after a filling meal. Leptin resistance is associated with excessive hunger and risk of obesity.

Ghrelin is released by the stomach and sends a signal to the brain that increases hunger. It has been shown that levels of ghrelin increase right before consuming a meal and decrease afterward. Ghrelin levels can be influenced by certain lifestyles and by stress. Studies have revealed a positive relationship with ghrelin and stress; thus, when stress rises and becomes significant, ghrelin levels also increase. Physical activities—such as weight lifting—have been shown to decrease ghrelin as well as food intake. Sleep deprivation has been associated with elevated ghrelin levels and therefore, increasing hunger (Adams, Greenway, Brantely, 2010).

Orexin, also known as "hypocretin," is produced by the hypothalamus. This neurotransmitter has various functions that include wakefulness, arousal, and appetite. Orexin increases feelings of hunger and has been shown to be inhibited by leptin and activated by ghrelin.

Hormones produced during the absorption of nutrients following digestion generally reduce feelings of hunger. These hormones include insulin, produced by the pancreas in response to elevations in blood sugar, and cholecystokinin, produced by the small intestine after a meal, in the presence of fats.

Prader-Willi Syndrome

Prader-Willi Syndrome is the most commonly known genetic cause of life-threatening obesity in children. It usually causes poor muscle tone, stunted growth, and a chronic feeling of hunger. It is a complex genetic disorder that causes the hypothalamus to dysfunction. This chronic feeling of hunger in turn causes the children to become obsessed with eating and with food. The amount that these children actually consume far exceeds physiological need. The lack of muscle tone results in the child only needing two-thirds of the normal calorie intake.

Sandy Wong

Research Issues

Dieticians and others who advise people on weight loss have been interested in research on hunger. Some popular weight-loss advice is based on the physiology of hunger. Dieters, for example, often are told to eat slowly so that hunger has time to fade. The fading of hunger is caused at least in part by the release of cholecystokinin by the small intestine when the organ detects the presence of fat. It takes at least 15 to 20 minutes for fat from a meal to reach the small intestine, which is why people are advised to eat slowly. Similarly, advice to get adequate sleep and manage stress is designed to reduce levels of the hormone "ghrelin."

See Also: Appetite; Obesity, causes.

Further Reading

Adams, C. E., Greenway, F. L., & Brantley, P. J. (2010, May 10). Lifestyle factors and ghrelin: Critical review and implications for weight loss maintenance. *Obesity Review, 12* (5), e211-e216.

Biological bases of hunger. (n.d.) *Boundless.* Retrieved from https://www.boundless.com /psychology/motivation/hunger/biological-bases-of-hunger/

Insel, P., Ross, D., McMahon, K., & Bernstein, M. (2014). *Nutrition.* Burlington, MA: Jones & Bartlett Learning.

Johnson, M. (2013, March 18). The magic of hunger. *U.S. News & World Report.* Retrieved from http://health.usnews.com/health-news/blogs/eat-run/2013/03/08/why-feeling-hungry -is-important

Palmer, S. (2009, April). Taking control of hunger. *Today's Dietitian.* Retrieved from http:// www.todaysdietitian.com/newarchives/040609p28.shtml

Prader-Willi Syndrome Association. (2012, November 12). Retrieved from http://www .pwsausa.org/

Hydrogenation

Hydrogenation is the process of adding hydrogen to a molecule, which then rearranges the molecule's chemical structure. Most often this occurs in organic molecules with a double bond between two carbons. The double bond becomes a single bond, leaving each carbon the opportunity to bind with an additional hydrogen atom. Although this phenomenon happens in nature, in the food industry it also occurs as part of a synthetic process using vegetable oils. Hydrogenated fats are desirable because their bonds are not as easily broken by oxygen; therefore shelf life is extended and taste is preserved longer. To initiate hydrogenation, oil typically must be heated to more than 300°F in the presence of hydrogen and a catalyst such as nickel, copper, or platinum. The level of hydrogenation can be controlled carefully through manipulation of temperature, pressure, agitation, and concentration of the catalyst. A by-product of hydrogenation is the creation of a fatty acid structure called a "trans fatty acid," or "trans fat"; during the process, a carbon-carbon double bond is not broken, but one of the hydrogens shifts position thus altering the shape of the fatty acid.

Increasing hydrogenation raises the boiling point of the oil and leads to a progressively more solid product when it reaches room temperature. As the oil becomes more hydrogenated, the concentration of mono- and polyunsaturated fats decreases and the concentration of saturated fats increases. Partially hydrogenated oil contains varying amounts of trans fat. Fully hydrogenated oil, such as margarine and shortenings, contains less trans fat. Due to the possible negative health effects of trans fat, the Food and Drug Administration now requires manufacturers to include all partially hydrogenated oils on the ingredient label, as well as the grams of trans fats contained in a serving of the product. Some products claim to be free of trans fat, but still list partially hydrogenated oils on their label. Although misleading, this practice is legal because the FDA considers foods with less than 0.5g of trans fat per serving to be free of trans fat.

Patricia M. Cipicchio

See Also: Trans fatty acids.

Further Reading

Brown, J. L. (2006). *Hydrogenated vegetable oils and trans fatty acids*. Penn State College of Agricultural Sciences Publications. Retrieved from http://pubs.cas.psu.edu/freepubs /pdfs/uk093.pdf

Clark, J. (2003). The hydrogenation of alkenes. *Chemguide*. Retrieved from http://www .chemguide.co.uk/organicprops/alkenes/hydrogenation.html

Haynes, F. (n.d.) *Do all foods listing hydrogenated oils contain trans fats?* About.com. Retrieved from http://lowfatcooking.about.com/od/faqs/f/hydrogenated.htm

Hyperglycemia

"Hyperglycemia" is the scientific term for high blood sugar. Fasting hyperglycemia is characterized by a blood glucose level of more than 130 mg per deciliter following an 8-hour fast. Postprandial hyperglycemia occurs when an individual continually has a blood glucose level that is greater than 180 mg per deciliter following meals (American Diabetes Association, 2013). A normal fasting blood glucose level should be less than 100 mg/dl and a random-sample blood glucose level should be less than 150 mg/dl. Occasional episodes of hyperglycemia can be benign, but frequent hyperglycemia can have extremely detrimental long-term consequences.

Diabetes is the most common cause of frequent hyperglycemia. This is because people with diabetes have difficulties producing or responding to insulin, a hormone produced by the pancreas that helps to regulate the amount of glucose that is removed from the blood by the body's cells. Certain medications (such as corticosteroids and protease inhibitors) and critical illnesses can produce acute hyperglycemia as well (American Diabetes Association, 2013). Critical illnesses such as myocardial infarction, stroke, hyperthyroidism, pancreatitis, pancreatic cancer, Cushing's syndrome, and unusual tumors create acute stress and can induce hyperglycemia. Hyperglycemia also occurs naturally during times of infection and inflammation, and the resulting blood sugar increase varies based on the person and type of response.

Although hyperglycemia has a host of symptoms, the most typical symptoms comprise what is called the "classic hyperglycemic triad." The symptoms are polyphagia, polydipsia, and polyuria, which mean "frequent hunger," "frequent thirst," and "frequent urination," respectively. Unexpected weight loss is another major symptom. Temporary hyperglycemia often is benign and asymptomatic. Blood glucose levels can rise well above normal for significant periods without causing any permanent effects or symptoms. Chronic hyperglycemia, however, spanning a period of years, can cause serious complications such as kidney, neurological, and cardiovascular damage, as well as damage to the retina. Acute hyperglycemia involving glucose levels that are extremely high is a medical emergency and can rapidly produce serious symptoms, including disorientation, mental confusion, dizziness, and (in severe cases) coma and even death.

Treatment of hyperglycemia begins with identifying its cause and, when possible, correctly the underlying problem. In people with diabetes—who are likely to experience hyperglycemia from time to time—treatment includes taking steps to improve glycemic control (control of blood sugar levels). People with diabetes must learn to recognize the symptoms associated with hyperglycemia and improve their glycemic control by increasing frequency of glucose testing, following a healthy diet, making lifestyle changes, and adjusting medications.

Lola Murray and Sonya Bhatia

See Also: Blood sugar regulation; Diabetes, type 1; Diabetes, type 2; Glucose; Hypoglycemia.

Further Reading

American Diabetes Association. (2013, June 7). *Hyperglycemia (High blood glucose)*. Retrieved from http://www.diabetes.org/living-with-diabetes/treatment-and-care/blood -glucose-control/hyperglycemia.html

Diabetes Health Center. (2012). *Diabetes and hyperglycemia*. WebMD. Retrieved from http://diabetes.webmd.com/diabetes-hyperglycemia

Inzucchi, S. E., Bergenstal, R. M., Buse, J. B., et al. (2012). Management of hyperglycemia in type 2 diabetes: A patient-centered approach. Position statement of the American Diabetes Association (ADA) and the European Association for the Study of Diabetes. *Diabetes Care, 35* (6), 1364–79. doi: 10.2337/dc12-0413

Stoppler, M. C. (2013). *Hyperglycemia*. MedicineNet. Retrieved from http://www .medicinenet.com/hyperglycemia/article.htm

Hypertension and Nutrition

"Hypertension" is the scientific term for high blood pressure. It is characterized by a person's resting blood pressure consistently being measured at 140/90 mmHg or greater while at rest. The normal resting blood pressure of a healthy individual is considered to be 120/80 mmHg or less. High blood pressure is the leading cause of strokes and heart failure, as well as one of the strongest risk factors for the development of heart disease. In 2008, these complications caused 7.5 million related deaths among adults worldwide, affecting about 40% of adults aged 25 and older

Main complications of hypertension

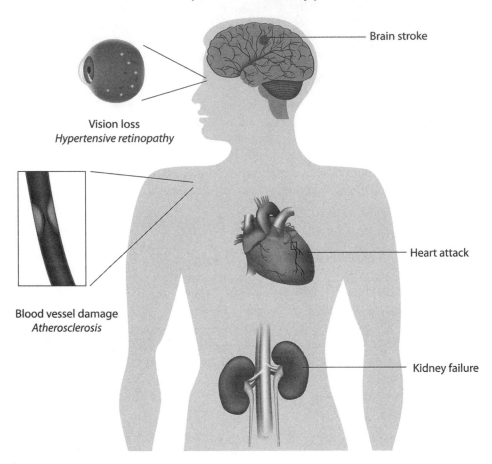

Hypertension is known as a "silent disease" because most people don't notice any symptoms. However, chronic, uncontrolled hypertension is associated with many health problems, including vision loss (hypertension retinopathy), blood vessel damage (atherosclerosis), heart attack, and kidney failure. (Shutterstock.com)

(WHO, 2014). The World Health Organization reports that the Americas had the lowest prevalence of high blood pressure readings, with about 35% of the population demonstrating an above-normal reading (WHO, 2014). The United States reports that hypertension affects about 30% of its adult population, with prevalence increasing with age and decreasing with education and income level (Keenan & Rosendorf, 2011).

Lifestyle change, including dietary change, is a central tool used in the prevention and treatment of hypertension. Increasing physical activity, reducing stress, and improving eating habits can reduce elevated resting blood pressure. One eating plan used to manage—and sometimes even reverse—hypertension is the DASH

(Dietary Approaches to Stop Hypertension) diet. The DASH diet emphasizes low salt intake with a high intake of vegetables and fruit and has been shown to lower blood pressure. Avoiding foods high in added fats and sugars also is beneficial to many people trying to reduce high blood pressure, as these foods can contribute to weight gain and increase the risk for high blood pressure.

Blood Pressure

Blood pressure is measured in millimeters of mercury, and is the measurement of the force exerted against the walls of the arteries as blood is pumped through them. The first number in a blood pressure measurement refers to systolic blood pressure, the pressure measured during systole, which is the contraction of the heart as it beats. The second number represents diastolic blood pressure, the pressure in the arterial system during diastole, the period between contractions. A number of factors influence blood pressure.

- Heart rate and the heart's force of contraction influence blood pressure. During exercise, for example, the heart must circulate a much higher volume of blood, thus the heart beats harder and faster and blood pressure rises; a normal and healthy response to exercise. Heart rate and the force of contraction also increase when a person feels stressed.
- The behavior of the arteries also influences blood pressure. The arteries have small muscles that alter their circumference, depending upon the need for blood in the tissues supplied by those arteries. During digestion, for example, the arteries that supply the digestive system become wider to accommodate increased blood flow. If the arteries do not widen appropriately, then the narrower artery passages create more resistance to blood flow, and blood pressure increases.
- Blood volume affects blood pressure. A greater blood volume increases blood pressure (when all other factors are equal). Fluid retention, such as that can resulting from a high intake of salt, can increase blood volume and blood pressure.

Blood pressure normally fluctuates throughout the day. Hypertension only is diagnosed when resting blood pressure is chronically elevated.

Physiological Effects of Hypertension

Over time, hypertension can lead to a number of harmful consequences. It contributes to artery disease because the greater pressure of the blood flowing through the arteries appears to cause damage to the artery lining. Hypertension seems to cause microscopic tears in the arteries that develop into scar tissue as the artery repairs itself. The scar tissue then can compromise the function of the artery lining, attracting substances such as LDL cholesterol that contribute to the formation of arterial plaque. Plaque buildup further worsens arterial function, increasing resistance to blood flow and thus increasing hypertension. Over time, plaque buildup causes arteries to become stiff and less responsive to the chemical signals that regulate vasoconstriction and vasodilation. High blood pressure also can cause vulnerable arteries to bulge and tear, creating a hemorrhage; this process is responsible for hemorrhagic strokes. Worldwide, hypertension is considered the leading risk factor for the development of cardiovascular disease and mortality. People with hypertension have a greater risk of developing kidney disease; having a heart attack; and experiencing heart failure, a stroke, retinal hemorrhage, visual impairment, and even early death.

Causes and Risk Factors

In fewer than 10% of cases hypertension is secondary to another health problem, such as kidney disease. The vast majority of hypertension is not connected to one single cause, but rather is considered a multifactorial illness, meaning that many different variables—including both inherited and lifestyle factors—contribute to its development and severity. Hypertension not secondary to another health problem is known as "essential hypertension." The term "essential" has an interesting history. In the mid-1900s, physicians and researchers had observed that blood pressure increases with age. It was hypothesized that this increase was essential, because aging arteries were less elastic. Experts thought increased blood pressure was required to accomplish adequate blood circulation. This hypothesis later was discarded, as scientists observed that age was not associated with increased blood pressure in many areas of the world.

Many factors influence a person's risk of developing hypertension. Although some of these factors are out of a person's control, many can be modified to reduce risk. An unbalanced diet that includes excess calories, added sugars, and is high in added fats and processed foods is linked to many of the conditions that increase the risks for developing high blood pressure. The risk factors known to increase the chances developing high blood pressure are listed below.

- Obesity
- Sedentary lifestyle
- Stress and anxiety
- Overconsumption of alcohol (more than one drink a day for women and more than two drinks a day for men)
- Excess salt in diet
- Diet low in fruits and vegetables
- Smoking
- Family history of hypertension
- Diabetes
- African-American ethnicity

Symptoms

Hypertension is a condition that presents with no symptoms. Occasionally, people with hypertension experience headaches, nosebleeds, or dizziness, but these symptoms are not reliable indicators of hypertension. Because hypertension typically has no symptoms, blood pressure is measured at most visits with health care providers, so that rising blood pressure can be detected and treated as early as possible.

Treatment

If resting blood pressure is only mildly or moderately elevated, patients might be able to reduce blood pressure significantly with lifestyle modification. Increasing physical activity and improving eating behaviors can help normalize blood pressure. If people are overweight, weight loss can also be beneficial. Learning to reduce feelings of stress that precipitate a fight-or-flight response can reduce the concentration of hormones that contribute to hypertension. When lifestyle measures alone do not lead to adequate control, or when people have difficulty implementing lifestyle change, medications can help reduce resting blood pressure.

Dietary Recommendations for Preventing and Treating Hypertension

Several dietary recommendations have been found to be helpful for preventing and treating hypertension, including the following.

Reduce Salt Intake

Greater salt intake has been associated with increased risk for hypertension in many studies. Research generally has found a modest but significant reduction in blood pressure when people with hypertension have decreased their salt consumption (He, Li, & MacGregor, 2013). Higher salt intakes also appear to contribute to increased blood volume.

U.S. public groups unanimously recommend fairly low salt intakes for the population at large. Myplate guidelines suggest that sodium intake not exceed 2,300 mg per day. People with hypertension—and those at high risk for the development of hypertension—are urged to keep sodium intake at less than 1,500 mg per day. Health Canada has similar recommendations (Government of Canada, 2012).

Increase Potassium Intake

Potassium, an important electrolyte mineral, is an essential component of the antihypertensive diet. Diets high in potassium have been shown to lessen the effects of sodium and thus aid in the control of blood pressure (American Heart Association, 2014). For this reason it is essential that foods rich in potassium be a component of a balanced diet. Potassium supplements, however, are not recommended because too much potassium can be harmful. The best way to achieve an adequate potassium intake is to consume plenty of vegetables and fruits, as suggested in the DASH diet. The recommended intake of potassium is 4,700 mg per day. Foods high in potassium include potatoes, bananas, spinach, and broccoli—plus many other fruits and vegetables.

Increase Magnesium Intake

Magnesium is another important mineral in the control and reversal of hypertension. Magnesium helps to maintain the optimum functioning of the artery lining, and aids the mechanics of vasodilation and vasoconstriction. A diet rich in magnesium has been found to reduce blood pressure the most when combined with high potassium intake and low sodium intake (Houston, 2011). Moreover, magnesium also has been found to increase the effectiveness of all antihypertensive medications (Houston, 2011). The recommended intake of magnesium is 320 mg per day for women and 420 mg per day for men. Magnesium is found in many nuts, and in spinach, cocoa, beans, and quinoa.

Increase Calcium Intake

Calcium plays an important role in vasodilation and vasoconstriction. The recommended intake of calcium is 1,000 mg per day for adults, and 1,200 mg per day for people 50 years of age and older. Calcium is found in dairy products including milk and yogurt, and in sardines, dark green vegetables such as broccoli, sesame seeds, and calcium-fortified food products.

Dietary Approaches to Stop Hypertension

The Dietary Approaches to Stop Hypertension (DASH) diet was created to help people reduce, treat, and prevent hypertension and maintain a balanced and healthy diet. If followed correctly, the DASH diet can reduce systolic blood pressure by 6 to 12 points (Mayo Clinic Staff, 2013). The DASH diet emphasizes the reduction of sodium intake by encouraging the consumption of fruits; vegetables; low-fat dairy; moderate intake of whole grains; lean meat; fish; poultry; and nuts, seeds, and legumes. In a typical DASH diet the allowed daily sodium intake is 2,300 mg; however, a lower sodium DASH diet is available, and its sodium allowance is 1,500 mg per day (Mayo Clinic Staff, 2013). The chart below illustrates approximate daily servings for each food group, for a 2,000-calorie daily intake.

It is important to note the serving sizes for foods in each group. In particular, the serving size for the meat group is extremely small (1 oz of meat). Most meat portions are typically much larger. The DASH diet also recommends that consumers choose whole-grain foods in the grain group and limit alcohol consumption. Men should not consume more than two alcoholic drinks a day, and women no more than one drink a day, as alcohol intake is linked to higher blood pressure.

Table 1. The DASH Eating Plan

Food Group	Servings	Serving Sizes
Grains	6 to 8	1 slice bread 1 oz dry cereal ½ cup cooked rice, pasta, or cereal
Vegetables	4 to 5	1 cup raw leafy vegetable ½ cup raw or cooked vegetable ½ cup vegetable juice
Fruits	4 to 5	1 medium fruit ¼ cup dried fruit ½ cup fresh, frozen, or canned fruit ½ cup fruit juice
Fat-free or low-fat milk and milk products	2 to 3	1 cup milk or yogurt 1 ½ oz cheese
Lean meats, poultry, and fish	6 or fewer	1 oz cooked meats, poultry, or fish 1 egg
Nuts, seeds, and legumes	4 to 5 per week	1/3 cup or 1 ½ oz nuts 2 Tbsp peanut butter 2 Tbsp or ½ oz seeds ½ cup cooked legumes (dry beans and peas)
Fats and oils	2 to 3	1 tsp soft margarine 1 tsp vegetable oil 1 Tbsp mayonnaise 2 Tbsp salad dressing
Sweets and added sugars	5 or fewer per week	1 Tbsp sugar 1 Tbsp jelly or jam ½ cup sorbet, gelatin 1 cup lemonade

Source: U.S. Dept. Health and Human Services (2006). *Your Guide to Lowering Blood Pressure.* http://www.nhlbi. nih.gov/health/public/heart/hbp/dash/new_dash.pdf

Other Dietary Recommendations

Caffeine raises blood pressure temporarily. Many people with hypertension benefit from reducing caffeine consumption (Mayo Clinic Staff, 2013). People who have diabetes in conjunction with hypertension usually benefit from a lower intake of grains than that recommended by the DASH diet, replacing those calories with healthful fats such as avocadoes and olive oil. This reduces the glycemic load of the diet, resulting in lower blood sugar and insulin levels. The Mediterranean diet and a variety of low-fat diet recommendations also have been found to reduce resting blood pressure in people with hypertension (Toledo et al., 2013).

Paula Sophia Seixas Rocha

Research Issues

A number of nutrients, phytochemicals, and herbs have been studied to determine whether they might help to normalize high blood pressure. It is too early to say exactly which substances might be most helpful and will not have long-term negative consequences. Substances that hold some promise include Coenzyme Q 10 (CoQ 10), marine omega-3 fatty acids, dietary fiber, probiotics, chocolate, garlic, and cinnamon.

EBSCO CAM Review Board. (2013). *Hypertension.* Retrieved from http://www.med.nyu.edu/content ?ChunkIID=21725

See Also: Calcium; Cardiometabolic syndrome; Cardiovascular disease and nutrition; Electrolytes; Magnesium; Mediterranean diet; Potassium; Sodium and salt.

Further Reading

American Heart Association. (2013, May 28). *What are the symptoms of high blood pressure?* Heart.org. Retrieved December 6, 2014, from http://www.heart.org/HEARTORG /Conditions/HighBloodPressure/SymptomsDiagnosisMonitoringofHighBloodPressure /What-are-the-Symptoms-of-High-Blood-Pressure_UCM_301871_Article.jsp

American Heart Association. (2014, August 14). *Potassium and high blood pressure*. Heart. org. Retrieved from http://www.heart.org/HEARTORG/Conditions/HighBloodPressure /PreventionTreatmentofHighBloodPressure/Potassium-and-High-Blood-Pressure _UCM_303243_Article.jsp

Government of Canada. (2012, June 8). *Sodium in Canada—food and nutrition*. Health Canada. Retrieved from http://www.hc-sc.gc.ca/fn-an/nutrition/sodium/index-eng.php

He, F. J., Li, J., & MacGregor, G. A. (2013). Effect of longer-term modest salt reduction on blood pressure. *Cochrane Database of Systematic Reviews 2013,* Issue 4. Art. No.: CD004937. DOI: 10.1002/14651858.CD004937.pub2

Houston, M. (2011). The role of magnesium in hypertension and cardiovascular disease. *Journal of Clinical Hypertension, 13* (11), 843–847. doi:10.1111/j.1751-7176.2011 .00538.x

Keenan, N. L., & Rosendorf, K. A. (2011, January 14). *Prevalence of hypertension and controlled hypertension—United States, 2005–2008*. Retrieved from http://www.cdc .gov/mmwr/preview/mmwrhtml/su6001a21.htm

Mayo Clinic Staff. (2013, May 15). *Nutrition and healthy eating*. MayoClinic.com. Retrieved from http://www.mayoclinic.com/health/dash-diet/HI00047

Toledo, E., Hu, F. B., Estruch, R., et al. (2013). Effect of the Mediterranean diet on blood pressure in the PREDIMED trial: Results from a randomized controlled trial. *BMC Medicine, 11,* 207. doi:10.1186/1741-7015-11-207

U.S. Department of Health and Human Services. (2006). *Your guide to lowering your blood pressure with DASH*. Retrieved from http://www.nhlbi.nih.gov/health/public /heart/hbp/dash/new_dash.pdf

World Health Organization. (2014). *Raised blood pressure*. WHO. Retrieved from http://www.who.int/gho/ncd/risk_factors/blood_pressure_prevalence_text/en/index .html